WRITING THE PULSE

Writing the Pulse

THE ORIGINS AND CAREER OF THE SPHYGMOGRAPH AND ITS AMERICAN MASTERS

Sandra W. Moss, M.D., M.A.

Copyright © 2018 by Sandra W. Moss, M.D., M.A.

Library of Congress Control Number:		2017917063
ISBN:	Hardcover	978-1-5434-6357-6
	Softcover	978-1-5434-6358-3
	eBook	978-1-5434-6359-0

All rights reserved. No part of this book may be reproduced or transmitted in any form or by any means, electronic or mechanical, including photocopying, recording, or by any information storage and retrieval system, without permission in writing from the copyright owner.

Print information available on the last page.

Rev. date: 03/24/2018

To order additional copies of this book, contact:
Xlibris
1-888-795-4274
www.Xlibris.com
Orders@Xlibris.com
746074

Contents

INSCRIPTIONS xi
NOTE xiii
DEDICATION xv
ACKNOWLEDGMENTS xvii
COVER xix
GLOSSARY xxi

CHAPTER 1: THE *TACTUS ERUDITUS:*
       AND THE WORKINGS OF THE BODY 1
CHAPTER 2: FROM SPHYGMOSCOPE TO
       SPHYGMOGRAPH: AND THE VISION OF
       ÈTIENNE-JULES MAREY 24
CHAPTER 3: "SPHYGMOGRAPHING NO END":
       THE SPHYGMOGRAPH IN BRITAIN 60
CHAPTER 4: "SPHYGMOGRAPHIC HIEROGLYPHICS":
       THE AMATEUR SCIENCE OF EDGAR
       HOLDEN 105
CHAPTER 5: ALONZO THRASHER KEYT:
       THE ELEGANT CHRONO-CARDIO-
       SPHYGMOGRAPH 165
CHAPTER 6: ERASMUS ALLINGTON POND:
       THE PRACTICAL PORTABLE
       SPHYGMOGRAPH 193
CHAPTER 7: THE SPHYGMOGRAPH IN AMERICA:
       RESEARCH, MARKETING, AND
       APPLICATION 217
CHAPTER 8: AN OPAQUE AND SLIPPERY TECHNOLOGY:
       THE VISIONS OF THE
       SPHYGMOGRAPH MEN 244

BIBLIOGRAPHY 279
INDEX 305

List Of Illustrations

Figure 1: Vesalius demonstration the anatomy of the arm 4
Figure 1a: Harvey demonstration of blood flow 4
Figure 2: Ivory pleximeter and percussion hammer (percussor) 8
Figure 3: Laennec stethoscopes 10
Figure 4: Cammann binaural stethoscope 11
Figure 5: Pulsilogium of Sanctorius 16
Figure 6: Hales: the rise and fall of arterial blood 20
Figure 7: Hutchinson spirometer 21
Figure 8: Landois "autosphygmogram" 26
Figure 9: Hérisson sphygmometer (sphygmoscope) 27
Figure 10: Scott Alison sphygmoscope 32
Figure 11: Poiseuille haemadynamometer 34
Figure 12: Ludwig kymograph 35
Figure 13: Vierordt sphygmograph 39
Figure 14: Vierordt sphygmograph with Ludwig kymograph 48
Figure 15: Marey sphygmograph (1859) 49
Figure 16: Marey sphygmograph (1881) 49
Figure 17: Detail of the Marey sphygmograph 50
Figure 18: Vierordt and Marey pulse tracings (sphygmograms) 52
Figure 19: Marey *sphygmographe à transmission* 54
Figure 20: Marey sphygmograph long tracings 55
Figure 21: Marey mechanical heart 56
Figure 22: Marey mechanical heart pulse tracing 56
Figure 23: Burdon-Sanderson modification of Marey sphygmograph ... 63
Figure 24: Burdon-Sanderson pulse tracings 66
Figure 25: Marey sphygmograph detail 68
Figure 26: Burdon-Sanderson "hard" and "soft" pulses 69
Figure 27: Garrod graph of sphygmosystole ratios 75
Figure 28: Marey hydraulic blood pressure device 85
Figure 29: Mahomed modification of the Marey sphygmograph 87
Figure 30: Components of the pulse wave 88
Figure 31: Mahomed high pressure pulse 88

Figure 32: Steell high and low tension pulses 93
Figure 33: Von Basch sphygmomanometer..94
Figure 34: Steell sphygmogram of atrial fibrillation 97
Figure 35: Steell patterned pulse irregularities 98
Figure 36: Knoll polygraph used by Mackenzie.......................................99
Figure 37: Portable Mackenzie clinical polygraph 100
Figure 38: Mackenzie ink polygraph venous and arterial tracings........101
Figure 39: Early Holden sphygmograph 136
Figure 40: Redesigned Holden sphygmograph......................................137
Figure 41: Holden sphygmograph detail..138
Figure 42: Holden sphygmograms of artifical heart and blood vessels 140
Figure 43: Holden 1874 monograph, *The Sphygmograph*, author's copy 145
Figure 44: Holden "sphygmographic hieroglyphics"............................162
Figure 45: Keyt sphygmometer (sphygmoscope) 167
Figure 46: Modified Keyt sphygmometer..169
Figure 47: Keyt sphygmograph recording a sphygmogram.................171
Figure 48: Keyt chrono-cardio-sphygmograph.....................................175
Figure 49: Keyt paired cardiac and arterial tracings 177
Figure 50: Keyt pulse tracings of child 178
Figure 51: Keyt serial tracings valvular heart disease 183
Figure 52: Keyt detail of cardio-carotid interval..................................186
Figure 53: Schematic of apexcardiogram 187
Figure 54: Pond early sphygmoscopes..195
Figure 55: Pond sphygmoscopes patent..196
Figure 56: Pond sphygmoscopes patent 197
Figure 57: Pond sphygmograph patented 1876 200
Figure 58: Pond sphygmograph patented 1878 201
Figure 59: Commercial Pond sphygmograph..202
Figure 60: Keyt chrono-cardio-sphygmograph patent....................... 208
Figure 61: Cardiologist Bishop with Mackenzie polygraph 234
Figure 62: Bishop complete cardiac evaluation 235
Figure 63: Dudgeon portable sphygmograph.......................................237
Figure 64: Riva Rocci sphygmomanometer...268
Figure 65: Einthoven electrocardiogram...274

WRITING THE PULSE:

THE ORIGINS AND CAREER OF THE SPHYGMOGRAPH

AND THE AMERICAN SPHYGMOGRAPH MEN

INSCRIPTIONS

"The pulse, as the external expression of circulation, has always been the beacon of physicians . . . The appreciation of the pulse is not necessarily confined to the medical touch. In a time not very far back, physicians had only the bulb of their fingers to perceive it. Then the detached second-hand of the watch came to their aid; and lastly, we have the 'pulse writer,' the sphygmograph, to add precision to perception, and at the same time register accurately the variations of pulse curves."

>Édouard Séguin, "Sphygmometry,"
>*Medical Record* (New York) 2 (1867/68): 243–44.

~~~~~~

In Arthur Conan Doyle's 1922 short tale of medical life, "The Doctors of Hoyland," the sphygmograph makes perhaps its only appearance in fiction. On first visiting the office of a new physician in town, young Dr. Ripley is shocked to learn that Dr. Verrinder Smith is a woman—and a very up-to-date one at that:

"On the other hand, there was much in the consulting-room to please him. Elaborate instruments, seen more often in hospitals than in the houses of private practitioners were scattered about. A sphygmograph stood upon the table and a gasometer-like engine, which was new to Doctor Ripley, in the corner."

>Arthur Conan Doyle, "The Doctors of Hoyland"
>*Tales of Adventure and Medical Life* (London: John Murray, 1922).

NOTE

To view a sphygmograph in action, see:
"Changing the Face of Medicine: Dr. Jacobi's Sphygmograph"
National Library of Medicine
https://cfmedicine.nlm.nih.gov/artifact/jacobi.html

Dedication

This book is dedicated to my husband of half a century, Rutgers University Professor Emeritus Robert A. Moss, whose lifelong devotion to academia, scientific research in chemistry, and teaching were a constant example to his colleagues and students. His prolific "extracurricular" writings in the fields of baseball history, Sherlockiana, and philately remain an inspiration to his children and grandchildren.

ROBERT A. MOSS
May 27th 1940 to November 27th 2017

Acknowledgments

The guidance of Professors Lisa Herschbach, Julie Livingstone, Stephen Pemberton, and Richard Sher, faculty members of the Graduate Program in the History of Technology, the Environment, and Medicine at Rutgers the State University of New Jersey and the New Jersey Institute of Technology is gratefully acknowledged. Their insights and experience informed my early work on the history of the sphygmograph. I am also indebted to Dr. W. Bruce Fye for a detailed reading of an early manuscript, with expert commentary. Dr. Charles S. Bryant read a later version and also offered helpful comments. Both readers are distinguished historians of medicine. Archivists and librarians at Special Collections, (Rutgers University, New Brunswick), Special Collections in the History of Medicine (University of Medicine and Dentistry of New Jersey, now Rutgers University Libraries), and The College of Physicians of Philadelphia have been of invaluable assistance over the lifetime of this project. The American Osler Society and the Medical History Society of New Jersey have been my intellectual homes; the members of both organizations remain perennial sources of inspiration and support for all my explorations into the history of medicine.

Cover

THREE AMERICAN SPHYGMOGRAPHS
Holden sphygmograph
Keyt chrono-cardio-sphygmograph
Pond portable sphygmograph

Glossary

Cardiograph: The cardiograph is a sphygmograph, adapted to register the pulsations of the heart against the chest wall, not to be confused with the electrocardiograph (see below). The rise and fall of the beating heart is detectable externally and produces a wave-like "cardiogram."

Electrocardiograph: The electrocardiograph is an instrument introduced early in the twentieth century to record the electrical conduction system of the heart (an electrocardiogram), often referred to familiarly as EKG (from German) or ECG. Injury to the heart muscle (as in a heart attack) or structural abnormalities (such as an enlarged heart) produce characteristic changes in the electrocardiogram .

Kymograph: Literally "wave writer," the kymograph is a laboratory instrument introduced in 1845 by Carl Ludwig, a pioneer of modern physiological research. The kymograph transmitted pressure changes within an artery to a moving strip of recording paper. This was the fundamental invention in the development of the graphic method for studying physiologic events. In modified form, it was incorporated into the design of the sphygmograph.

Polygraph: The polygraph, invented by British cardiologist James Mackenzie, in the 1890s was a combination sphygmograph (an index of left heart function) and venous pulse wave sensor (an index of right heart function). The polygraph permitted simultaneous recording of arterial and venous impulses, revealing mechanisms of cardiac failure and arrhythmias.

Sphygmogram: The sphygmogram is the tracing produced by a sphygmograph, just as the electrocardiogram is the tracing generated by an electrocardiograph.

Sphygmograph: The sphygmograph is literally a "pulse writer," a device that transmits the pulsations of the artery to a moving strip of paper or glass, thus producing a pulse tracing with dimensions of vertical displacement and horizontal passage of time.

Sphygmology: Sphygmology is the study of the pulse by means of palpation of the artery. Pulse study was the particular skill of the learned physician, and much of it was based on classical authority. The "learned touch" of the physician (the tactus eruditus) referred to pulse palpation.

Sphygmomanometer: The sphygmomanometer (the familiar blood pressure cuff) was introduced in its present form late in the nineteenth century. Attempts to determine arterial tension by means of the sphygmograph were subjective and impractical. The sphygmomanometer produced reliable and reproducible numerical readings of the blood pressure.

Sphygmometer: The sphygmometer, a forerunner of the sphygmograph, was a simple device for transmitting the pulsations of the artery to a calibrated hollow glass tube by means of a reservoir of colored water or alcohol (it is similar to a thermometer in design). The observer(s) could easily see the fluid rise and fall in the tubing as the bulb at the bottom of the sphygmometer was pressed against an artery. There was no recording device.

Sphygmoscope: The sphygmoscope is another name for the sphygmometer.

Chapter 1

The *Tactus Eruditus:* And the Workings of the Body

The subject of this book, a device called the sphygmograph (literally "pulse writer"), was an instrument for recording the pulse waves on a moving strip of paper. The rocky history of the sphygmograph can be seen as part of what historian Kenneth Lipartito refers to as an "active [part] of the technological narrative."[1] In the mid-nineteenth century, the sphygmograph took its place in the technological narrative and began its troubled half-century odyssey through medical research, medical practice, and the medical literature.

In the eighteenth and early nineteenth centuries, physicians reimagined the workings of the body through advances in diagnostic techniques and technologies. This fundamental transformation in the way physicians experienced the body was largely a change in their experience of space as they sought to see with their mind's eye the interior landscape of the body in sickness and health. Since there was little of therapeutic benefit to offer, master diagnosticians could predict during life the anatomic abnormalities—such as pneumonia or fluid collections—that would be revealed at the inevitable autopsy. Proof of disease resided in pathological anatomy. The insights provided by the stethoscope and the microscope, as well as the "technology" of autopsy, were largely spatial in nature.

In time, new technologies—"instruments of precision"— allowed physicians to study normal and pathological physiological events—that is,

---

[1] Kenneth Lipartito, "Picturephone and the Information Age: The Social Meaning of Failure," *Technology and Culture* 44 (2003): 57.

bodily functions such as cardiac arrhythmias, high blood pressure, lung dysfunction, and elevated body temperature that might not be discoverable upon interviewing the patient or discernable at autopsy or visible under the microscope. With the transfer of these new technologies for the study of physiologic events from the laboratory to the bedside, the hegemony of anatomic pathology was challenged. Instruments of registration such as the sphygmograph and the spirometer—with their aura of measurable objectivity and the visible permanent records they created—expanded the spectrum of disease states and altered the practice of medicine.

Stanley Joel Reiser, a historian of medical technology, refers to such nineteenth-century instruments as the spirograph or spirometer (for recording respiratory excursions) and the sphygmograph (for recording the rise and fall of the arterial pulse) as "the time and space machines of medicine," a new set of technologies that "metamorphosed the biological rhythms and motions of the body into graphical formats."[2] These new space and time instruments of medicine did not develop in a vacuum. Their utility and appeal were a reflection of revolutionary challenges to ancient systems of Western medicine embodied in Hippocratic and Galenic teachings that had become ossified as dogma in the course of fifteen centuries. The challenges came from many quarters, initiated emphatically (and flamboyantly) by the radical Swiss physician and iconoclast, Paracelsus, who was said to have publicly burned the works of Galen and other classical authors in 1527.[3] Although they successfully challenged the hegemony of a stagnant academic medicine, Paracelsus and his followers exhausted their energies in pursuit of an iatrochemical concept of therapeutics and various vitalistic formulations.

DE HUMANI CORPORIS FABRICA: THE VESALIAN REVOLUTION

In 1543, the brilliant anatomist Andreas Vesalius published the first edition of his revolutionary study of human anatomy entitled *De Humani Corporis Fabrica*. For almost fifteen hundred years, physicians had "known" human anatomy by studying the writings of the Greco-Roman physician

---

[2] Stanley Joel Reiser, "The Technologies of Time Measurement: Implications at the Bedside and the Bench," *Annals of Internal Medicine* 132 (2000): 34.

[3] Roy Porter, *The Greatest Benefit to Mankind: A Medical History of Humanity* (New York: W. W. Norton & Co., 1997), 202–3. Theophrastus Philippus Aureolus Bombastus von Hohenheim (1493–1542), who styled himself "Paracelsus" (surpassing Celsus, a first century Roman author of medical works), challenged academic medicine, championed empiricism, and developed medical practices based largely on alchemy.

Claudius Galen. Indeed, Vesalius himself was a Galenist in his formative years. Vesalius's revolution was radical in its boldness and deceptively simple in concept. In the relatively liberal atmosphere of the medical school at Padua, this young Flemish-born physician conducted anatomical dissections *with his own hands* and carefully recorded what he saw *with his own eyes*.

His choice of a title—*De Humani Corporis Fabrica*—was more revealing than it might seem at first glance. In 1943, four hundred years after the appearance of the *Fabrica*, British medical historian and Vesalius scholar Charles Singer explained that *fabrica* refers neither to "fabric" nor to "mechanism." Rather, *fabrica* is etymologically related to the notion of a factory, an artisan's workshop, a place where "something is going on," something is fabricated. To Vesalius, wrote Singer, the body was a "piece of workmanship by the Great Craftsman."[4] Thus, Vesalius, who dissected dead bodies, was writing about the "workings" of the living human body, amalgamating structure and function, anatomy and physiology. In the fourth book of *De humani corporis fabrica* Vesalius challenged Galen's notion that the right and left ventricles were connected by pores too tiny to be seen by the human eye. He also correctly elucidated the anatomy of the cardiac veins.

DE MOTU CORDIS: HARVEY AND THE CIRCULATION OF THE BLOOD

The application of Vesalian anatomical studies to cardiac physiology reached its apotheosis in the work of William Harvey, formerly a student at Padua, who demonstrated the circulation of the blood. Harvey published his *Exercitatio anatomic de motu cordis et sanguinis in animalibus* (*An Anatomical Essay Concerning the Movement of the Heart and Blood in Animals*; familiarly *De motu cordis*) in 1628. Historian of medicine Roy Porter believes that Harvey's revolutionary work not only reconceptualized cardiac physiology, but "convinced later investigators that medical science had to be put on a new footing."[5] The heart, arteries, and veins were transformed into the circulatory system.

---

[4] Charles Singer, "To Vesalius on the Fourth Centenary of His *De Humani Corporis Fabrica*," *Journal of Anatomy* (London) 77 (1943): 261–63. Although Vesalius is little read today, his work continues to electrify modern students of history, medicine, and art through the illustrations attributed to Jan Stevan von Calcar, a student of Titian, who was engaged by Vesalius to render drawings from the dissected cadavers.

[5] Porter, *The Greatest Benefit*, 211–16; quotation, 211. Harvey and his predecessors reached their conclusions through vivisection experiments.

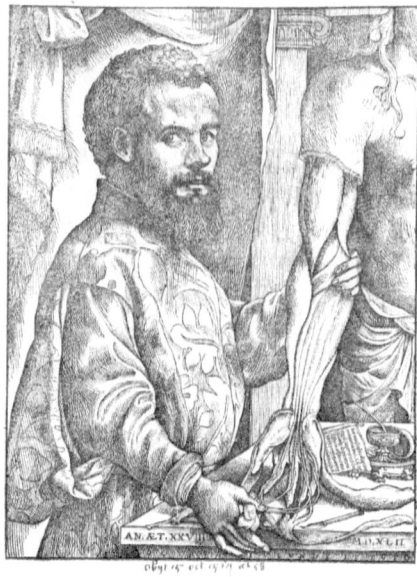

Figure 1: Andreas Vesalius demonstrating the anatomy of the arm. The tendons rather than the arteries dominate the detailed anatomy. *De Humani Corporis Fabrica*, 1843; artist (attributed) Jan Stephan van Calcar.

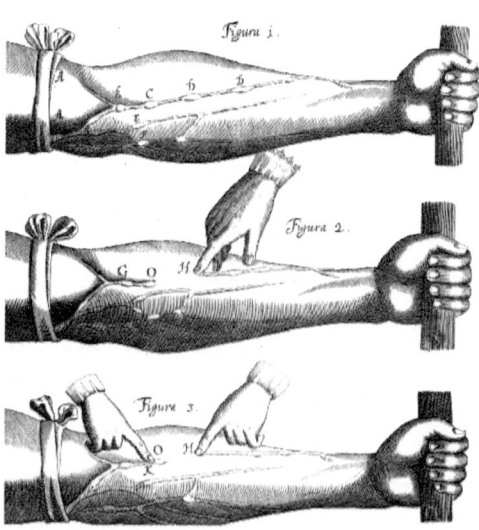

Figure 1a: William Harvey's demonstration of venous blood flow, showing venous valves that function to direct venous flow toward the heart. *Exercitatio anatomica de motu cordis et sanguinis in animalibus (De motu cordis)*, 1628.

Harvey did not invent the circulation out of whole cloth. In the decades after the appearance of Vesalius's anatomy, anatomists such as Michael Servetus and Andrea Cesalpino explored the circulation of the blood through the pulmonary vessels. Fabrizio d'Acquapendente, one of Harvey's teachers at Padua, had discovered the venous valves; the fact that venous blood could flow only in one direction—toward the heart—was a vital clue for Harvey. The final proof that the arterial and venous circulations were connected was provided in 1661 (just a few years after Harvey's death) by Marcello Malphigi, professor of medicine at Pisa, who used a microscope to visualize the tiny capillaries postulated by Harvey, but invisible to his unaided eye.[6]

DE SEDIBUS ET CAUSIS MORBORUM: MORGAGNI AND ANATOMIC PATHOLOGY

The concept that the heart could be the seat of disease had its modern origins in the systematic work of Giovanni Battista Morgagni, professor of anatomy at Padua, who published his monumental study of clinical pathology, *De sedibus et causis morborum per anatomen indagatis* (*The Seats and Causes of Diseases Investigated by Anatomy*), in 1761. Morgagni identified major pathologic processes in the heart and its vessels, including myocardial degeneration and hypertrophy, valvular disease, atherosclerosis, and vascular anomalies.[7] Disease, concluded Morgagni, resided in human organs. Symptoms were, as Morgagni remarked, the "cry of the suffering organs."[8] Disease models based on classical theories of fluctuating humoral balance and imbalance were beginning to be seen as sterile and unrelated to the increasingly hegemonic evidence of the autopsy room. Newly minted rationalistic theories of neurovascular tonicity, codified by William Cullen at Edinburgh and canonized in America by his student, Benjamin Rush, also lacked the explanatory power to satisfy nineteenth-century demands for empirical evidence at the bedside and in the autopsy room.

While not rejecting this localized anatomical theory of organ-based disease, physicians in the nineteenth century also began to redefine some diseases in terms of physiological dysfunction (pathophysiology) rather

---

[6] Ibid., 223–24.
[7] Ibid., 263.
[8] Sherwin B. Nuland, "The New Medicine: Anatomical Concept of Giovanni Morgagni," in *Doctors: The Biography of Medicine* (New York: Knopf, 1988; Vintage Books, 1989), 147.

than structural anatomic abnormality. An irregular pulse, rapid respiratory rate, or elevated body temperature were not discoverable at autopsy.[9] Sickness could be better understood in the interlocking frameworks of morbid anatomy *and* pathophysiology.

FROM "NATURAL" TO "NORMAL"

A critical conceptual reformulation was the epistemological leap from diagnosis and prognosis based on the specificity of each patient's "natural" balanced state of health—a potentially unstable condition influenced by environment, temperament, heredity, and climate—to a notion of the "normal" based on studies of groups of individuals.[10] An uneven process, this new definition of health was accompanied by changing philosophies of therapeutics, in which interventions were chosen with an eye to restoring normality rather than resetting a disordered balance. These nineteenth-century revolutions in medical perception were bracketed by the new clinical methods of the French school early in the century and the rise of the germ theory, with its tidy etiological models, near the end of the century.

THE NEW TECHNOLOGIES OF BEDSIDE CARDIOVASCULAR DIAGNOSIS

Innovations in medical technology began slowly in the eighteenth century, gathering momentum and maturity in the nineteenth century. In contrast to the instant and often uncritical embrace of new medical technologies in recent decades, diagnostic innovations and instruments gained acceptance more slowly and unevenly in past centuries.[11] Although some clinicians welcomed diagnostic technologies as superior to subjective impressions filtered through patients' sensibilities, others were suspicious of reductionist technologies that seemed to distance them from the patient. Critics questioned the overdependence on devices that could blunt the

---

[9] Stanley Joel Reiser, *Medicine and the Reign of Technology* (Cambridge: Cambridge University Press, 1978), 91.

[10] John Harley Warner, *The Therapeutic Perspective: Medical Practice, Knowledge, and Identity in America, 1820–1885* (Princeton: Princeton University Press, 1997), 85–87.

[11] For a discussion of the rapid acceptance of new medical technology, see David A. Grimes, "Technology Follies: The Uncritical Acceptance of Medical Innovation," *Journal of the American Medical Association* 269 (1993): 3030–33.

ancient "art" of the physician. The dialogue continued through the nineteenth century. While no longer framed as a conflict between "art" and "science," technology-based medical practice continues to generate debate today.

PERCUSSION: THE TAPPING FINGER

In 1761, Leopold Auenbrugger, in what was then the medical backwater of Vienna, described percussion, a technique for tapping the chest to elicit diagnostic information (similar to the technique for locating wall studs). Percussion represented a new process of translation, in which the physician was required to "transform auditory patterns quickly into their visual analogues." A certain pattern and quality of percussion sounds, for example, led the knowledgeable examiner to mentally visualize lung consolidation or pleural effusion, disorders made familiar through the performance of autopsies. The fingers informed the ear, which in turn brought forth a mental image of anatomical disturbance. Auenbrugger's technique was not popularized until his work was translated and expanded upon in 1808 by Jean-Nicolas Corvisart, a leading light of the French clinical school.[12]

The necessary element for the popularity of percussion was not the new technique itself, but the intellectual ferment of clinicopathological study in Paris. Diagnosis and confirmation at the inevitable autopsy were the primary functions of the hospital physician in the new French school of medicine. Such therapy as existed was not seriously expected to alter the outcome.

Although Auenbrugger described percussion using only the fingers of the examiner ("immediate" percussion), French physician Pierre Adolphe Piorry introduced "mediate percussion," a technique in which a small disc of ivory (a plessimeter, or pleximeter) was interposed between the chest wall and the physician's tapping finger. Such "mediate percussion" was believed to enhance the percussion tone. Some physicians replaced the tapping finger with a small hammer. However, within a few years, a finger

---

[12] Reiser, *Medicine and the Reign of Technology*, 20–22, quotation, 21. The oft-retold and entirely plausible story is that young Auenbrugger learned percussion by tapping on the casks in his father's inn in order to determine the level of beer or wine remaining; Ralph Major, *Classic Descriptions of Disease*, 3rd ed. (Springfield, IL: Charles C. Thomas, 1945), 563. Corvisart gave full credit to Auenbrugger. Sherwin B. Nuland, "Without Diagnosis There Is No Rational Treatment: René Laennec, Inventor of the Stethoscope," in *Doctors*, 205.

of the non-tapping hand, when laid against the chest wall, was found to give the best results.[13] In this case, technology failed to improve the quality of the information to be gained by use of the examiner's fingers, a diagnostic technique still used by physicians today in detailed physical examination of the chest.

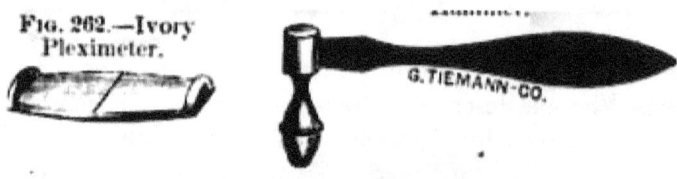

Figure 2: Ivory pleximeter and percussion hammer (percussor). George Tiemann & Co., *American Armamentarium Chirurgicum*, ca. 1879, 1:82.

Percussion moved the manual maneuvers of the physician to a central place in diagnosis. It put the physician in closer contact with the "suffering organs." While observation of the patient and attention to his recitation of symptoms remained important, percussion required no translation by the patient; the physician's tapping fingers communicated directly with the interior of the body.[14]

AUSCULTATION: THE HEART SPEAKS

With René T. H. Laennec's introduction of the stethoscope in 1816 and the subsequent clinicopathological correlations described in his 1819 treatise, *De l'ausculation médiate*, physical diagnosis took on unprecedented objectivity. The physician could learn something intimate about the patient's heart and lungs that the patient himself could neither observe or relate.[15] Like the percussor, the auscultator, "undistracted by the motives and beliefs of the patient" could rely on what "he believed to be objective,

---

[13] Mahlon H. Delp and Robert T. Manning, *Major's Physical Diagnosis*, 7th ed. (Philadelphia: W. B. Saunders, 1968), 9.

[14] Reiser, *Medicine and the Reign of Technology*, 20.

[15] The full title of Laennec's classic work is *De l'ausculation médiate, ou traité du diagnostic des poumons et du coeur, fondé principalement sur ce nouveau moyen d'exploration* (*On Mediate Auscultation, or A Treatise on the Diagnosis of Diseases of the Lungs and Heart Based Principally on the New Method of Investigation*).

bias-free representations of the disease process."[16] Stressing the translations from one "language" to another, Reiser formulates the new process of diagnosis: "Laennec devised a method in which nonverbal sounds became the signals of disease and a new instrument, the stethoscope, became essential to broadcast their presence."[17] As Laennec and his colleagues confirmed at autopsy the pathological anatomy corresponding to the sounds heard through the stethoscope, a further translation from sound to visual image became imprinted on the physician's mind. In Reiser's apt formulation, "the ear became an eye."[18]

Often, new technologies ran ahead of a sound understanding of underlying physiological processes. The application of the stethoscope to the reading of lung disease was quickly confirmed by Laennec, who both invented the instrument and correlated clinical findings with pathological anatomy. However, the stethoscope was also used to examine the heart. The mechanisms of normal and abnormal heart sounds were not fully elucidated until well into the twentieth century.[19]

Laennec's first stethoscope (1816) was simply a rolled-up paper tube. It seems he found it difficult and possibly embarrassing to properly listen to the breath sounds of a plump young woman by the standard method of laying his ear directly upon her chest. Laennec, recalling a "well-known acoustic phenomenon," quickly formed a tube by rolling up a sheaf of paper, placing one end on the patient's chest and the other against his ear. The scene, as described by Laennec in an 1819 treatise, remains one of those "great moments in medicine," celebrated in artists' renderings and histories of medicine.[20]

The classic stethoscope constructed by Laennec some months later was a wooden tube with a hollow central channel. One end was pressed over the chest and the other against the ear of the examiner. Some monaural (one ear) stethoscopes had a flange at one or both ends. "Mediate" auscultation with the stethoscope replaced "immediate" auscultation, in which the ear of the examiner was placed upon the patient's chest.

---

[16] Reiser, *Medicine and the Reign of Technology*, 38.

[17] Ibid., 28.

[18] Ibid., 30.

[19] Ibrahim R. Hanna and Mark E. Silverman, "A History of Cardiac Auscultation and Some of Its Contributors," *American Journal of Cardiology* 90 (2002): 259–67. The normal sounds are the familiar "lubb-dupp" generated by valve closures; abnormal findings include such sounds as murmurs, clicks, and gallops.

[20] Jacalyn Duffin, *To See with a Better Eye: A Life of R.T.H. Laennec* (Princeton: Princeton University Press, 1998), 122–30, reference to Laennec's treatise, 122.

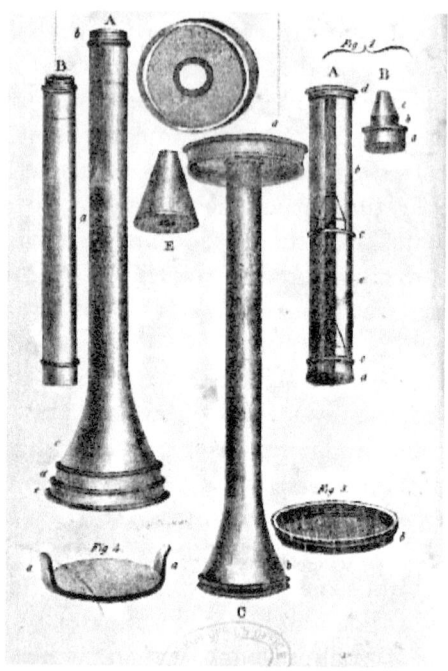

Figure 3: Laennec stethoscopes. Frontispiece, R. T. H. Laennec, *A Treatise on the Disease of the Chest and of Mediate Ausculation* (New York: Samuel S. and William Wood, 1838); English translation of third French edition of the 1819 Laennec, *De l'ausculation médiate, ou traité du diagnostic des poumons et du coeur, fonde principalement sur ce nouveau moyen d'exploration.*

An early and possibly the first binaural (two ear) stethoscope was designed and produced by George Cammann in New York City in mid-century, although there were other claimants. Cammann described his "self-adjusting stethoscope" in the *New York Medical Times* in 1855. Some physicians continued to use the monaural stethoscope until the turn of the twentieth century.[21] The familiar binaural stethoscope, often draped around the physician's or nurse's neck as he or she proceeds from patient to patient on rounds, remains an iconic emblem of the medical profession two centuries after Laennec rolled up his sheaf of paper to examine a young woman's chest in a Parisian hospital.

---

[21] Paul B. Sheldon and Janet Doe, "The Development of the Stethoscope: An Exhibition Showing the Work of Laennec and His Successors," *Bulletin of the New York Academy of Medicine* 11 (1935): 608–28; "Self-adjusting Stethoscope of Dr. Cammann," *New York Medical Times* 4 (1855): 140–42.

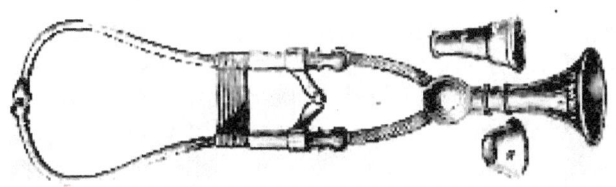

Figure 4: Cammann binaural stethoscope (invented ca. 1855, with later modifications). George Tiemann & Co., *American Armamentarium Chirurgicum*, ca. 1879, 1:82.

Busy practitioners were, in general, conservative; the books in their libraries were often classic works by authors of earlier decades and even earlier centuries. Certainly in America, and probably in Europe, there were many men in practice who had only the most rudimentary preparation, who neither sought nor acquired new knowledge after apprenticeship and brief attendance at an inferior medical college, and who were oblivious to new technologies.

But many American physicians, generally the best educated and the best read, rapidly adopted the stethoscope. As early as the 1820s, James Jackson of Boston was teaching the new methods of auscultation at a private medical school.[22] General acceptance of the stethoscope by midcentury was attested to by the release of multiple editions of Austin Flint Sr.'s 1868 *Compendium of Percussion and Auscultation, and of the Physical Diagnosis of Diseases Affecting the Lung*.[23] After the Civil War, medical supply catalogues offered a plethora of monaural and binaural stethoscopes.

THE THERMOMETER: EMBRACING NUMBERS

New concepts and representations of disease entwined new technologies. With the introduction of the clinical thermometer in the

---

[22] Thomas Neville Bonner, *Becoming a Physician: Medical Education in Britain, France, Germany, and the United States, 1750–1945* (Baltimore: Johns Hopkins University Press, 1995), 180.

[23] Austin Flint Sr. held prestigious medical professorships at a number of American schools, including the Bellevue Hospital Medical College. His *Treatise on the Principles and Practice of Medicine; Designed for the Use of Practitioners and Students of Medicine* was a leading American textbook, going through seven editions beginning in 1866; Howard A. Kelly and Walter L Burrage, *American Medical Biography* (Baltimore: Norman Remington Co., 1920), 394–95.

mid-nineteenth century, physicians could redefine traditional subjective concepts of "fever." The clinical thermometer was part of a revolution in the physician's reading of the body. The thermometer, urged into medical practice by the work of Leipzig professor Carl Wunderlich in the 1860s, allowed descriptive qualities such as hot flushed skin to be transformed into a discrete objective number readable from a hollow glass tube filled with an expanding fluid such as mercury or alcohol. At the same time, the concept of a "fever" as an illness characterized by a constellation of signs and symptoms was gradually replaced by a reductionist definition of fever as an elevated temperature.

Temperature charts or graphs, upon which readings were plotted serially over the course of the illness, carried diagnostic and prognostic import. Hand-drawn temperature graphs were first added to the written medical record at the Massachusetts General Hospital in Boston in 1867; printed graphs appeared a few years later.[24] With advances in diagnosis, the clinical chart, with its plots of temperature, pulse rate, and such later additions as blood pressure and fluid intake and output, was a prime example of the translation of physiologic and pathophysiologic events into the language of numbers and graphs, an inscription of change over time—a "data-organizing technology" that was "the first technology to establish the significance of time in the practice of medicine."[25]

THE *TACTUS ERUDITUS* OF THE LEARNED PHYSICIAN

Counting the pulse was a relatively late endeavor in the history of pulse study. But studying the pulse dated back in to ancient times. The pulse was a nuanced and emotionally resonant physiological manifestation of human and animal life. Historian Shigehisa Kuriyama refers to "the stirrings of the arteries." People across many cultures and all ages were curious about the pulse because they were curious about themselves, their sicknesses, and their chances of death or recovery; they hoped or believed that the

---

[24] Warner, *Therapeutic Perspective*, 155–56. The Commercial Hospital of Cincinnati, for example, did not use temperature graphs until 1878.

[25] Reiser, "Technologies of Time Measurement," 32–34. For Reiser's discussion of the "translation of physiological actions into the language of machines," see Reiser, *Medicine and the Reign of Technology*, 91–121 (Wunderlich's successful promotion of the medical thermometer, 115–17).

pulse held answers to these human dilemmas.[26] Although interpretations varied radically, physicians across time and cultures sensed or reasoned that the pulse revealed secrets about the workings of the body. The fact that the pulse disappeared when a person died must have been a powerful inducement to explore or imagine its workings.

Before turning to the sphygmograph, an instrument for recording the movements of the pulse over time, it is necessary to consider sphygmology, the traditional European study of the pulse, often referred to by nineteenth-century writers as the *tactus eruditus* (learned touch) of the physician.

The pulse has occupied the professional attention of Western physicians since antiquity; characteristics such as rate, regularity, forcefulness, fullness, and the palpable profile or shape of the pulse were carefully noted.[27] The pulse was a window into the vital processes; skill and professional authority were required to detect and interpret its messages. An American physician called the pulse one of the great "sign-bearers of diseases" and the "beacon of physicians."[28]

Classical pulse study distinguished *pulsus frequens* and *pulsus rarus* (referring to slow or fast rate, though without a numerical value), *pulsus celer* and *pulsus tardus* (referring to the time occupied by each beat relative to the duration of each pulse interval), *pulsus magnus* and *pulsus parvus* (referring to the degree to which the artery dilates in length and breadth), *pulsus durus* and *pulsus mollis* (referring to hardness or softness and compressibility of the artery). Thus, in phthisis (tuberculosis) and hysteria, the skilled practitioner of the past could, so he claimed, detect *pulsus frequens, celer et parvus*, while in an inflammatory fever he would find *pulsus frequens, magnus et celer*, and in eruptive fever, *pulsus frequens, magnus et mollis*.[29]

---

[26] Shigehisa Kuriyama, *The Expressiveness of the Body and the Divergence of Greek and Chinese Medicine* (New York: Zone Books, 1999), 18.

[27] A complex pulse lore was an integral feature of non-Western medicine as well; however, such pulse lore remained static and was not a factor in advances in sphygmology in Europe or America.

[28] É[douard] Séguin, *Medical Thermometry and Human Temperature* (New York: William Wood & Co., 1876), xxii; É[douard] Séguin, "Sphygmometry," *Medical Record* (New York) 2 (1867): 248.

[29] John Burdon-Sanderson, *Handbook of the Sphygmograph: Being a Guide to Its Use in Clinical Research, to Which is Appended A Lecture Delivered at the Royal College of Physicians on the 29th of March 1867 on the Mode and Duration of the Contraction of the Heart in Health and Disease* (London: Robert Hardwicke, 1867), 13–16. His "Lecture on the Characteristics of the Arterial Pulse in Their Relation to the Mode and Duration of the Contraction of the Heart in Health and Disease" was originally published in three parts in the *British Medical Journal* 2 (1867): 19–22, 39–40, 57–58.

JOHN BURDON-SANDERSON ON THE PULSE

John Scott Burdon-Sanderson, an 1851 graduate of the medical college of the University of Edinburgh and a former student of famed Paris physiologist Claude Bernard, was a rising practitioner, public health officer, hospital man, medical school lecturer, and private scientist in London by the mid-1860s.[30] Burdon-Sanderson confessed in 1867 that the subtler distinctions in pulse interpretation were unclear to him and his contemporaries and had passed into disuse. He neatly sidestepped the onus of calling into question the teachings of his mentors, claiming that present fingers lacked the well-developed *tactus eruditus* of the past.[31] He admitted quite frankly that palpation of the pulse was open to great variation among observers, despite the detailed descriptions and classifications taught to medical students and reported by experienced physicians.

In a paragraph studded with exclamation marks, Burdon-Sanderson expressed his frustration. One can almost see him leaning over his lectern and demanding of the assembled members of the Royal College of Physicians: "How difficult—how impossible—is it for the skilled physician to impart this [i.e. pulse] knowledge to his less-experienced junior!" and "How difficult to describe to the student what you feel when you place your finger on the wrist!" and "How various the opinions given by different physicians as to the same pulse!"[32]

Burdon-Sanderson's remarks on the pulse were made in connection with his early and enthusiastic embrace of the sphygmograph, giving him something of a professional and personal interest in pointing out the pitfalls of traditional pulse study. However, he by no means rejected pulse palpation, as long as claims for its usefulness were not exaggerated. In his 1867 *Handbook of the Sphygmograph*, Burdon-Sanderson noted that pulse palpation, even in the face of the new technology of the sphygmograph, was not to be entirely discarded: "In certain rare instances we may find out what is the matter by feeling a patient's pulse, just as by looking at the countenance, but in general we may be content if by means of it we can discover the condition

---

[30] Terrie M. Romano, *Making Medicine Scientific: John Burdon Sanderson and the Culture of Victorian Science* (Baltimore: Johns Hopkins University Press, 2002), 39–40, 49.
[31] Burdon-Sanderson, *Handbook of the Sphygmograph*, 13–16. The title appears also as *Hand Book* in some catalogues. John Burdon-Sanderson is variously referred to as Sanderson, Burdon Sanderson, or Burdon-Sanderson. The latter is used in this chapter.
[32] Burdon-Sanderson, *Handbook of the Sphygmograph*, 66.

of the circulation."[33] In effect, Burdon-Sanderson was articulating a redefinition of pulse palpation. No longer was it the learned physician's mystical window into the hidden organs of the body; rather, it was one clue to the state of the circulatory system.

COUNTING THE PULSE: THE PULSILOGIUM OF SANCTORIUS

The utility of counting the number of pulse beats per unit time was not obvious to early students of physical diagnosis, nor had they the technology to count the pulse rate accurately and assign it a number. We have seen earlier in this chapter that learned physicians, from antiquity until well into the nineteenth century identified *pulsus frequens* and *pulsus rarus* (referring to slow or fast rate) in addition to noting qualities such as the fullness of the pulse and its apparent contour under the educated finger. In the second century, Galen, the Greco-Roman physician, anatomist, and prolific writer, taught that pulses were specific to diseases. The doctrine would not lose its currency in western medicine for almost two millennia.

The concept of counting the pulse and assigning it a number apparently occurred to several early scientific men including Galileo and Johannes Kepler. However, the first machine designed to time the pulse for medical purposes is credited to Sanctorius of Padua (also known as Santorio Santorio), a Venetian physician who, in the early decades of the seventeenth century invented a device that he called the pulsilogium. There is evidence that the prototype of Sanctorius's device was in fact conceived and constructed by Galileo, though never applied to medical diagnosis. The pulsilogium utilized a leaded weight hanging from a cord, which was made to swing in harmony with the pulse (probably palpated at the wrist); a fast pulse required a shorter cord, while a slow pulse required a longer cord. Thus the length of the cord, measured on a scaled ruler, indicated the pulse rate. This clever device, despite Sanctorius's vision, does not seem to have found any application in clinical medicine.[34]

---

[33] Ibid., 19.
[34] N. H. Naqvi and M. D. Blaufox, *Blood Pressure Measurement: An Illustrated History* (New York: Parthenon, 1998), 21; Sanctorius's description of his pulsilogium is quoted by these authors in English translation from *Commentaria in Primam Fen Primi Libri Cononis Avicennae* (Santorius 1625). See also Reiser, *Medicine and the Reign of Technology*, 96–97.

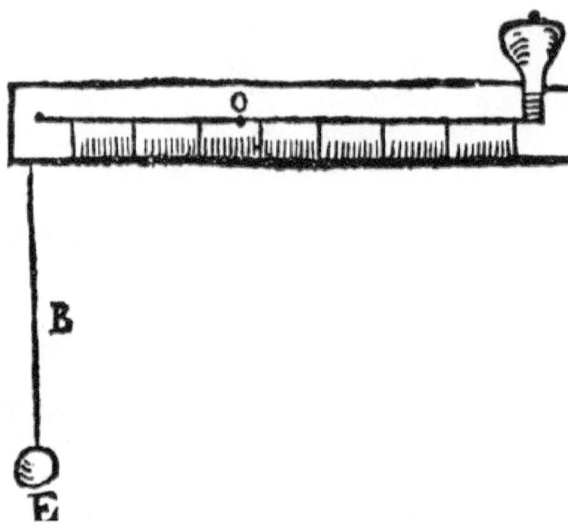

Figure 5: Pulsilogium of Sanctorius, an early device for measuring the rate of the pulse by adjusting the length of a weighted string until it swung in time with the pulse. The length of the string, measured on a calibrated ruler, equaled the pulse rate; Sanctorius, *Commentaria In Primam Fen Primi Libri Cononis Avicennae*, 1625).

JOHN FLOYER: *THE PHYSICIAN'S PULSE-WATCH*

The clock occupies a central place in histories of Western technology. In medieval times, the clock was a representation and affirmation of order in the universe. Poorly understood or mythologized phenomena of nature such as night and day could be represented in arithmetic terms.[35] In *Technics and Civilization*, Lewis Mumford links time-keeping, together with a new awareness of expanded space and accelerating time, to a compulsion to reduce human experience to numbers: "In time-keeping, in trading, in fighting, men counted numbers; and finally, as the habit grew, only numbers counted."[36]

---

[35] Arnold Pacey, *Technology and World Civilization* (Cambridge: Massachusetts Institute of Technology Press, 1990), 96–98. See also Lewis Mumford for a consideration of the central role of the clock as the "key-machine of the modern industrial age" and its origins in monastic life. Lewis Mumford, *Technics and Civilization* (New York: Harcourt Brace & Co., 1934; reprint, 1963), 12–18; quotation 14. Page citations are to reprint edition.

[36] Mumford, *Technics and Civilization*, 22.

Although medicine never lost its subjective and social dimensions, a reduction of disease and health to numerical data at the bedside and later in the laboratory increasingly dominated the thinking of clinicians and researchers. Arnold Pacey, a historian of technology, sees the seventeenth century as a time when "the habit of thinking about processes in terms of machines spread from ideas about clocks and the universe [e.g., astronomy] to the study of the human body."[37] Thus, physicians began to think of the heart in terms of a pump that beats with a certain regularity. For astute forward-thinking physicians long accustomed to palpating the *pulsus frequens* and *pulsus rarus*, the practice of timing the pulse by a clock was a logical step.

Although a number of seventeenth-century physicians and scientists experimented with timing the pulse, it was John Floyer of Staffordshire who invented a clock that ran for exactly one minute and which was conveniently portable. In his book, *The Physician's Pulse-Watch*, Floyer wrote:

> I have for many years try'd pulses by the minute in common watches and pendulum clocks, when I was among my patients; after some time I met with the common sea minute-glass . . . and by that I made most of my experiments. But because this was not portable I caused a pulse-watch to be made which run [sic] 60 Seconds. I placed it in a box to be more easily carried, and by this I now feel Pulses.[38]

Floyer, who used as his model the Galenic concept of a characteristic pulse for individual disease states, tabulated various pulse rates in health and disease, and concluded that the "most natural magnitude" of the pulse was seventy to seventy-five per minute. Intensive investigations into the pulse as it varied with factors such as climate, seasons, geography, age, illness, diet, and activity—together with his own assessment of Galenic and Chinese pulse lore—are a testament to Floyer's status as a careful medical scientist of the early eighteenth century. He intended that his study of the pulse, with the aid of his pulse-watch (or "minute-glass"), should contribute to therapeutics. In the title page of his treatise, he declared: "A new mechanical device is propos'd for preserving health, and prolonging

---

[37] Pacey, *Technology and World Civilization*, 98.
[38] John Floyer, "Preface," *The Physician's Pulse-Watch* (London: S. Smith and B. Walford, 1707).

life and for curing diseases."[39] "Our life," declared Floyer, "consists in the circulation of blood," and it was the "physician's business to regulate the circulation." He believed that by "rais[ing] deficient [i.e. slow] pulses" and "depress[ing] and sink[ing] the number of exceeding pulses," he could improve therapeutics.[40]

WILLIAM WITHERING: *AN ACCOUNT OF THE FOXGLOVE*

In practice, the pulse rate was not routinely "taken" by medical consultants until the nineteenth century.[41] One outstanding exception was William Withering, the observant Birmingham physician who studied the effects of foxglove leaf (*digitalis purpurae*) in dropsy (massive fluid retention, most often due to congestive heart failure; less commonly due to kidney or liver disease). In his seminal 1785 monograph, *An Account of the Foxglove and Some of Its Medical Uses*, Withering mentioned a slow pulse rate of thirty-five per minute under the heading of "Effects, Rules, and Cautions," evidence that he relied on his pulse watch:

> The foxglove when given in very large and quickly-repeated doses, occasions sickness, vomiting, purging, giddiness, confused vision, objects appearing green or yellow; increased secretion of urine, with frequent motions to part with it; slow pulse, even as slow as 35 in a minute, cold sweats, convulsions, syncope [fainting], death.[42]

---

[39] Floyer, *Physician's Pulse-Watch*, title page. A biography of Floyer is found in Jacob Rosenbloom, "The History of Pulse Timing with Some Remarks on Sir John Floyer and his Physician's Pulse Watch," *Annals of Medical History* 4 (1922): 97–99; S. Weir Mitchell, *The Early History of Instrumental Precision in Medicine: An Address before the Second Congress of American Physicians and Surgeons, September 23rd, 1891 by the President of the Congress* (New Haven: Tuttle, Morehouse, &Taylor, 1892), 21–24; "The Early History of Instrumental Precision in Medicine. An Address Before the Second Congress of American Physicians and Surgeons, September 23, 1891, by the President of the Congress," *Transactions of the Congress of American Physicians and Surgeons* 2 (1892): 177–80.

[40] Floyer, "Preface," *Physician's Pulse-Watch*.

[41] Mitchell, *The Early History of Instrumental Precision in Medicine*, 23–24; J. Worth Estes, *Hall Jackson and the Purple Foxglove: Medical Practice and Research in Revolutionary America, 1760-1820* (Hanover, NH: University Press of New England, 1979), 153.

[42] William Withering, *An Account of the Foxglove and Some of Its Medical Uses* (Birmingham: M. Swinney, 1785), 184. Reprinted in facsimile in J. K. Aronson, *An*

SEEING THE PULSE: STEPHEN HALE'S *HAEMASTATICKS*

Over many centuries, intellectually curious physicians had made isolated attempts to translate the workings of the cardiovascular system into a visual process occurring in real time. A much-celebrated experiment by clergyman and enthusiastic experimentalist Stephen Hales of Teddington is often cited as the first measurement of the blood pressure. Within the field of study he called "haemastaticks," Hales observed and measured the pulsations of blood in an artery. At some date between 1707 and 1711, Hales cannulated the crural (femoral) artery in a living horse, using a brass pipe connected to a vertical glass tube. Hales recorded arterial pressure as height, the principle behind the now-obsolete twentieth-century blood pressure cuffs with calibrated columns of mercury. He appears to have observed (but not understood) the exaggerated fall in blood pressure that is seen with deep inspiration, a normal physiological phenomenon not understood at the time: "Then untying the ligature on the artery, the blood rose in the tube eight feet three inches perpendicular above the left ventricle of the heart.... When it was at its full height, it would rise and fall at and after each pulse two, three, or four inches; and sometimes it would fall twelve or fourteen inches."[43]

Although witnesses to trauma since prehistoric times had been aware that blood spurted from severed arteries, Hales literally *visualized* the pulsations of the artery in a controlled fashion. In the 1830s, as will be described in greater detail in the next chapter, the sphygmometer, a device which transmitted the external pulsations of the radial artery at the wrist to a column of liquid, allowed physicians to *see* the human pulse. Such diagnostic instruments allowed several physicians to observe simultaneously a physiological event, watching together as the column of liquid moved up and down with each pulse beat.

Account of the Foxglove and its Medical Uses, 1785–1985 (London: Oxford University Press, 1985). Derivatives and synthetic forms of digitalis remained mainstays of clinical cardiology well into the twentieth century and, though less commonly used in recent decades, are still prescribed for congestive heart failure and atrial fibrillation.

[43] Stephen Hales, *Statistical Essay Containing Haemastaticks: An Account of Some Hydraulic and Hydrostatic Experiments Made on the Blood and Blood-Vessels of Animals* (London: W. Innys and R. Manby, 1733), 1–2.

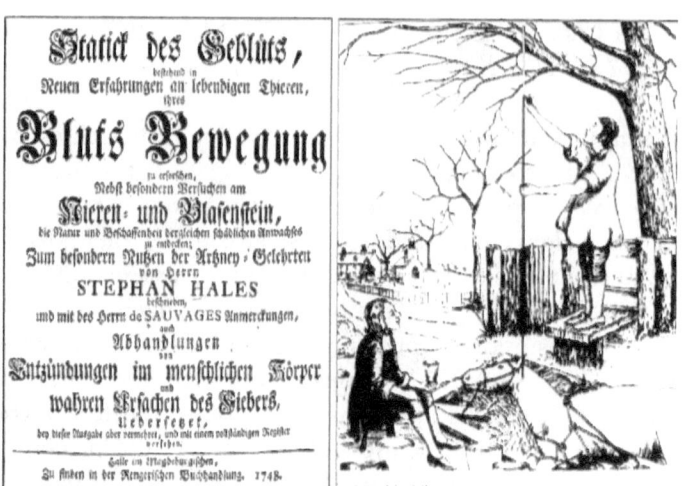

Figure 6: Clergyman Stephen Hales observing the rise and fall of arterial blood in a cannulated artery in a horse, considered the first numerical measurement of blood pressure (1733). The illustration does not appear in Hales' original *Statistical Essays*. The woodcut appears to have been made in 1748 in connection with a German-language version of Hales' *Haemastaticks*. The image has been much reproduced (even colorized) without attribution. Note that the image shows a carotid artery cannulation rather than the crural artery (in the leg) mentioned in the text.

RESPIRATORY TIME AND SPACE: HUTCHINSON'S SPIROMETER

In the related field of respiration, John Hutchinson of England invented the spirometer, a device for measuring the capacity of the lungs. The strength or volume of a subject's forced expiration (starting from maximum inspiration) was transmitted to a graduated monitor, giving a numerical value in cubic inches for the "vital capacity." Hutchinson's work, reported in 1846, is remarkable for its carefully tabulated correlation of over two thousand spirometric readings on healthy subjects with such variables as height, weight, habitus, gender, age, body temperature, posture (standing or sitting), and profession (from Grenadier Guards to pugilists and wrestlers). Hutchinson attended to the reproducibility of results and the identification of preclinical disease. He demonstrated that breathing, another deeply resonant and fundamental human function, could be reduced to meaningful numbers with practical applications in clinical medicine.[44]

---

[44] Reiser, *Medicine and the Reign of Technology*, 91–93. John Hutchinson, "On the Capacity

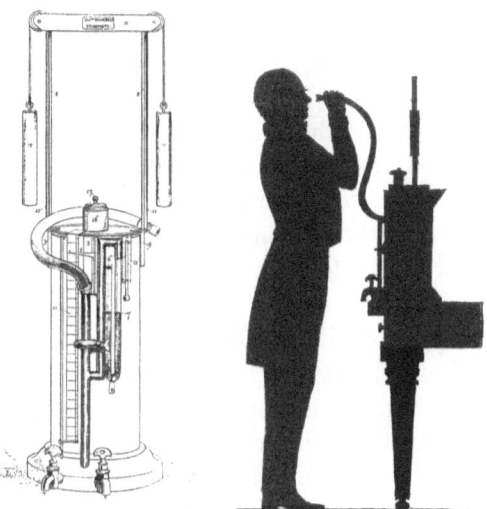

FIGURE 7: John Hutchinson's spirometer for recording respiratory excursions and lung capacity. "On the Capacity of the Lungs, and on the Respiratory Functions, with a View of Establishing a Precise and Easy Method of Detecting Disease by the Spirometer." *Medico-Chirurgical Transactions*, 2d ser., 29 (1846), 234, 236.

THE PARTIAL ECLIPSE OF PULSE STUDY

Advances in anatomic pathology and the enthusiastic embrace of the stethoscope temporarily diverted attention from pulse study, which seemed to be mired in old rationalistic theories of disease causation. One of the great British masters of the sphygmograph and the first to identify essential hypertension (high blood pressure not due to disease of the kidneys), Frederick Akbar Mahomed, reflected on the role of the stethoscope in "throwing aside" the study of the pulse:

> The study of morbid anatomy [i.e., autopsy and biopsy findings] has thrown cold water upon our study of functional disorders and symptoms, and deservedly so, for it has

---

of the Lungs, and on the Respiratory Functions, with a View of Establishing a Precise and Easy Method of Detecting Disease by the Spirometer," *Medico-Chirurgical Transactions*, 2nd ser., 29 (1846), 137–252. The dynamic term, "vital capacity," is still used today in clinical spirometry.

demonstrated the gross fallacies and errors into which such observations led our predecessors, and it has taught us the invaluable lesson of accepting nothing without anatomical proof. There are certain things, however, which morbid anatomy cannot show us, at any rate, not at present. . . . Unfortunately, when we obtained the stethoscope we threw aside the pulse; the stethoscope indicated structural changes which we could demonstrate after death, the pulse told us of functional conditions which we could not discover by dissection, and of the existence of which we could offer no scientific or irrefragable proof.[45]

The good clinician can still deduce a great deal from pulse palpation. The very act of taking the patient's wrist and encircling it within the examiner's fingers is an oddly intimate yet unthreatening act of sanctioned professional contact between physician and patient. Remnants of Latin persist in the modern description of the pulse under the physician's finger. For example, the terms *pulsus parvus et tardus* of aortic stenosis, *pulsus alterans* of left heart failure, and *pulsus paradoxus* of severe lung disease remain in textbooks today. In some cases, descriptive terms such as "bounding" and "thready" have appeared in place of older Latin terms. Despite a general campaign to obliterate eponyms from modern medical textbooks, the characteristic bounding pulse of aortic valvular insufficiency (leakage) is still referred to as Corrigan's pulse or "water-hammer" pulse—an example of what a modern diagnostician calls the "curious attachment to obsolete points of reference."[46]

---

[45] Frederick Akbar Mahomed. "Some of the Clinical Aspects of Chronic Bright's Disease." *Guy's Hospital Reports*, 3rd ser., 24 (1879): 364–65. The unusual and unjustly neglected career of Mahomed and his critical role in the modern understanding of blood pressure are described in J. Stewart Cameron and Jackie Hicks, "Frederick Akbar Mahomed and His Role in the Description of Hypertension at Guy's Hospital," *Kidney International* 49 (1996): 1494; Mahomed's critical work with the sphygmograph and his elucidation of essential hypertension are discussed in Chapter 3.

[46] Janice L. Willms, Henry Schneiderman, and Paula S. Altranati, *Physical Diagnosis: Bedside Evaluation of Diagnosis and Function* (Baltimore: Williams & Wilkins, 1994), 337. Dominic John Corrigan of Dublin wrote a classic description of aortic valvular insufficiency ("leaky" valve) and its characteristic pulse in 1832. A water hammer was a thick glass tube half filled with water in which a vacuum was created by boiling prior to sealing the glass tube; sudden inversion of the tube produced a knocking sensation as the water fell against the lower end of the tube. See Delp and Manning, eds., *Major's Physical Diagnosis*, 138.

In contrast to the pulse-savvy physicians of the nineteenth century, the modern examiner frequently neglects the subjective quality of the peripheral pulses. Determination of rate, now relegated to nurses and aides (and increasingly to electronic monitors), is often the sole pulse examination a patient experiences. Nevertheless, cardiology textbooks continue to stress examination of the pulse, including the palpable "shape" of the wave, as an integral part of the cardiovascular examination. In 2001, authors of an authoritative American cardiology textbook wrote: "The frequency, regularity, and *shape* of the pulse wave and the character of the arterial wall should be determined." The point was illustrated with schematics of pulse waves in health and in a variety of cardiac abnormalities.[47]

The next chapter examines the technological pathway that led up to the invention of the sphygmograph and the intellectual dialogue that surrounded its journey from the laboratory to the bedside. The groundwork was laid by physiologist Carl Ludwig in Germany at mid-century. But the flashpoint of invention was in 1860s Paris in the laboratory of a remarkable researcher who reflected and interpreted a European sensitivity to new concepts of energy and what has been called "the human motor."[48] The subsequent British narrative of the sphygmograph, beginning in the late 1860s, identified the challenges that a handful of American sphygmographers would face a decade later.

---

[47] Eugene Braunwald and Joseph K. Perloff, "Physical Examination of the Heart and Circulation," in *Heart Disease: A Textbook of Cardiovascular Medicine*, 6th ed., ed. Eugene Braunwald (Philadelphia: W. B. Saunders, 2001), 51–52. (italics added)

[48] Anson Rabinbach, *The Human Motor: Energy, Fatigue, and the Origins of Modernity* (Berkeley: University of California Press, 1990).

Chapter 2

From Sphygmoscope to Sphygmograph: And the Vision of Ètienne-Jules Marey

The sphygmograph was the nineteenth-century centerpiece of the "time and space machines" of cardiology. The word sphygmograph comes from the Greek σφυγμoς (pulse or beat) and γραφειν (to write). Ètienne-Jules Marey of Paris, "physician, physiologist, pioneer of medical measurement, cardiologist, aviation pioneer, student of hydraulics, and photographic and cinema pioneer," was the central figure in the development of the sphygmograph.

Social historian Anson Rabinbach locates Marey at the epicenter of emerging European modernity in the last third of the nineteenth century—"the archimedean point at which social and cultural modernity intersected."[1] Marey's fertile mind grasped the transformative role of graphic inscription in the study of cardiovascular physiology. With minor modifications, the sphygmograph Marey designed in the early 1860s was the basis for most of the machines introduced in the forty-year career of the instrument. As one physiologist recalled in 1902, "the transmission of movement was in the air, and Marey made the air subservient to the transmission of movement."[2]

---

[1] Anson Rabinbach, *The Human Motor: Energy, Fatigue, and the Origins of Modernity* (Berkeley: University of California Press, 1990), 87.
[2] William Stirling, *Some Apostles of Physiology: An Account of Their Lives and Labours* (London: Waterlow, 1902), 93.

The sphygmograph was linked to many of the key themes of late-nineteenth-century medicine: the role of medical technology, the self-image of physicians, tensions between elite physicians and general practitioners, the patient's perception of his encounter with the physician, and the source and location of professional authority. Because it was a device to investigate the pulse, the sphygmograph tapped into a nuanced and emotionally resonant physiological manifestation of human existence.

The sphygmograph did not spring fully realized from a medical world without interest in technologies of pulse study. Like most medical technologies, Marey's sphygmograph was part of a longer technological narrative. There were imaginative men who used the knowledge available to them to make a series of preliminary steps toward a practical "pulse writer"—men who laid the groundwork for the truly monumental imagination of Étienne-Jules Marey. In order to understand the sphygmograph and its reformulation of physiologic space and time, it is necessary to examine, if only briefly, some fundamental advances in understanding and diagnosing the workings of the body, particularly the cardiovascular system.[3]

SEEING THE PULSE: PLUMBING THE ARTERIES

Before physicians could "write the pulse," they learned to "see the pulse" in real time. The earliest efforts to visualize the pulsations of the arteries involved what modern physicians would characterize as invasive methods. As noted in the previous chapter, Stephen Hales studied the pulse early in the eighteenth century by introducing a hollow tube into the artery of a horse and observing the fluctuations of the blood column with each cardiac cycle. A few surgeons recorded intraarterial pressures in humans during surgeries such as amputations. In the early 1870s, Leonard Landois, a German physiologist, solved a dispute about the shape of the pulse by means of what he termed a "haemautogram," in which the blood spurting from an animal's surgically severed artery was captured on a moving strip of paper.[4] Though this was technically a sphygmogram—a permanent recording of a pulse wave—the utility of such a technique was obviously limited.

---

[3] For an excellent overview and commentary, see Stanley Joel Reiser, *Medicine and the Reign of Technology* (Cambridge: Cambridge University Press, 1978), 91–121.

[4] Leonard Landois, *A Text-book of Human Physiology; Translated from the Seventh German Edition* (Philadelphia: P. Blakiston, Son & Co., 1892), 119.

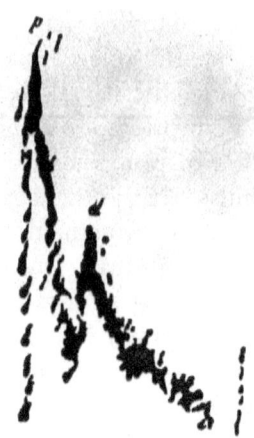

FIGURE 8: Leonard Landois's "Autosphygmogram [Haematosphygmogram] from Posterior Tibial Artery of a Dog," Leonard Landois, *A Text-book of Human Physiology*, 7th German ed., translated with additions by William Stirling, 4th English ed. (Philadelphia: P. Blakiston, Son & Co., 1892), 119.

What was needed for clinical use was a non-invasive technique (to borrow a modern term) for pulse study outside the vivisection laboratory and the operating room, by which useful information about the pulse could be obtained without cannulating or opening an artery.

THE HÉRISSON "SPHYGMOMÈTRE"

Beginning in the mid 1830s, a number of European physicians built devices designed to visualize the cyclical excursions of the pulse. Sphygmometer is a general term for an instrument that displays the rise and fall of the pulse, used interchangeably in the nineteenth century with sphygmoscope, a term that emphasized the visualization of the pulse as it rose and fell.

The earliest sphygmometer for measuring and visualizing pressure over an intact human artery (in contrast to a cut artery at surgery or a cannulated artery requiring an incision into the artery) was a rudimentary instrument devised in 1834 by Jules Hérisson in France. Hérisson's *sphygmomètre* (he did not use the term sphygmoscope) was the "first device to visually portray and numerically measure the rise and fall of the pulse beat without requiring the puncture of an artery."[5]

---

[5] Reiser, *Medicine and the Reign of Technology*, 98–99.

Hérisson simply attached a graduated glass tube to an inverted mercury-filled cup covered by a taut leather membrane. When the membrane was pressed over the radial artery at the wrist, pulsations were transmitted to the column of mercury in the vertical glass tubing. Although there was no recording device and therefore no permanent record, observers could see the mercury column fluctuate. Since the glass tube was calibrated, an upper and lower number (not to be confused with the upper and lower numbers of the modern blood pressure machine) could be assigned to the moving column of mercury. Hérisson also applied the device over the cardiac impulse on the chest wall, thus revealing to the physician "all the movements of this central organ, and when appled to an artery it indicates all the movements of the pulse."[6]

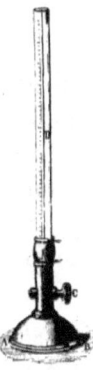

FIGURE 9: Hérisson sphygmometer (sphygmoscope). Jules Hérisson. Le Sphygmomètre: *instrument qui traduit à l'oeil toute l'action des artères* (Paris, 1854), front matter; also in Étienne-Jules Marey, *La circulation du sang à l'état physiologique et dans les maladies* (Paris: G. Masson, 1881), 208.

The title of Hérisson's monograph, *Le sphygmomètre, instrument qui traduit à l'oeil toute l'actiones artères* (*The Sphygmometer, Instrument that Translates to the Eye all the Actions of the Arteries*) emphasizes the *translation* of the pulse from the tactile to the visual. The pulse ceased to be a private matter between a single physician and his patient. Now a group of

---

[6] E. S. Blundell, "Preface," in Jules Hérisson, *Le sphygmomètre: instrument qui traduit à l'oeil toute l'action des artères (The Sphgymometer, an Instrument Which Renders the Action of the Arteries Apparent to the Eye): Being a Memoir Presented to the Institute of France, by Dr. Julius Hérisson with an Improvement of the Instrument and Prefatory Remarks by the Translator, Dr. E. S. Blundell* (London: Longman, Rees, Orme, Brown, Green, and Longman, 1835), iii–xvi, quotation from main text, 5.

physicians could observe the oscillations of the pulse simultaneously and offer a semiquantitative report. For example, he described a pulse that was "feeble, irregular, intermittent, unequal . . . The column of mercury in the sphygmometer falls below its level, 1, 2, and even 3 degrees, in proportion to the extent of the obstacle."[7]

Hérisson used his sphygmometer on a variety of patients, observing not only the height of the column of mercury, but the pattern of oscillations. He also correlated his observations in life with autopsy findings, a critical step in understanding the cause and course of disease. For example, twenty-seven patients close to death from heart failure ("inexpressible anguish, the patient no longer breathes, he is smothered, and death menaces him every moment") were found at autopsy to have "concentric and excentric hypertrophies of the left ventricle and its dilatations" due to some obstruction between the ventricle and the aorta (a "forced excitement of its valves and orifices").[8]

Hérisson's work was of sufficient interest to warrant translation into English within a year by English physician E. S. Blundell. Rather optimistically, Blundell predicted in his preface that the sphygmometer was a promising "new means of combating disease." Equally important was the potential value of the sphygmometer in "elucidat[ing] those points which the Stethoscopist is not able to reach . . . and thus furnish[ing] the Stethoscopist with a powerful auxiliary in enabling him to indicate, with unerring precision, not only the seat, nature, and extent of the disease, but also the slightest disturbance to the central circulation." For the student, "in his daily rounds through the wards of the public hospitals" and the "country practitioner" requesting consultation, the device would also prove useful.[9]

In an appended note on his own improvements to the Hérisson sphygmometer, Blundell conveyed his dismay upon discovering that the Paris-made instrument that he had purchased was not built to Hérisson's specifications.[10] Although Blundell could not know it at the time, it was a

---

[7] Ibid., 26.

[8] Ibid., Clinical descriptions of these and other cardiac patients on pages 26–27; table of observations on pages 29–30 of Blundell's translation. Hérisson did not specify aortic valve stenosis (narrowing), which was the most likely (modern) diagnosis in most patients in this group.

[9] Ibid., iii–xvi. Blundell appended a "Description of the Improvements of the Instrument," explaining his own changes in the stopcock.

[10] Ibid., "Description of the Improvements of the Instrument," 42–43. Blundell's "improved sphygmograph" was available for purchase in London.

harbinger of future technical difficulties with the sphygmograph and the thorny problem of standardization.

An American physician, Joseph Nancrede, published a translation with a Philadelphia publishing house in the same year (1835). He had been sent a copy of Hérisson's text and "one of the instruments, the first that have crossed the Atlantic." In his brief preface, Nancrede hailed Hérisson's sphygmometer as "an additional means of facilitating the healing art, and at the same time imparting to them [i.e., the medical profession] an exactness, in which they are too often confessedly defective." Nancrede reported that Hérisson's invention had generated a "very great sensation" in Paris, where the press "teems with its praises."[11]

Hérisson himself promoted his sphygmometer as an aid to written consultation. At a time when consultation required either a lengthy case description by letter or inconvenient travel, the general practitioner armed with a sphygmometer could convey to a "distant physician of celebrity" a quantitative measurement of the pulse of the patient; "[T]he instrument being the same every where, the measure formed at St. Petersburg [i.e., by the provincial Russian physician] will be perfectly understood in Paris" [i.e., by the celebrated specialist].[12]

Hérisson, eager to apply his invention at the bedside, used his sphygmometer as a guide to therapy in non-cardiac cases of impending "apoplexy" (an antiquated descriptive term for a catastrophic stroke-like event) due to "cerebral congestion." If the pulse "passed beyond the degree of impulse necessary to equilibrium," he bled the patient, either with leeches or by opening a vein. He followed these apoplectic patients (for whom he prescribed a healthful regimen) with his sphygmometer; he found them much improved, "maintain[ing] their circulation at that degree of moderation which the sphygmogmeter never fails to indicate."[13]

Not every physician was dazzled by Hérisson's sphygmometer. David Badham, an English physician writing from Paris in 1835, challenged Hérisson's assumption that the peripheral pulse was a reliable indicator of the state of the heart or of the cerebral circulation. He himself had observed

---

[11] Joseph G. Nancrede, "Preface," in Jules Hérisson, *The Sphygmometer. An Instrument which Exhibits to the Eye the Entire Action of the Arteries; The Usefulness of this Instrument in the Study of all Diseases; Researches on the Diseases of the Heart and on the Means of Discriminating Them; A Memoir Presented to the Institute of France by Dr. Julius [sic] Herisson, of Paris; Translated from the French by Joseph G. Nancrede, M.D.* (Philadelphia: Grigg and Elliot, 1835).

[12] Blundell translation of Hérisson, *Le sphygmomètre*, 14.

[13] Ibid., 12–13 (footnote).

sphygmometric discrepancies between the left and right radial arteries in the same patient at the same time; obviously, both readings could not reliably indicate cardiac action. In patients known to have lost a great deal of blood, he sometimes observed an unexpectedly wide fluctuation in the mercury in the sphygmometer. With remarkable insight, Badham wrote: "it ought to be inquired whether the motive force of one part of the arterial system, in disease, does indeed bear a constant proportion with that of a distant and internal part of the economy." He referred to his own previous work in which he postulated "inherent independent action occasionally exercised by the arteries themselves." From a practical point of view, Badham concluded that vigorous bloodletting for incipient apoplexy, as recommended by Hérisson based on his sphygmometric observations, was ill-advised.[14]

Variations on Hérisson's instrument were constructed over the next few decades, culminating in a small portable device introduced in England in the 1890s for use by clinicians. The professional reception ranged from overoptimistic predictions of a great breakthrough in diagnosis to the remarks of a critic who called it "one of the most silly and ridiculous baubles that was ever attempted to be foisted on the attention of the profession." In his negative review of Blundell's translation of Hérisson's monograph on the sphygmometer, a writer for the *Medico-Chirurgical Review and Journal of the Medical Sciences* charged:

> A complicated apparatus to be fixed on the arm or on the chest, to indicate the action of the heart and arteries—an action that will vary from Alpha to Omega while the apparatus is being applied, and which, after all, will not convey one-hundredth part the information to the *experienced* practitioner, which the finger [on the pulse] will indicate! To the *inexperienced*, it will only prove an ignis fatuus [will o'the wisp] and lead him into sloughs and ditches.

The reviewer missed the larger point—the utility of translation from touch to sight—calling Hérisson's sphygmometer "a complicated piece of machinery for *seeing* the pulse, when it can be *felt* by the finger—the touch in this case, as in many others, being a thousand times less deceptive

---

[14] David Badham, "A Few Remarks on the Sphygmometer," *London Medical Gazette* 16 (1835–36): 265–68. Later studies in neurovascular physiology would confirm that the cerebrovascular circulation, for example, far from being a passive conduit for blood pumped from the heart, is controlled by complex neuroendocrine and neurovascular factors.

than the sight. But enough of the bauble."[15] Although Hérisson seems to have been forgotten, his sphygmometer, a simple mechanical device, was periodically reinvented. The American experience will be discussed in a future chapter.

THE SCOTT ALISON SPHYGMOSCOPE

In Britain, Somerville Scott Alison did considerable work with sphygmoscopes (he preferred the term sphygmoscope over *sphygmomètre* or sphygmometer) of his own design as early as the late 1830s, constructing devices for observing the rise and fall of the cardiac impulse in the chest and arterial impulses in peripheral arteries. For cardiac studies, Scott Alison applied an inverted cup filled with "spirits of wine or other liquid" and covered by an india rubber membrane over the cardiac impulse in a seated subject. A one-foot long hollow calibrated glass tube was attached to the upper end of the cup and the rise and fall of the liquid observed and measured. The rather unwieldy apparatus was fixed to a stand.[16]

For study of the arteries, Scott Alison built and tested what he referred to as a "hand sphygmoscope." At the outset, he was unaware of Hérisson's apparatus and monograph, which he later acknowledged in his 1856 paper in the *Proceedings of the Royal Society*: "Since this instrument [the hand sphygmoscope] was contrived, the author has learned that a sphygmometer of much the same construction was invented some twenty years ago by Mons. le Docteur Hérrison, and that a memoir upon it was presented to the Institute of France." He pointed out that Hérisson used mercury rather than alcohol or water in the glass tubing and "gold-beater's skin" (ox intestine, used by goldsmiths, and less elastic than Scott Alison's india rubber) as the sensing membrane.[17]

---

[15] Review of *The Sphygmometer: An Instrument Which Renders the Action of the Arteries Apparent to the Eye &c.* by Jules Hérisson, *Medico-Chirurgical Review and Journal of Practical Medicine* n.s. 27 (1835): 159–60; italics in original.

[16] Somerville Scott Alison (reported by G. O. Rees), "A Description of a New Sphygmoscope, an Instrument for Indicating the Movements of the Heart and Blood-Vessels; With an Account of Observations Obtained by the Aid of that Instrument," *Proceedings of the Royal Society of London* 8 (1856–57): 18–26; Somerville Scott Alison, *The Physical Examination of the Chest in Pulmonary Consumption* (London: John Churchill, 1861), 344–46.

[17] Scott Alison, "Description of a New Sphygmoscope," 22 (footnote).

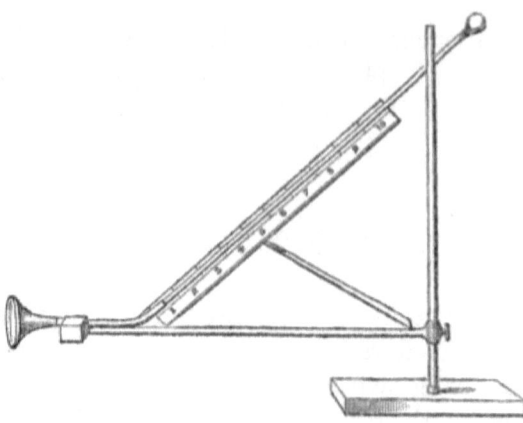

FIGURE 10: Scott Alison's sphygmoscope for examining the cardiac impulse
Somerville Scott Alison, "A Description of a New Sphygmoscope, an Instrument for Indicating the Movements of the Heart and Blood-Vessels; With an Account of Observations Obtained by the Aid of that Instrument," *Proceedings of the Royal Society of London* 8 (1856–57): 19.

The most novel application of Scott Alison's sphygmoscope was his demonstration of the sequential timing of the cardiac impulse (ventricular contraction) and the transmitted pulse in a peripheral artery such as the carotid or radial. Simultaneous manual palpation of the cardiac impulse and the pulse did "not admit of a distinct difference in respect to time being made out. It has been to this very defect that the erroneous idea, that the beat of the heart and the beat of the pulse are synchronous, or nearly so, has owed its origin and continuance." With one sphygmoscope over the heart and a second over the radial artery, he showed that the "movements in the two instruments at the same instant are always opposed." As fluid rose in the cardiac sphygmoscope, it fell in the arterial sphygmoscope and vice versa. This held true in twenty subjects with varying pulses. Scott Alison concluded that the heartbeat alternated with the pulse, an incomplete analysis at best. He found that two sphygmoscopes placed simultaneously over a proximal artery (such as the carotid in the neck) and a distal artery (such as the radial at the wrist or dorsalis pedis in the foot) rose and fell simultaneously.[18] This was an incorrect observation, limited by the insensitivity of his equipment (the pulse is transmitted from the heart to the limbs in a fraction of a second). Alison seems to have imagined the

---

[18] Ibid., 23–24.

pulse as a sort of panarterial beat linked inversely to the cardiac beat, rather than as a wave front moving from the center to the periphery.

The fatal limitation of the sphygmoscope (sphygmometer) was the lack of a permanent written or inscribed record of the pulse wave. The rise and fall of the pulse could be seen by observers standing near the subject and described in writing. A later worker with more advanced technology wrote that sphygmoscopes "may be regarded as ingenious toys, but the sphygmograph [with its permanent inscribed pulse curve] is the only instrument that can be recommended for determining accurately and permanently the true character of the pulse."[19] The solution would come in the middle decades of the nineteenth century.

REGISTRATION: THE LUDWIG KYMOGRAPH

The critical invention that reconfigured the representation of physiological events was the kymograph, the revolving drum recorder introduced in the winter of 1846–47 by German physiologist Carl Friedrich Ludwig. The infinitely useful kymograph (literally "wave writer") was a sophisticated device designed to translate physiological events into visual inscriptions with dimensions of space and time. Ludwig's student William Stirling traced the origins of the kymograph to his master's "epoch making" conversion of the hemodynamometer of physiologist Jean Léonard Marie Poiseuille into his "kymographion of 1847, the instrument that first recorded the beating of the heart."[20]

Poisseuille's hemodynamometer was a U-shaped glass tube with a horizontal arm leading to the cannulated artery. The glass tubing was marked off at regular intervals on both vertical arms and partly filled with mercury. Blood from the cannulated artery of an experimental animal entered the tube through the sidearm, forcing the mercury to descend in one vertical arm and ascend in the other; the level of the ascendent mercury corresponded to the pressure in the artery. The experimenter read off the level of the mercury column and recorded the pressure.[21]

---

[19] Robert E. Dudgeon, *The Sphygmograph: Its History and Use as an Aid to Diagnosis in Ordinary Practice* (London: Baillière, Tindall, & Cox, 1882), 28.

[20] Stirling, *Some Apostles of Physiology*, 107.

[21] "The Haemodynamometer," *Lancet* 1 (1838–39): 278; J. L. M. Poiseuille, "Researches on the Forces of the Aortal or Left Side of the Heart," *Edinburgh Medical and Surgical Journal* 32 (1829): 30–31.

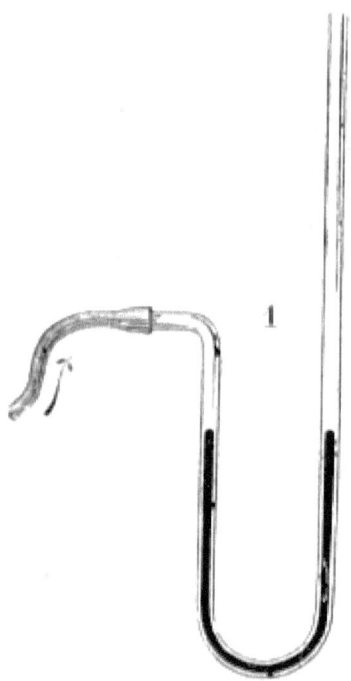

FIGURE 11: Poiseuille's "haemodynamometer." Poiseuille designed his "haemodynamometer" ca. 1829 to determine the pressure of blood inside the (punctured) artery of an experimental animal. The pressure exerted by the blood is equal to the height of the column of blood in the tall branch of the "U" tube minus the height of the blood column in the short branch. In this image, the artery has not yet been punctured, so the columns are equal. Étienne-Jules Marey, *La circulation du sang à l'état physiologique et dans les maladies* (Paris: G. Masson, 1881), 169.

Ludwig, seeking to make a permanent record of the pulse, placed a small float on the column of mercury in a Poiseuille hemodynamometer. The mercury moved up and down in its glass column as tiny pulsations were transmitted from the heart or cannulated artery of an experimental animal. The float was connected by a lever (with a wide sweep) having at its tip a stylus or other writing point. The stylus rested on smoked paper affixed to a rotating drum (revolving cylinder) and, with each tiny fluctuation in the mercury column, scratched a magnified wavy line onto the paper, creating a permanent record. With the introduction of the kymograph, physiologic events such as the pulse, respiratory excursions, muscle contractions, and the impulse of cardiac contraction against the chest wall—were translated to a graphic form in which the dimension of time was represented by the horizontal axis, while the physiologic event was inscribed on the vertical axis as the drum rotated. The result was a series of waves or curves in which height and shape were read as inscriptions of the "workings of the body."

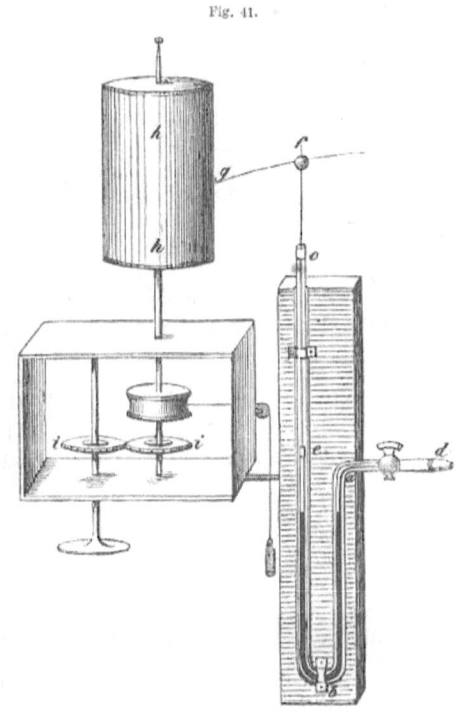

FIGURE 12: Ludwig's kymograph (wave writer). Carl Ludwig, *Lehrbuch der Physiologie des Menschen* (1856), II:85.

Historians of physiology have never ceased to celebrate the power of Ludwig's vision. Stirling recalled in 1902 that Ludwig "had the genius to cause the float to write on a recording cylinder, and thus at one *coup* gave us his kymograph or wave writer, and application of the graphic method to physiology."[22] Wrote one modern author: the kymograph was "the forerunner of all graphic recording instruments used in physiology."[23] Called "the characteristic instrument of physiology in

---

[22] Stirling, *Some Apostles of Physiology*, 85.
[23] E. M. Tansey, "The Physiological Tradition," in *Companion Encyclopedia of the History*

the second half of the nineteenth century," Ludwig's kymograph became the "prime instrumental intermediary between the physiologist and his experiment."[24]

In addtion to making a permanent inscription of a physiological event in an experimental animal, the kymograph operator, by changing the rate of rotation of the drum, could bring out various details—seemingly "slowing down and magnifying hitherto indistinguishable or unobservable biological events." The kymograph and "numerous families of derivative instruments" became the key elements in a wide variety of physiological experiments involving the neurological, muscular, pulmonary, and cardiovascular systems.[25] The Ludwig kymograph, because of its size, never achieved portability; nor did Ludwig intend that it be a device for bedside clinical application.

Historian of physiology Merriley Borrell highlighted both the creation ("autograph") and the utility ("permanence") elements of the kymographic tracings. The term "autograph" seems particularly apt, not only in the literal sense of "self writing," but in the secondary dictionary sense of a permanent manuscript in the author's own handwriting:

> The resultant tracing produced an actual autograph of these minute and transient fluctuations. Moreover, each record or tracing [preserved on the smoked paper peeled off the drum] could be compared with others generated under different experimental conditions. Every oscillation and physiological response—invisible to the [unaided] senses—was preserved and measurable.[26]

The earliest efforts by Ludwig and others to study the form and pressure of the pulse wave required direct cannulation of an artery, either during vivisection experiments on animals or in anesthetized patients undergoing amputations. The pulses in the interior of the artery were transmitted to a mercury manometer and thence to the kymograph. The impact of the kymograph on basic medical research was highlighted some years ago by its apt comparison to the impact of the telescope on astronomy.

---

of Medicine, ed. W. F. Bynum and Roy Porter (London: Routledge, 1993), 129.

[24] Robert G. Frank, "American Physiologists in German Laboratories, 1865–1914," in *Physiology in the American Context, 1850–1940*, ed. Gerald L. Geison (Bethesda, MD: American Physiological Society, 1987), 34.

[25] Merriley Borrell, "Extending the Senses: The Graphic Method," *Medical Heritage* 2 (1985): 114, 116.

[26] Ibid., 117.

It was both elegant and simple. In Borrell's words, the kymograph made it possible to "see the unobservable."[27]

LA MÉTHODE GRAPHIQUE

The new instruments of precision, beginning with the kymograph, intersected with what the French called *la méthode graphique* (the graphic method) to create a permanent record of physiological events such as the arterial pulse and the beating of the heart against the chest wall. With his invention of the kymograph in 1846–47, Ludwig introduced graphic registration into the physiology laboratory—the permanent inscription of bodily functions over time.[28] The familiar wavy lines of monitors in cardiac wards, neonatal units, intensive care units, ambulances, operating rooms, and emergency wards have their origins in the *méthode graphique*, as does the ubiquitous electrocardiogram.

Ludwig was confident that the workings of the body would be revealed in the physiology laboratory, much as the laws of physics and chemistry were being discovered in their respective laboratories. Rabinbach, in *The Human Motor: Energy, Fatigue, and the Origins of Modernity*, explains how the mid-nineteenth-century scientific concept of *Kraft* (energy) spilled over exuberantly from physics into the physiology laboratory, as well as into political, economic, and military spheres. Ludwig and others, most notably Hermann von Helmholtz, a physician, physiologist, and physicist who formulated the law of conservation of energy, saw the human or animal body as a "field of forces to be investigated and measured by medical technologies designed for that purpose." In Rabinbach's terms, Helmholtz "did not demote the living creature to the machine; he transposed the character of an energy-converting machine to the body." These investigations into energy and force in the context of physics and biology were linked to social phenomena such as labor power and human work and, ultimately, constructs of fatigue.

Rabinbach characterizes Étienne-Jules Marey, the inventor of the practical sphygmograph (discussed in detail later in this chapter),

---

[27] Comment on astronomy by Paul Cranefield, "Foreword," in *Two Great Scientists of the Nineteenth Century: Correspondence of Emil Du Bois-Reymond and Carl Ludwig*, ed. Estelle Du Bois-Reymond and Paul Diepgen (Baltimore: Johns Hopkins University Press, ca. 1982), viii; paraphrased in Borrell, "Extending the Senses," 116; 114, 117; phrase "see the unobservable," Borrell, "Extending the Senses," 114.

[28] W. Bruce Fye, "Carl Ludwig and the Leipzig Physiological Institute: 'A Factory of New Knowledge,'" *Circulation* 74 (1986): 925.

as a Helmholtzian, perhaps because it was Marey who most cogently demonstrated in a practical way the workings of the new mechanical body, a social and cultural nexus of the laws of physics and the human body. Most telling to physiologists searching for the workings of energy within the body was the discovery of electrical activity in the nerves and muscles. The new physiologists also began to frame their studies of metabolism in terms of heat production and energy conservation.[29] *La méthode graphique* illuminated and expanded these increasingly interconnected worlds of the physics laboratory and the physiology laboratory.

In her analysis of Marey's impact, Borrell concludes that Marey promoted and conflated dual meanings of the graphic method: "the power of graphics to display quantitative information" typified in medicine by growth and fever charts, and the inscribed curves of physiological processes such as the pulse and neuromuscular activity indication "actual movement through space" over time.[30]

Most importantly for medicine, "Marey adapted the invasive procedures used for experimental work to the noninvasive requirements of practitioners." At the same time, he applied the techniques of the chemistry and physics laboratories to the physiology and biological laboratories. Marey himself proclaimed that the graphic method made the "illusions of the observer, the slowness of descriptions, and the confusion of facts" disappear. Yet he was mindful that the the new technologies of registration (such as the sphygmograph) introduced artifacts and created problems of standardization; these problems would plague the sphygmograph throughout its four-decade career.[31]

THE VIERORDT SPHYGMOGRAPH—THE "PULSE WRITER"

The sphygmograph, a hybrid of the sphygmometer and the kymograph, produced a visual image of the pulse wave without direct cannulation of the

---

[29] Rabinbach, *Human Motor*, 61, 66–67. Helmholtz invented the ophthalmoscope, one of the first and most influential of the new diagnostic technologies, in 1851; he also invented the myograph, an instrument to study and record the contractions of muscles, in 1849.

[30] Merriley Borrell, "Marey and D'Arsonval: The Exact Sciences in Late Nineteenth-Century French Medicine," in *From Ancient Omens to Statistical Mechanics: Essays on the Exact Sciences Presented to Asger Aaboe*, ed. J. L. Berggren and B. R. Goldstein (Copenhagen: University Library, 1987), 230.

[31] Ibid., 228, 231.

artery, thus opening the door to the study of pulse pressure and dynamics in the human subject. Karl Vierordt, professor of physiology at Tübingen, introduced the first sphygmograph in 1854. What Vierordt had in fact set out to construct was an instrument for measuring the pressure of the blood in the artery beneath the intact skin. A cup filled with variable weights was pressed upon the radial artery. A system of levers transmitted the pulsations to a Ludwig kymograph, where a stylus recorded the excursions of the pulse on smoked paper mounted on the turning drum. The end result was not a measure of blood pressure, as Vierordt had intended, but rather a recording of pulse waves—a sphygmograph producing a sphygmogram. Vierordt's sphygmograph utilized the same principle as Hérisson's sphygmometer: the application of pressure upon the artery to detect pulsatile motion.[32]

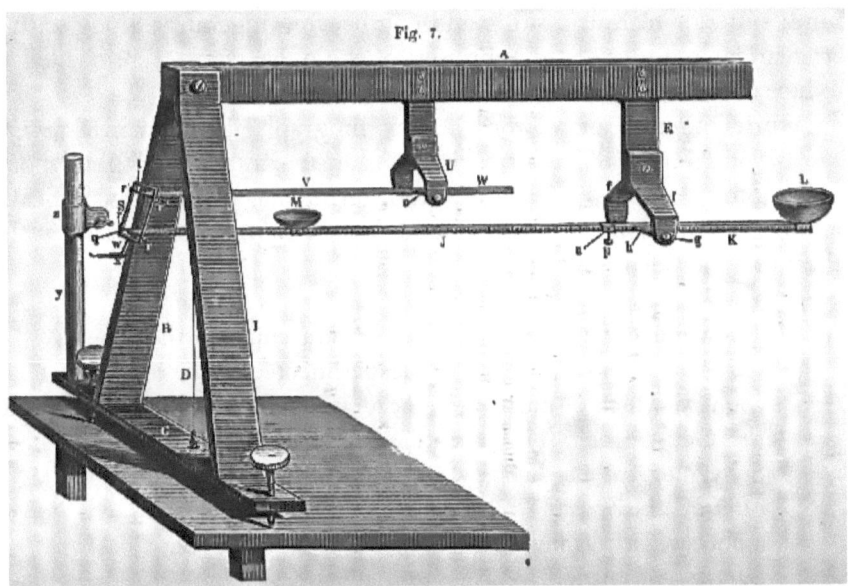

FIGURE 13: The Vierordt sphygmograph (pulse writer). Karl Vierordt, *Die Lehre vom Arterienpuls in Gesunden und Kranken Zustanden* (Braunschweig: Vieweg, 1855), 22.

---

[32] Karl Vierordt, "Die bildliche Darstellung des menschlichen Arterienpulses," *Archiv für Physiologische Heilkunde* 13 (1854): 284–87 (transl."The Visual Representation of the Human Arterial Pulse"); Karl Vierordt, *Die Lehre vom Arterienpuls in Gesunden und Kranken Zuständen* (transl. *The Teaching of the Arterial Pulse in Healthy and Sick States*), (Braunschweig: Vieweg, 1855); Reiser, *Medicine and the Reign of Technology*, 101.

Vierordt's sphygmograph was unwieldy, finicky, and insensitive.[33] The most serious limitation, beside the weight and size of the machine, was excessive damping of the lever movement (the short end of the lever was pressed against the artery, while the long end extended to the recording device). An incomplete understanding of cardiovascular physiology led Vierordt to adjust the instrument in such a fashion that subtle components of normal wave forms were dampened. Vierordt, by using counterweights to erase curves in the downstroke of the pulse wave, obliterated important movements of the artery that later sphygmographers, using better instruments, studied closely. Robert E. Dudgeon, British inventor of a practical portable sphygmograph, commented some decades later that Vierordt "took great pains to furnish us with a meaningless tracing."[34] Nevertheless, the basic concept (if not the fine tuning) was sound; superior technical skills and engineering ingenuity, along with a better understanding of the subtleties of the pulse wave, were needed to produce a usable sphygmograph.

A brief note about Vierordt's sphygmograph appeared in *Scientific American* in March 1855. Correspondent Dr. A. Zumbruck of Baltimore, in a letter to the popular science and engineering magazine, enthusiastically (but mistakenly) claimed priority for an American inventor working at the behest of a physician:

> Allow me to state that there has been a machine for the same purpose, invented, made, and experimented with, in this country, which is much more accurate and ingenious than the German one. The invention of this instrument called Sphygmograph i.e. Pulse-writer, was occasioned by the wish of Dr. C. Hering, of Philadelphia, to have a machine for such a purpose. It was invented by Mr. E. F. Hilgard, U.S. Coast Survey, and made in Washington about a year ago. It is an electro magnetic machine, recording on the same strip of paper the time and the number of beats of the pulse; it is, in fact, a

---

[33] Marey's description of Vierordt's sphygmograph appears in Étienne-Jules Marey, *La circulation du sang à l'état physiologique et dans les maladies* (Paris: G. Masson, 1881), 209–11; reproduced (in French, with expert commentary in English) in H. A. Snellen, *E. J. Marey and Cardiology: Physiologist and Pioneer of Technology, 1830–1904* (Rotterdam: Kooyker Scientific Publications, 1980), 130–32.

[34] Robert G. Frank, "The Telltale Heart: Physiological Instruments, Graphic Methods, and Clinical Hopes," in *The Investigative Enterprise*, ed. William Coleman and Fredrick L. Holmes (Berkeley: University of California Press, 1988), 216; Dudgeon, *Sphygmograph*, 17.

Morse's recording telegraph instrument, with two levers, two magnets, two batteries, and a clock. The current of one battery is broken by the stroke of the pendulum of a clock, each stroke making a dot. The current of the other battery is broken by the pulse. To a splint fastened to the arm of the person whose pulse is to be recorded, a lever is attached, one end of which rests on the pulse, so that each beat of the pulse. . . . breaks the circuit and makes a dot.

Thus the time interval and pulse beat were recorded simultaneously. The operator was able to conduct an experiment by which he followed the pulse rate after the administration of drugs such as alcohol.[35] In fact, the American had invented a novel and useful pulse counter, but not a true "wave writer" (sphygmograph). In contrast, Vierordt's over-dampened pulse wave was of no diagnostic value (beyond rate), but it was nevertheless a recorded wave and his invention was indeed a true sphygmograph.

CURRENTS IN FRENCH MEDICINE AND PHYSIOLOGY

By mid-century French academic medicine was moving from its emphasis on clinical observation of patients confirmed by post-mortem examination toward the German model of experimental medical science. A second, and more hesitant transition was the move away from the vitalism of the early leaders of French physiology, most notably Claude Bernard. Bernard was critical of reductionist approaches to the biological organism, stressing the distinction between the methods of physics and physiology—the mechanistic and the vitalistic.

Étienne-Jules Marey, introduced at the beginning of this chapter and the subject of the remainder of the chapter, believed that the workings of the body were potentially discoverable through applications of the laws and methods of physics and chemistry to the physiology laboratory. But he stopped short of rejecting vitalism altogether, perhaps hedging his bets because he instinctively understood that even the best of contemporary technology could not expose all the secrets of the animal organism. Early

---

[35] L. A. Geddes, *Handbook of Blood Pressure Measurement* (New York: Springer Scientific, 1991), 145 (Geddes quotes from Vol. 10 (old series) of *Scientific American*, which appeared in 1855, but misquotes the date as 1955), A. Zumbruck, "The Sphygmograph or Pulse Writer," *Scientific American* 10, no. 28 (1855): 219.

in his career, he wrote: "We are forced, in the name of logic, to apply the methods of physics and chemistry to the study of the phenomena of life; and it is only after having unprofitably used all these procedures, that we will be correct in invoking the existence of extra-physical causes for the explanation of vital phenomena."[36] Like heavenly bodies moving in space within the confines of Newtonian physics, the animal body and its components were subject to laws. Rather than celestial time, Marey was concerned with physiologic time. He saw the cardiovascular system as a straightforward mechanical construction—a pump and pliable tubes. Later researchers would correct such an oversimplified view of cardiovascular physiology by demonstrating the dependence of arterial pressure on endocrine and neurological factors.

THE MAREY SPHYGMOGRAPH: DISCOVERING THE *FABRICA*

As a young medical graduate in Paris at the end of the 1850s, Marey found practice uncongenial and turned instead to the fledgling and unstructured field of physiology. His personal preference had been a career in engineering, but his father insisted upon medicine. In his 1878 book, *La méthode graphique*, Marey reviewed the various applications of graphic analysis to diverse fields such as geography, economics, history, politics, physics, chemistry, meteorology, and medicine.[37] Clearly, Marey was in close touch with many of the social and scientific currents of his time.

The conjunction of interests was profoundly productive; a student said of Marey in 1904 that he was "never really a physiologist or a doctor in the usual sense of those terms, but above all, an engineer of life." ("Marey ne fut jamais en réalité un médecin, ni même un physiologiste, dans le sens où ce terme est communément employé: il fut avant tout un ingénieur de la vie.")[38] Working independently, Marey set up a laboratory in an old building once used by the Comédie Française. His earliest work, dating from 1857, was a study of the circulatory system using novel instrumental

---

[36] Ètienne-Jules Marey, *Du mouvement dans les fonctions de la vie: leçons faites au Collége de France* (Paris: Germer Bailliére, 1868), 39; on vitalism see Rabinbach, *Human Motor*, 64–66, 88.

[37] Snellen, *E. J. Marey*, 171.

[38] Rabinbach, *Human Motor*, 88, 90. "Engineer of Life" translated by Rabinbach from René Quinton, "E. J. Marey," *La Revue des Idées: Études de Critique Générale* 1 (1904): 484.

methods for recording and displaying the actions of the heart and blood vessels.[39]

It is useful to think of Marey's work in terms of the metaphor of the *fabrica* as used by Vesalius in his anatomic opus (see Chapter 1). Marey sought to discover the workings—the *fabrica*—of the "human motor," a task too complex for the unaided human senses, however experienced and well educated. Speaking in Brussels in 1876, Marey expressed his concern that, in the laboratory and at the bedside, subjectivity was an ever-present danger. Later users of medical technologies such as the sphygmograph would refer to this inherent bias of the observer or examiner as "the personal equation."

"TO SEE WITH A BETTER EYE": FROM LAENNEC TO MAREY

In his work with the sphygmograph, and later (and better known) experiments in human and animal motion, Marey relied on technology to allow him to "see with a better eye," the phrase used by French diagnostician Jean Nicolas Corvisart in 1806. Corvisart taught that a physician experienced in the art of medicine and skilled in the diagnostic science of the day (palpation and percussion in the case of cardiology) would "see, with a better eye, the nicest phenomena of life and predict more remotely the kind of disease which threatens an individual." Corvisart's profundity of thought was enhanced at the turn of the nineteenth century by his close study of chest percussion, a procedure which extended what he called the *coup d'oeil* (gaze or glance) of the diagnostician. The stethoscope invented by Corvisart's pupil René T. H. Laennec a decade later, was truly a "better eye."[40]

Marey intended that the sphygmograph would be a new "better eye" with which to expose the workings of the body. The sphygmograph reconfigured the blood vessels in the mind of the physician as structures which produced a visual, graphic image. At the same time, it reorganized the mental image of the entire cardiovascular system. Since the time of Harvey, the pulse was, in a sense, the messenger of the beating heart. In

---

[39] For a succinct account of Marey's career, see Snellen, *E. J. Marey*, 11–21.

[40] J. N. Corvisart, *An Essay on the Organic Diseases and Lesions of the Heart and Great Vessels* (1806), trans. Jacob Gates, ed. C. E. Horeau (Philadelphia: Anthony Finlay; Boston: Bradford and Reed, 1812), 19; Jacalyn Duffin, *To See with a Better Eye: A Life of R. T. H. Laennec* (Princeton NJ: Princeton University Press, 1998), epigraph, 33.

the physician's mind, the state of the pulse reflected the state of the organ that pumped the blood. With the sphygmograph, the palpable pulse and, by extension, the audible heart, became visible. It seemed self-evident to Marey that a visual and permanent record of pulse waves offered increased objectivity:

> In the laboratory, as at the bedside of the patient, the skill of the individual, his practiced tact, and the subtlety of his perceptive powers, played too large a part. To render accessible all the phenomena of life—*movements which are so light and fleeting, changes of condition so slow or rapid, that they escape the senses*—an objective form must by given to them, and they must be fixed under the eye of the observer, in order that he may study them and compare them deliberately.[41]

A familiar example of this change in the concept of the body is the typical behavior of physicians and cardiac patients today. A doctor making his rounds on a cardiac patient will check the heart monitor at the nursing station and the latest twelve-lead electrocardiogram in the patient's paper or electronic chart *before* proceeding to the bedside. His mental image of the patient's heart is formed before he walks into the room. The modern patient, now conditioned to the relevant technology, might open with some variation of "How is my cardiogram?" rather than "How am I doing?" In many cases, the cardiogram *seems* to "make" the decision as to whether the patient is discharged or stays in the hospital.

Marey, writes Rabinbach, was "among the first French physiologists to use [the metaphor of the machine for the functions of the animal organism] as the central metaphor to redefine the life sciences."[42] Marey's interest was in developing methods of physiological study that would be useful to physicians, although he himself never practiced clinical medicine. He also sought to replace vivisection with a better method of "seizing the delicate movements by which the circulation of the blood is transmitted externally."[43]

---

[41] Étienne-Jules Marey, "Lectures on the Graphic Method in the Experimental Sciences, and on Its Special Application to Medicine," *British Medical Journal* 1 (1876): 1 (italics added).

[42] Rabinbach, *Human Motor*, 90.

[43] Marey, *La circulation du sang*, ii. The complete sentence in French is: "Cherchant à substituer aux vivisections des moyens propres à mieux faire saisir les mouvements délicats par lesquels se traduit au dehors la circulation du sang."

MAREY'S "*LANGUE INCONNUE*"—THE UNKNOWN LANGUAGE OF PHYSIOLOGICAL TIME

Although Marey, in the course of his career, sought to construct a broad "science of the economy of the body," he began with the sphygmograph—a relatively simple device for inscribing what he considered a moving mechanical system, namely, the heart (pump) and blood vessels (tubes). At this early point in his career, Marey drew on physics and engineering for his conceptual models. Movement remained the focal point for much of his later work as well. A modern biographer wrote of Marey's later investigations of human and animal movement: "Marey's interest was broadened to the study of physiologial changes varying with time and place, i.e., movements as the chief expression of life."[44]

Marey was no mere technician; he was something of a philosopher of science as well. Rabinbach cites Marey's disparagement of constructivism: "One pretends to *construct* a science, and one searches for the cornerstone which must support the entire edifice, [but] what guarantees that it is truly the base of the edifice?" Marey continued, "I would be more inclined to compare the study of natural science with the work of archeologists who decipher inscriptions written in an unknown language" ("une langue inconnue").[45] In the introduction to his 1885 work, *La méthode graphique dans les sciences expérimentales et principalement en physiologie et en médicine*, Marey wrote:

> Science has before it two obstacles that impedes its progression: firstly the defect of our senses in discovering realities (truths, facts), and then the inadequacy of language to express and transmit the truths that we acquired. The object of scientific methods is to rid ourselves of these obstacles; the graphic method [*la méthode graphique*] achieves this dual goal better than all other methods. In fact, in delicate research, this method seizes the nuances that escape other methods of observation; when it is a question of revealing the progress of a phenomenon, the graphic method translates the phases of it with a clarity that language does not possess.[46]

---

[44] Snellen, *E. J. Marey*, 7.
[45] Marey, *Du mouvement dans les fonctions de la vie*, 24; English translation in Rabinbach, *Human Motor*, 94. Italics in original.
[46] Étienne-Jules Marey, *La méthode graphique dans les sciences expérimentales et principalement en physiologie et en médicine* (Paris: G. Masson, 1878), i. Translation courtesy L. Bergner.

In Marey's view, then, descriptive language based on the information available to the unaided senses, cannot be the basis of proper and progressive scientific research into biological phenomena. In the second half of the nineteenth century, the language of technology would become the voice of physiology.

Marey saw what he termed the "*langue inconnue*" (unknown language) of physiological time (Rabinbach's "interior rhythms of the body") and compared graphic inscription of physiological phenomena to the maps of the geographer. He was the "pioneer of modern medical notation—graphic inscription—as a diagnostic tool," advancing "the increasingly complex technologies of registration and measurement beyond the limits of the senses."[47] He expressed most eloquently the transcendence of graphic registration over the human senses:

> Not only are these instruments destined to replace the observer, and in his place, perform their function with an incontestable superiority; they will become irreplaceable in their domain. When the eye can no longer see, the ear cannot hear, or touch cannot feel, or even when our senses appear to deceive us, these instruments perform like a new sense with astonishing precision.[48]

Time was refigured by a tracing of the pulse—it could be retarded or accelerated, compressed or expanded, depending on the settings of the recorder. The pulse recording could be read as it was being acquired at the bedside. It could be displayed at a conference of physicians or before a class of medical students. It could be enclosed in a written case report and studied in a distant city by a consultant. It erased the barriers of language. It could be viewed in the latest edition of medical journal or in a new book about cardiovascular physiology.[49]

TECHNICAL ASPECTS OF THE MAREY SPHYGMOGRAPH

In contrast to the neuromuscular system and metabolic systems, both of which fitted in nicely with the new European constructions of energy,

---

[47] Rabinbach, *Human Motor*, 93–95.
[48] Marey, *La méthode graphique*, 108; cited and translated by Rabinbach, *Human Motor*, 95.
[49] The observaton concerning retardation and acceleration of time is taken from Frank, "Telltale Heart," 218.

the cardiovascular system seemed more mechanical, less thermodynamic or electrical. Charles François-Franck, student and collaborator of Marey, distinguished between the cardiovascular and other human systems: "There are general laws which preside over the apportionment of the nervous activity in the different points of the system as there are mechanical laws governing the circulation of the blood in the vascular system."[50] However, according to cardiologist and Marey biographer Snellen, Marey and François-Franck seemed to be vaguely aware that the circulatory system might also be subject to neural influences, particularly pressure on the carotid artery, a neural phenomenon now known as the "carotid sinus reflex."[51] The neuroelectrical infrastructure of cardiac conduction would not attract much attention until the electrocardiograph was invented at the turn of the twentieth century. Twentieth-century research would show that metabolic factors, including an array of hormones (such as adrenalin) and electrolytes (such as potassium), also impact the cardiovascular system. The heart and vessels are far more complicated than a simple mechanical model allows.

The mechanical device that linked the workings of the body to Marey's concept of graphic inscription was Ludwig's kymograph. It is unclear whether Marey actually studied under Ludwig (or even visited his laboratory) during a trip to Germany prior to beginning work in Paris in 1860, but it is possible that he learned about the kymograph in Germany.[52] Karl Vierordt's primitive sphygmograph (1854) incorporated a modified kymograph.[53] Similarly, Marey's myriad laboratory studies often incorporated the kymograph.[54]

Marey introduced his new sphygmograph in 1859 in a lengthy article, entitled "Recherches sur le pouls au moyen d'un nouvel appareil enregistreur: le sphygmographe" ("Pulse Research Using a New Recording Device: The Sphygmograph") in *Comptes rendus des séances de la Société de*

---

[50] Quoted in English translation in Rabinbach, *Human Motor*, 67. Charles François-Franck, "Nerveux (Physiologie)," *Dictionnaire encyclopédique des idées médicales* (Paris: P. Asselin, G. Masson, 1878): 12:572.

[51] Snellen, *E. J. Marey*, 147. The "carotid sinus reflex," in which pressure applied over the carotid artery causes slowing of the heartbeat, is mediated by stimulation of pressure-sensitive neuroreceptors in the wall of the carotid artery; impulses transmitted via the spinal cord stimulate the vagus nerve, which slows the pulse rate.

[52] Frank, "American Physiologists in German Laboratories," 34.

[53] Marey, *Circulation du sang*, 210.

[54] There are multiple illustrations in Marey's *La Circulation du Sang* showing a kymograph in use during a physiological experiment; see Snellen, *E. J. Marey*, 32, 57, 81, 108.

biologie et de ses filiales. The following year, the article was reprinted as a monograph.[55]

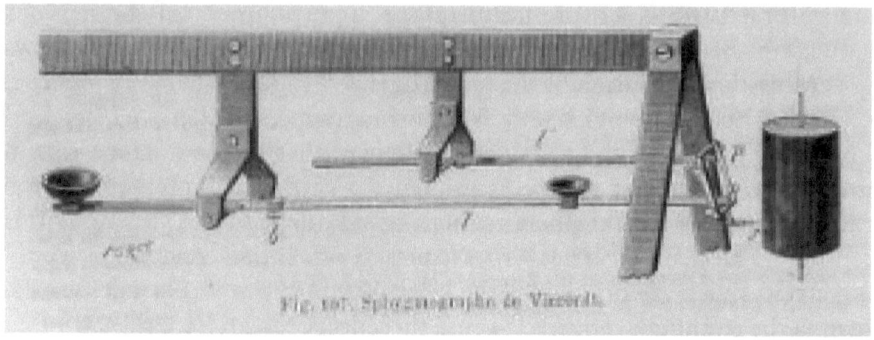

FIGURE 14: Vierordt sphygmograph connected to a Ludwig kymograph. The relative size of the two instruments is unclear; if correctly to scale, the Vierordt sphygmograph was clearly extremely bulky. Étienne-Jules Marey, *La circulation du sang à l'état physiologique et dans les maladies* (Paris: G. Masson, 1881), 210.

Finding the Vierordt sphygmograph to be sound in principle but lacking in *utilité pratique*, Marey devised a sphygmograph that was sensitive, reasonably portable, and capable of providing a pulse contour that was "many times richer in details" than that of Vierordt.[56] Marey's "sphygmograph élastique," as he called it, featured an adjustable compressing spring connected to a set of levers. The system of levers transmitted the delicate movements of a thin ivory plate that rested on the radial artery. The instrument was strapped to the subject's forearm to provide a steady pressure and prevent fortuitous wrist movements. The Marey sphygmograph recorded pulse waves on a moving strip of paper or smoked glass propelled by a clockwork mechanism. From a practical point of view, the number of recorded pulse waves was limited to about ten by the length of the moving strip of paper or glass.

---

[55] Étienne-Jules Marey, "Recherches sur le pouls au moyen d'un nouvel appareil enregistreur: le sphygmographe," *Comptes rendus des séances de la Société de biologie et de ses filiales*, 3rd ser., 1 (1859), 281–309; "Recherches sur le pouls au moyen d'un nouvel appareil enregistreur," *Gazette Médicale de Paris*, 3rd ser., 15 (1860): 225–36, 236–42, 298–301.

[56] Snellen, *E. J. Marey*, 133.

From Sphygmoscope to Sphygmograph:
And the Vision of Étienne-Jules Marey

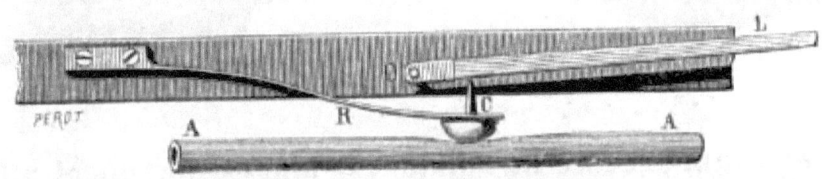

g. 108. Théorie du sphygmographe à ressort. — A A, artère; R, ressort qui la comprime; C, couteau qui souleve le levier L; O, centre de mouvement du levier.

FIGURE 15: Schematic of the mechanism of the Marey sphygmograph: AA (artery); R (spring that compresses the lever); C (knife edge that raises the lever L); O (center of movement of the lever). Étienne-Jules Marey, *La circulation du sang à l'état physiologique et dans les maladies* (Paris: G. Masson, 1881), 213.

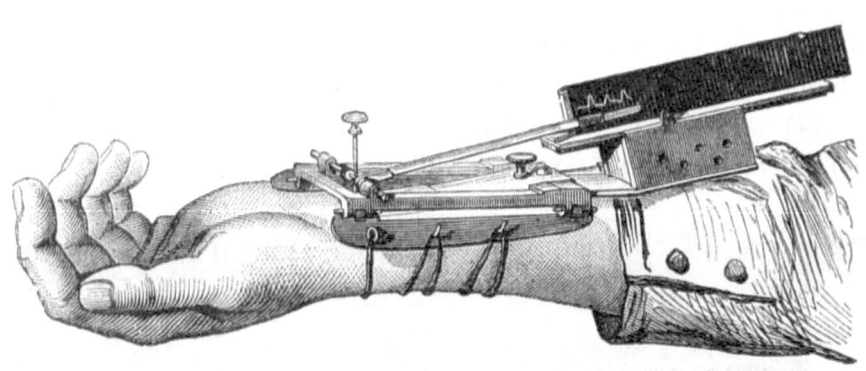

FIGURE 16: The Marey sphygmograph as it appeared in 1881, two decades after its invention. There is little if any apparent redesign. The instrument is attached to the forearm with restraining cords to maintain constant pressure and prevent movement of the wrist. The lever amplifies the minute excursions of the pulse with each heartbeat, recording the details of the pulse wave on the moving paper or smoked glass. Étienne-Jules Marey, *La circulation du sang à l'état physiologique et dans les maladies* (Paris: G. Masson, 1881), 214. Note: To see a Marey type sphygmograph in use, see a dynamic visual presentation by the National Library of Medicine at https://cfmedicine.nlm.nih.gov/artifact/jacobi.html.

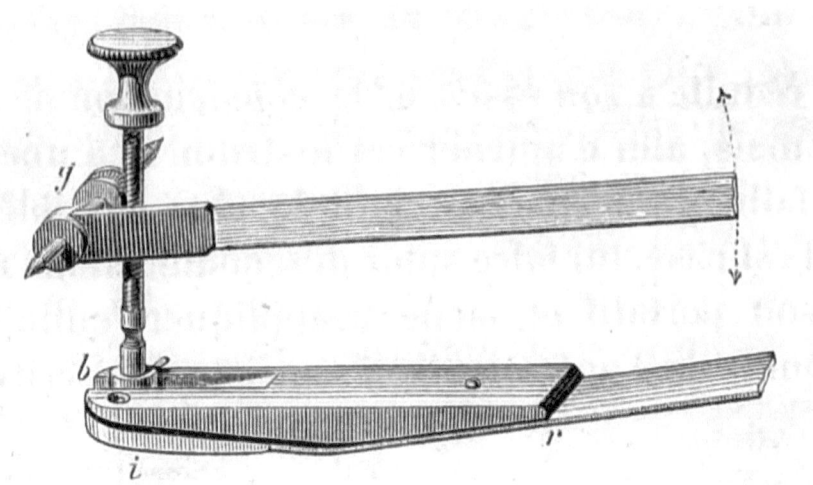

FIGURE 17: Detail of the Marey sphygmograph showing the thin plate that rests upon the artery and the screw for altering the pressure applied to the artery. Étienne-Jules Marey, *La circulation du sang à l'état physiologique et dans les maladies* (Paris: G. Masson, 1881), 214.

> **Note: To see a Marey type sphygmograph in use, refer to a dynamic visual image by the National Library of Medicine at https://cfmedicine.nlm.nih.gov/artifact/jacobi.html.**[105]

Marey's sphygmograph was one of "the first complex, sophisticated, and practicable instruments for measuring bodily function."[58] It was, said a biographer, the "hallmark of [his] ingenuity of technique."[59] Because his instrument was so influential in Europe and the United States, it is worth quoting Marey's original description in translation and with bracketed annotations (see figures 15–17):

> Our first concern [*préoccupation*] was to give to the new instrument all necessary sensitivity, which could only be realized with an extremely light lever ["L"]. As, on the other hand, it

---

[57] "Changing the Face of Medicine: Dr. Jacobi's Sphygmograph," National Library of Medicine, https://cfmedicine.nlm.nih.gov/artifact/jacobi.html (accessed 6 August 2017).

[58] Rabinbach, *Human Motor*, 93.

[59] Snellen, *E. J. Marey*, 14.

was necessary to exert rather considerable pressure on the artery in order to detect [*obtenir*] the pulsation, we used a completely independent component [*pièce*] consisting of [*formée par*] a long steel spring ["R"], which can apply a small ivory plate ["bb"] to the artery with a force that can be increased at will [*graduer à volonté*] with a regulating button [*un bouton de réglage*, "V"]. The movements that this [ivory] plate receives from the arterial pulsations are transmitted to the lower part of the lever ["L"] rather near its center of motion, so that the free end [of the lever, which has the inscribing device or writing tip] can move to a sufficient extent [*dans une étendue suffisante*] to amplify and record the arterial pulsations. The whole apparatus is mounted [*établi*] on a sort of armband ["BB"] which is adjusted to the forearm and can keep everything perfectly steady. Finally, the [pulse] tracing is received on a small plate of [smoked] glass or metal ["P"] that a clockwork movement runs parallel to the lever with a known speed ["H", i.e., the clockwork "H" propels the strip of paper or smoked glass mounted on "P" past a recording stylus at the tip of lever "L"], which serves to evaluate the pulse frequency. The instrument having a length of only 18 centimeters and a weight of 240 grams, is as portable as [the operator] desires.[60]

The innovative lever mechanism was far more sensitive than that of Vierordt, although Marey was also aware of the risk of adventitious transcriptions of portions of the pulse wave due the momentum of the lever itself.[61] To emphasize the great advantage of his sphygmograph, Marey included paired images of the pulse tracings recorded with both the Vierordt and Marey sphygmographs.

The top example in Figure 18 is a rather featureless "tracing of the pulse in a state of health" recorded by Vierdordt. It is easy to recognize the isochronism [equal time intervals] of the periods of ascent and descent of the lever, a trait common to all the outlines given by the German physiologist." In the bottom example in Figure 18 are segments of different tracings made by Marey and mounted end-to-end for purposes of illustration with the caption: "All these forms are physiological types gathered in weaker and weaker conditions of tension," referring either to the palpable firmness of the pulse or to the pressure applied to the artery by the screw connected to the ivory plate resting on the artery.

---

[60] Marey, "Recherches sur le pouls," 283–84; translation courtesy Lynn Bergner.
[61] Snellen, *E. J. Marey*, 133.

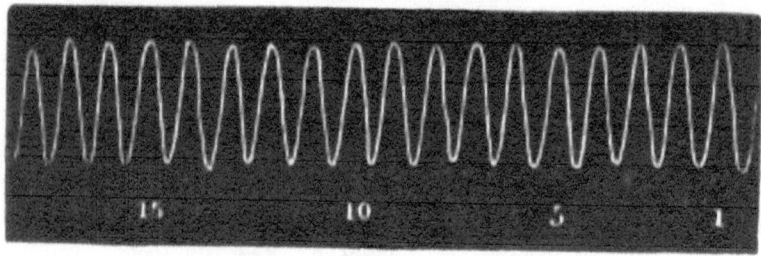

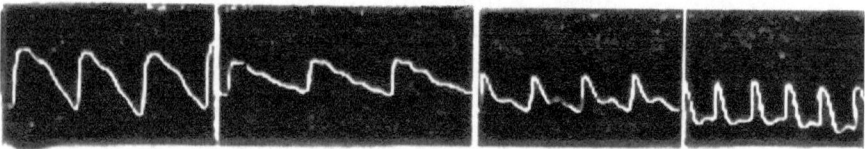

FIGURE 18: Top image: pulse tracing with Vierordt sphygmograph, showing featureless pulse waves that give little more information than a physician would deduce by simply palpating the pulse. It does provide a permanent record of heart rate. Bottom tracing: pulse tracings made with the Marey sphygmograph and mounted end-to-end for illustration. The tracings show fine details of pressure within each pulse cycle as the artery transmits the blood pumped by the heart. The upstroke of the pulse is much quicker than the downstroke (relaxation phase). Étienne-Jules Marey, "Recherches sur le pouls au moyen d'un nouvel appareil enregistreur: le sphygmographe," *Comptes rendus des séances de la Société de biologie et de ses filiales*, 3rd ser., 1 (1859), 284.

It is apparent that the upstroke of the pulse is far quicker than the relaxation phase, in contrast to the "isochronism" of the Vierordt tracings. Clearly, the Marey tracings, which presage all future sphygmographic tracings by other investigators, are far richer than the overdamped tracings of Vierordt. Marey, however, justly paid tribute to Vierordt: "We have thought it necessary to preserve for our instrument the name of sphygmograph which Vierordt has given to his. This name will remind us that the German physiologist is the author [originator] of the use of a lever which alone makes it possible to obtain tracings of the pulsations of the arteries of man."[62]

---

[62] Marey, "Recherches sur le pouls," 284–85; translation courtesy Lynn Bergner.

STUDIES WITH THE MAREY SPHYGMOGRAPH

Marey recorded pulse waves in a variety of diseases. But it was the development of the instrument itself that occupied his attention. It was left for later clinicians and students of the sphygmograph to analyze the physiological correlates of the pulse wave contour in health and disease. Marey's interest was in designing an instrument to "help in research on the normal and pathological characteristics of the circulatory system."[63]

The original Marey sphygmograph, sometimes referred to as *le sphygmographe à pression élastique*, was first mentioned in a French journal in 1859. In the same year, Marey presented his sphygmograph to the Académie des Science. The response was evidently positive and his personal fame was advanced by a request for a demonstration of the instrument at the court of Napoleon III. His discovery of an irregular pulse in a courtier was punctuated by the unfortunate man's sudden death some days later.[64]

Marey subsequently devised (or more precisely improved upon existing devices) a *sphygmographe à transmission*, in which a specially designed sensor (*tambour à levier*, also described as a pneumatic capsule) mounted on the sphygmograph at the wrist allowed transmission of the wave through an air-filled tube to a recording kymograph (or polygraph if simultaneous events were being recorded) a few feet away. This allowed a longer tracing on a greater length of recording paper, an important requirement for studying abnormalities of cardiac rhythm. (The short recording surface on his self-contained *sphygmographe à pression élastique* permitted a recording of no more that about six to ten beats depending on the heart rate.)

In a recording of about twenty-five beats (probably about twenty seconds) using his transmission sphygmograph, Marey recorded what is now called "sinus arrhythmia," the normal slight increase in pulse rate during inspiration and slight decrease during expiration. This phenomenon is now known to be regulated by neurovascular pathways. An astute clinician can detect this normal variation by palpating the pulse of a patient instructed to breathe deeply. "*Cette periodicité*," wrote Marey, "ètait reglée par le rythme des mouvements respiratoires." ("This periodicity is regulated by the respiratory movements.")

---

[63] Reiser, *Medicine and the Reign of Technology*, 101.
[64] Rabinbach, *Human Motor*, 89–90, cites the Napoleon vignette in "Nécrologie—Marey," *Revue Scientifique* 1:22 (1904): 673.

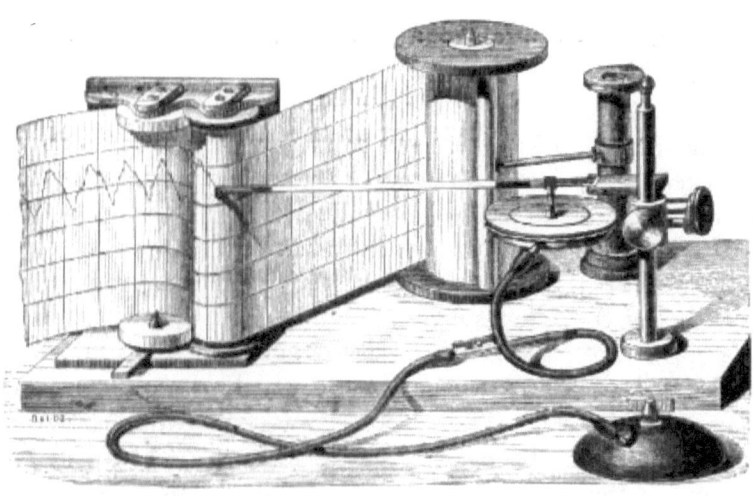

FIGURE 19: Marey's "sphygmographe à transmission." The transmitting sphygmograph transmits the arterial pulsation to an inscribing lever situated at a distance; the tracing of a large number of pulse waves is recorded on a long strip of paper mounted on the kymograph. Étienne-Jules Marey, *La circulation du sang à l'état physiologique et dans les maladies* (Paris: G. Masson, 1881), 222.

Marey also recorded simultaneous tracings of the cardiac impulse and the radial pulse, referred to as "*double tracés des coeur et de pouls inscrits simultanément*," on a kymograph adapted to record two simultaneous physiologic events (a polygraph). One sensor (possibly an adapted transmission sphygmograph) was placed on the left anterior chest wall over the apex of the heart and a second sensor (a transmission sphygmograph) was mounted over the radial artery in the wrist. He observed that the pulse irregularities mirrored irregularities in cardiac contractions. While this was a trivial observation evident to anyone conversant with the rudiments of cardiovascular physiology—the heart pumps blood into the arteries and if the heart beat is irregular, the pulse will follow—he succeeded in demonstating the power of simultaneous tracings. Other investigators, including the American Alonzo Thrasher Keyt (see Chapter 5) would interest themselves in the detailed measurement of minute delays between ventricular contraction and transmission of the impulse to peripheral arteries in an attempt to diagnose cardiovascular disorders.[65]

---

[65] Marey, *La circulation du sang*, 221–24.

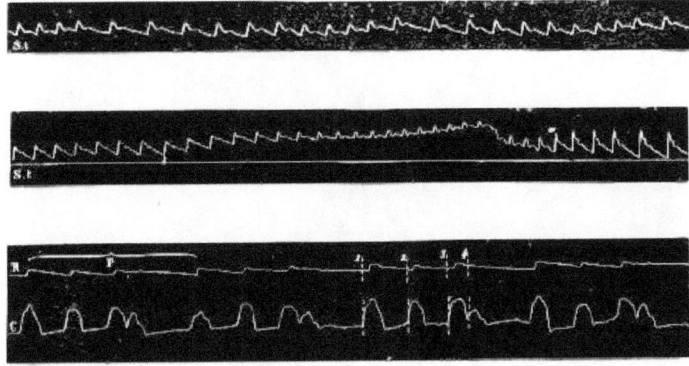

FIGURE 20: Three long recordings of the pulse using Marey's transmitting sphygmograph. Top tracing: "Long pulse traces showing periodic changes in pulsation frequency. These irregularities were insensible to touch; their rhythm was regulated by breathing." Bottom tracing: "Double traces of the heart and the pulse inscribed simultaneously on the polygraph. The heart shows irregular systoles (beats) which result in irregularities of the pulse." Étienne-Jules Marey, *La circulation du sang à l'état physiologique et dans les maladies* (Paris: G. Masson, 1881), 223.

MAREY'S MODEL HEART AND CIRCULATORY SYSTEM

In the poorly understood cardiac cycle, Marey found a fertile field for his technical skills. To assist in his studies of cardiac physiology, he constructed an ingenious (and quite beautiful) mechanical model of the heart—or more precisely, the left atrium and ventricle with attached arteries—in which a rubber chamber was encased in a thread mesh, the latter gathered in fascicles that could be controlled by the operator. The end result was an artificial heart with alternating *resserrements* (contractions) and *relâchements* (relaxations) as in life.

When Marey pressed specially constructed pressure transducers against the front of the artificial heart; the atrial and ventricular impulses were transmitted to a Ludwig type drum kymograph. Marey found that his artificial heart produced tracings almost identical to those he recorded on the chest wall overlying a human heart. Referred to as "cardiograms," such pressure tracings should not be confused with the modern electrocardiogram.[66]

---

[66] Ibid., 142–44; translation, L. Bergner; Snellen, *E. J. Marey*, 95–96.

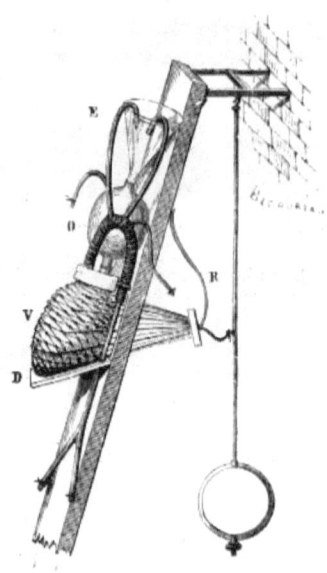

FIGURE 21: Marey's artificial left atrium (O) and left ventricle (V) encased in a silk mesh connected to a pulley. Moving the pulley up and down caused the mesh to tighten and relax, imitating the pumping of the animal or human heart. Étienne-Jules Marey, *La circulation du sang à l'état physiologique et dans les maladies* (Paris: G. Masson, 1881), 142.

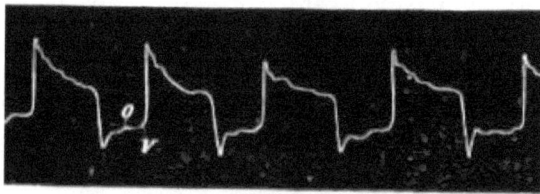

FIGURE 22: Tracing of the pulsations of the Marey's mechanical heart. The atrial contraction ("o") and ventricular contraction ("v") appear almost identical to "cardiographs" obtained by placing a sensor over a human heart. Étienne-Jules Marey, *La circulation du sang à l'état physiologique et dans les maladies* (Paris: G. Masson, 1881), 143.

To better study the pulsations of the arteries, Marey experimented with rigid and elastic tubing, observing how two side-by-side conduits ("arteries")—one a rigid tube of glass and the other an "elastic" tube of rubber—responded to waves of fluid imitating cardiac contractions. The entry of fluid into both tubes was controlled by a simple hand-operated lever. The rigid tube simply poured out waves of fluid at the distal ("artery") end with the intermittent timing identical to that of the fluid introduced intermittently at the proximal ("heart") end. Output was a simple reflection of input. The elastic tube, in contrast, poured out a continuous and regular flow at the distal end when the fluid was introduced in the same intermittent manner at the proximal end. Marey concluded that under the influence of arterial elasticity, blood flow is gradually regulated as the blood flows downstream. The "elastic" artery refined the input.[67]

IMPACT OF THE MAREY SPHYGMOGRAPH

Although Marey was not affiliated with a medical school, the quality of his work and his position as one of new generation of physiologists led to his election to the Collège du France in 1866. He published a second physiology textbook, *La circulation du sang a l'état physiologique et dans les maladies*, in 1881, adding new material (from his own investigations and the work of others) and attempting to make cardiac physiology, as registered by his non-invasive mechanical devices, more applicable to medical practice.[68]

The respected firm of Breuget (Paris) manufactured and marketed Marey's sphygmograph, which was eagerly purchased by European and American physiologists, as well as ambitious clinicians. Some likely had the instrument shipped to them and others, especially in the United States, seemed to have asked colleagues and friends to bring an instrument back from their European studies and travels. Although the basic instrument remained the same, tinkerers everywhere felt compelled to modify and (they hoped) improve upon Marey's design. Charles Ozanam of the Parisian medical faculty credited Louis-Jules Béhier, a Parisian pathologist and professor of medicine, with perfecting the Marey sphygmograph (1868) and noted several other early modifiers from France and England.[69]

A most productive innovator was the British master Frederick Akbar Mahomed of Guy's Hospital in London, who used his modifed Marey sphygmograph to elucidate essential hypertension several decades before the introduction of the blood pressure cuff (see Chapter 3). Edgar Holden

---

[67] Marey, *La circulation du sang*, 163–64; Snellen, *E. J. Marey*, 116.
[68] Snellen, *E. J. Marey*, 23–24; Rabinbach, *Human Motor*, 87, 100–103.
[69] Charles Ozanam, *Le circulation et le pouls: histoire, physiologique, séméiotique, indications thérapeutic* (Paris: J. B. Baillière et Fils, 1886), 401–4.

of New Jersey published an article introducing his modified design in 1870, claiming its superiority to the Marey sphygmograph (see Chapter 4). In 1873, Holden published a major book on his work with the sphygmograph; the frontispieces of the book were full-page facing images of the Marey sphygmograph and the Holden sphygmograph, looking quite similar except for the omission of restraining straps on the Holden model and modest tweaks to the tension spring and writing apparatus. In time, sphygmographs of novel design operating on an entirely different mechanical principle—namely hydraulics rather than springs—would gain popularity.

Despite their mechanical and theoretical shortcomings, the time and space machines transformed the ways in which physicians experienced the healthy and sick human body. Events indistinguishable to the palpating finger resting on the artery or to the eye observing the fluttering heart of a vivisected animal could be figuratively stretched out on a moving surface and become readable, measurable, portable objects of study. The tracings could be shown to a colleague, displayed at a lecture, mailed to a consultant, or published in a journal. In a fundamental transformation of medical authority, the pronouncements of the learned physician became subject to what we would now term peer review.

HUMAN AND ANIMAL TIME AND MOTION STUDIES

During the second phase of his career, Marey transformed his cardiovascular work into a more general study of human and animal motion, the common thread being his preoccupation with *la méthode graphique*, specifically the registration of movements. Marey's earlier tracings of the heartbeat and pulse progressed logically to his later studies of photographed bodily motion, a process he called "chronophotography." Marey and the Anglo-American Eadweard Muybridge, whose sequential photographs of horses and humans in motion are familiar to all students of photography, strongly influenced one another. In Rabinbach's view, Marey's vascular and other laboratory investigations with the sphygmograph as well as his later photographic studies of movement in living animals were part of a desire to discover the "economy of the body" by breaking down motion—whether the pulsation of an artery or the progress of a galloping horse or human runner—into its fundamental building blocks.[70]

---

[70] Rabinbach, *Human Motor*, 87, 100–103.

MAREY AND VIVISECTION

Because it was "non-invasive," reasonably comfortable for the patient, and satisfying to the dedicated diagnostician, Marey's sphygmograph entered elite medical practices on both sides of the Atlantic. His reputation in France and abroad rested "almost entirely on his ability to construct devices that could detect and measure aspects of the organism without disturbing it." In the research environment of the late-nineteenth century, Marey's "non-invasive" physiological instruments stood in stark contrast to the vivisectionist practices of the day.

Recently, Kenton Kroker, in a thesis investigating sleep research and its origins in nineteenth-century physiology, commented on Marey's attitude toward vivisection. Marey considered vivisection crude, limited to "lay[ing] bare the phenomenon simultaneously with the organ which is the seat of it; it reveals to our senses only what they are capable of perceiving." Marey, continues Kroker, "wanted to ground physiology in a new observational practice—one that would 'renounce' vivisection, replacing it with apparatus capable of examining living organisms in their undisturbed conditions."[71]

Not only did the Marey sphygmograph and its associated devices reconfigure the physiology laboratory and bring physiology and *la méthode graphique* out of the laboratory to the bedside and examining room, but they also cracked opened a door to alternatives for vivisection and a new experimental ethos.

---

[71] Kenton Kroker, "From Reflex to Rhythm: Sleep, Dreaming, and the Discovery of Rapid Eye Movement, 1870–1960" (doctoral thesis, Institute for the History & Philosophy of Science & Technology, University of Toronto, 2000), 35–36, http://www.collectionscanada.gc.ca/obj/s4/f2/dsk2/ftp02/NQ53765.pdf (accessed 17 February 2017). It is not clear if Marey also found some merit in the arguments of the antivivisectonists in their fight against unspeakable cruelty to unanesthetized animals in the name of science.

Chapter 3

"Sphygmographing No End": The Sphygmograph in Britain

THE EARLY NEWS FROM FRANCE

In 1860, the *Lancet* briefly reviewed Marey's article in the *Gazette Médicale*. The initial reaction was at best lukewarm: "The French instrument . . . can only indicate the frequency or the more or less regularity of the pulse. It may be doubted whether these instruments [i.e. the Vierordt and Marey sphygmographs], though very ingenious, will ever prove actually useful in practice." However, a few months later, a *Lancet* "special correspondent" reported from Paris that Marey's novel sphygmograph, recently reported to the French Academy of Sciences, was "highly ingenious."[1] Interestingly, one of the earliest international articles describing the use of Marey's instrument was by D. K. Koschlakoff in St. Petersburg, Russia, who published a lengthy article in the German literature in 1864 ("Untersuchungen über den Puls mit Hülfe des Marey'schen Sphygmographen").[2]

---

[1] "The Sphygmograph, or Register of the Arterial Pulse," *Lancet* 1 (1860): 435; "Parisian Medical Intelligence," *Lancet* 2 (1860): 599.

[2] D. K. Koschlakoff, "Untersuchungen über den Puls mit Hülfe des Mareyschen Sphygmographen," (trans. "Investigations of the Pulse with the Help of the Marey Sphygmograph.") *Archiv für Pathologische Anatomie und Physiologie und für Klinische Medicin* 30 (1864): 149–76; translation of title, courtesy Robert A. Moss.

TINKERING

Constructing sphygmographs, or, more accurately, making slight changes to existing instruments, became something of a cottage industry among motivated European physicians. In the late nineteenth century, tinkering and inventing, often conducted privately, was a popular pastime. "It is characteristic of that period and of the inventors it produced," observed a Marey scholar, "that there was a widespread surge of new technical advancements, one supporting and paving the way for another, tumbling over each other as it were. This meant rivalry and fights over priority."[3] This was certainly true of the sphygmograph men.

Those who adapted and used the sphygmograph accepted, implicitly or explicitly, a similar set of challenges: building a better instrument and extolling its virtues; interpreting the wave forms and establishing the parameters of the normal pulse wave; taking and interpreting tracings in a wide variety of cardiac and non-cardiac diseases; identifying medical cases in which the sphygmograph proved helpful; attempting to elucidate the hazy concept of arterial pressure; and, almost universally, listing the limitations of the technology and caveats about its misuse.

One important consideration was the issue of patient comfort. Most inventors tried to design their modifications to minimize both the time required for making a tracing and the hyperextension of the immobilized wrist. British sphygmograph inventor (and marketer) Robert Ellis Dudgeon pointed out that the Marey sphygmograph (and its various modifications), by "its size and formidable appearance [is] apt to alarm the patient." Byrom Bramwell in Newcastle took care to explain to the patient the harmless nature of the instrument. He emphasized the point by explaining that one of his patients "left the hospital rather than have the instrument applied."[4]

BURDON SANDERSDON: BRITISH SPHYGMOGRAPH PIONEER

In late 1864, two young London physicians, John Scott Burdon-Sanderson, physician to the Hospital for Consumption, assistant physician

---

[3] H. A Snellen, *E. J. Marey and Cardiology: Physiologist and Pioneer of Technology, 1830-1904: Selected Writings in Facsimile with Comments and Summaries, a Brief History of Life and Work, and a Bibliography* (Rotterdam: Kooyker Scientific, 1980), 8.

[4] Robert E. Dudgeon, *The Sphygmograph: Its History and Use as an Aid to Diagnosis in Ordinary Practice* (London: Baillière, Tindall, & Cox, 1882). 19; Byrom Bramwell, "Examination of the Pulse," *Edinburgh Medical Journal* 26 (1880): 522.

to the Middlesex Hospital, public health officer, and medical school lecturer, and Francis E. Anstie, senior assistant physician to Westminster Hospital, were using the sphygmograph in hospital practice. Burdon-Sanderson, who was probably the first British sphygmographer, had studied with the young French physiologist Claude Bernard in 1851. There is no evidence that Burdon-Sanderson returned to Paris to observe the sphygmographic experiments of Marey a decade later. His biographer suggests that he may have read about the instrument in the *Lancet* in 1860 and subsequently obtained Marey's publications.[5]

Burdon-Sanderson's initial enthusiasm led him to spend many hours experimenting with his Marey sphygmograph (manufactured in Paris by the firm of Brégeut), working at home as well as at University College and on the wards of several hospitals. According to his wife, who often assisted him in his experiments with the sphygmograph, Burdon-Sanderson found time in a busy schedule for "sphygmographing no end."[6] Consistent with his French training in experimental physiology, Burdon-Sanderson performed studies of the velocity of transmission of vibrations and the production of "successive movements, identical with those of the pulse, in elastic tubes containing liquids."[7] These investigations echo similar studies by Marey.

The instrument had barely crossed the Channel before Burdon-Sanderson began making modifications. Finding that the "bandages" used by Marey at the wrist failed to hold the instrument firmly against the artery should the patient's wrist move, he added a small brass block and elastic band designed to fix the apparatus firmly over a tendon in the wrist. The human subject lay supine with the forearm affixed by "strong elastic bands" to a padded board that kept the wrist in full extension. He also adjusted the pressure applied to the artery by adding weights to a pan affixed to the frame. Finally, he substituted smoked glass (and a needle point) for paper (and a pen) in the recording strip; the resulting etching onto the smoked

---

[5] Terrie M. Romano, *Making Medicine Scientific: John Burdon Sanderson and the Culture of Victorian Science* (Baltimore: Johns Hopkins University Press, 2002), 26–28, 80–81.

[6] Ibid., 77, 89. Quoted from letter written by Ghetel Burdon-Sanderson.

[7] John Burdon-Sanderson, *Handbook of the Sphygmograph: Being a Guide to Its Use in Clinical Research, to Which is Appended A Lecture Delivered at the Royal College of Physicians on the 29th of March 1867 on the Mode and Duration of the Contraction of the Heart in Health and Disease* (London: Robert Hardwicke, 1867), vi; John Burdon-Sanderson, "Lecture on the Characters of the Arterial Pulse, in Relation to the Mode and Duration of the Contraction of the Heart in Health and Disease," *British Medical Journal* 2 (1867): 19–22, 39–40, 57–58. The three-part lecture as it was reprinted in the *Handbook* is renumbered sequentially from 49 to 83.

glass surface was found to be far more reliable than making a tracing with a finicky pen on a slip of paper. The smoked glass tracings also lent themselves to display during lectures using the "magic lantern" and in publications using photographs.[8]

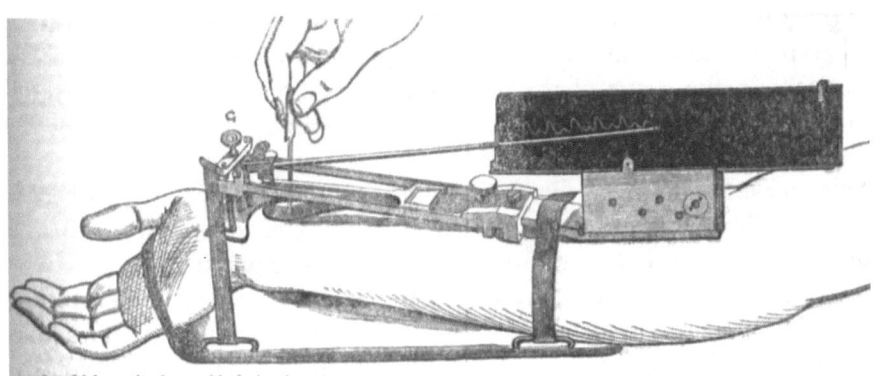

FIGURE 23: Modified Marey sphygmograph based on recommendations of John Burdon-Sanderson and others, as described by Francis Anstie. Note especially the elastic bands holding the extended wrist against a pad resting on the bed. Hyperextension of the wrist appears somewhat uncomfortable. Francis E. Anstie, "On Certain Modifications of Marey's Sphygmograph," *Lancet* 1 (1868): 783.

"THE PULSE IS ARMED WITH A PEN"

By 1865, the *Lancet* editorialist was far more enthusiastic, declaring, "There are few things more interesting in the recent history of Medicine than the remarkable ingenuity with which physical means of research have been brought to bear on the hidden secrets of the body in health and disease." In an effort to convey the revolutionary concept to the reader (there was no illustration of the instrument), the writer explained: "The sphygmograph of Marey is an exquisitely designed instrument, by the aid of which *the pulse is armed with a pen*, and at every beat writes its own diagram, and registers its own characters."

According to the editorial, Anstie, Burdon-Sanderson's colleague, had "determined . . . without loss of time, to direct the attention of English physicians to the immense field of fruitful observation which lies open to the investigation of observers who are willing to devote time and patience

---

[8] Burdon-Sanderson, *Handbook*, 5–10.

to the development of M. Marey's brilliant invention." He demonstrated the instrument before the Medical Society of London in late 1865. It was, said the editorialist, "an instrument of precision, of remarkable beauty and wide range of usefulness." Many early sphygmograph men found evidence—or at least were guardedly hopeful—that the varying shapes of the pulse waves correlated with specific illnesses such as typhoid fever and typhus and would served as a guide to both diagnosis and prognosis. Changes in the shape of the pulse wave suggested decreases in arterial "tonicity" and the persistence of such an abnormal pulse wave presaged a poor prognosis.[9]

A subsequent *Lancet* editorial in 1866, anticipating new sphygmographic studies by Burdon-Sanderson and Anstie, optimistically predicted that "a rich harvest of pathological discovery awaits those practical workers who are now applying the new physical methods to morbid phenomena." The great hope, destined to be restated for at least a decade, was that the tracings would not only "clear up some difficult problems in the physiology of the circulation," but would be diagnostic in clinical practice and "illustrate the diseases to which they referred."[10]

EXPLORING THE FRONTIERS

Accordingly, in 1866, a two-part article, under the title "On the Application of Physical Methods to the Exploration of the Movement of the Heart and Pulse in Disease," was authored by Burdon-Sanderson and co-edited with Anstie. The science was still young and its details uncertain. Even at this early date, Burdon-Sanderson grasped the limitations of the sphygmograph—his predictions and caveats would prove correct, both with regard to general disease diagnosis and to targeted cardiovascular diagnosis:

> It is perfectly true that by the sphygmograph we become familiar with differences and peculiarities of the pulse so minute that the most delicate and practised fingers would fail to recognized them; but the difficulty lies in the fact that the

---

[9] "Physicians and Physicists," *Lancet* 2 (1865): 599. Since the editorial asserts that only Anstie and Burdon-Sanderson had "taken the matter up in this country [England]," it is likely that one or both of these London physicians wrote or oversaw the unsigned editorial. Italics in quotation ("the pulse is armed with a pen") added.

[10] "The Pulse in Health and Disease," *Lancet* 2 (1866): 501.

record is written in a language which we are are only beginning to understand.... If anyone imagines that he will discover in pulse-curves invariable characteristics of particular disease, he is entirely mistaken.... Even in diseases of the arterial system, to the discrimination of which the sphygmograph is more directly applicable than to any other diagnostic question, the form of the tracing may be modified by a large number of circumstances.... He who attempts to found a diagnosis on the indications of the sphymgograph... will probably fall into errors which he would otherwise have avoided.

Burdon-Sanderson and Anstie anticipated that the sphygmograph would be most useful as a guide to prognosis, aiding in determining, say, a "failing" pulse in the presence of serious illness. Among the sphygmogram strips published with the article were interesting paired carotid artery/radial artery tracings. Having studied the behavior of fluids in artificial arteries, Burdon-Sanderson was aware that an artery close to the heart would give more reliable indications of the heart's action. The carotid artery in the neck was the closest accessible artery to the heart. It is not clear exactly how he obtained his carotid tracings with "successive [but not simultaneous] applications of the sphygmograph to the carotid and radial arteries." He may simply have pressed the instrument gently over the pulsating artery in the neck, since use of the restraining cords would have been impossible at that location.[11]

In the second article in the series, the current limited understanding of the physiology of the pulse was considered. Burdon-Sanderson began by elegantly stating the advantage of the sphygmograph in pulse study: "The ordinarily received doctrine of the pulse, as stated in physiology text-books, affords no sufficient or intelligible explanation of the varieties of pulse which can be detected by the practised finger, and are represented by corresponding variations in the spygmographic tracing."[12]

---

[11] John Burdon-Sanderson, "On the Theory of the Pulse," (No. 1 in a series "On the Application of Physical Methods to the Exploration of the Movement of the Heart and Pulse in Disease"), *Lancet* 2 (1866): 517–18.

[12] John Burdon-Sanderson, "On the Varieties of Pulse in Disease" (No. 2 in a series "On the Application of Physical Methods to the Exploration of the Movement of the Heart and Pulse in Disease"), *Lancet* 2 (1866): 688.

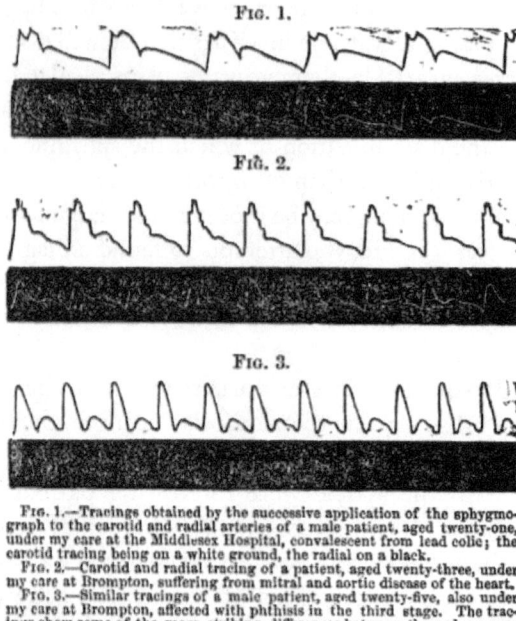

FIGURE 24: Burdon-Sanderson's investigations into the function of the aortic valve and the transmission of the pulse wave using three paired (but not simultaneous) tracings of the carotid and radial pulses in a single individual. The carotid tracings are inscribed in black on a white background; the radial tracings are inscribed on white on a black background and are obscured in the scanned image. "On the Theory of the Pulse" (No. 1 in a series "On the Application of Physical Methods to the Exploration of the Movement of the Heart and Pulse in Disease"). *Lancet* 2 (1866): 518.

HANDBOOK OF THE SPHYGMOGRAPH: A CAUTIONARY NOTE

By 1867, Burdon-Sanderson's *Handbook of the Sphygmograph* was ready for publication.[13] In his introduction, he took a instructive tone, hinting at the inevitable frustrations that awaited aspiring sphygmographers:

---

[13] The handbook might have been ready a year earlier, but Burdon-Sanderson was preoccupied by his obligations to the Royal Commission on the Cattle Plague from 1865 to 1866. Romano, *Making Medicine Scientific*, 81.

> I offer this little book to my fellow-workers in the hope that it may help them to overcome those preliminary difficulties which are apt to be encountered in the application of any new method of research, and that, in this way it may tend to prevent the loss of time that might be more usefully employed in collecting and recording observations.[14]

Although he was already aware that the sphygmograph had serious technical limitations, Burdon-Sanderson understood its greatest virtue: the sphygmographic tracing was "a permanent record—as faithful as a photograph—of the transient phenomena of life."[15] In the *Handbook* and his appended lecture to the Royal College of Physicians, he emphasized the clinical rather than the experimental applications of the sphygmograph. The fold-out frontispiece (with permission of Marey's publisher and recaptioned in English) was taken directly from plates used in Marey's 1863 *Physiologie médicale de la circulation du sang* and shows the system of levers in detail.[16]

PROCEED WITH CAUTION

In 1867, in lectures before the Royal College of Physicians (and appended to his *Handbook of the Sphygmograph*), Burdon-Sanderson continued to advise clinicians to approach the sphygmograph with caution:

> The tendency to force theories to practical ends before they have had time to be established, is one of which we have many instances in the history of medicine. Let us remember that no theory ought to be applied to the issues of practical life, until it has been subjected to scientific criticism, and received as a scientific truth. Let us, therefore, avoid being in too great a hurry to introduced the sphygmograph into the consulting-room for if, with so imperfect a knowledge as we at present possess of first principles, we endeavour to use those principles in diagnosis, we shall not only discredit ourselves, but the method by which we profess to be guided.[17]

---

[14] Burdon-Sanderson, *Handbook*, v.
[15] John Burdon-Sanderson, "On the Theory of the Pulse" (No. 1): 517.
[16] Étienne-Jules Marey, *Physiologie médicale de la circulation du sang* (Paris: Adrien Delahaye, 1863), 4, 180, 181.
[17] Burdon-Sanderson, "Lecture on the Characters of the Arterial Pulse, in Relation to

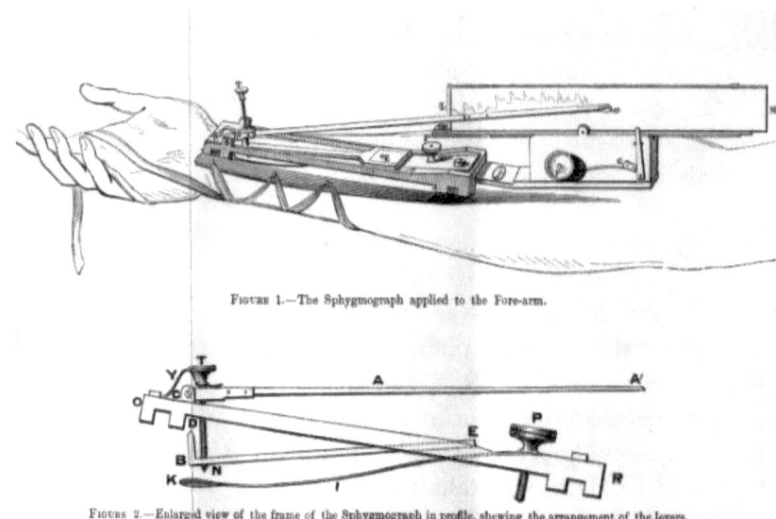

FIGURE 1.—The Sphygmograph applied to the Fore-arm.

FIGURE 2.—Enlarged view of the frame of the Sphygmograph in profile, showing the arrangement of the levers.

FIGURE 25: Images from Étienne-Jules Marey, *Physiologie médicale de la circulation du sang* (Paris, Adrien Delahaye,1863), 180–81, reproduced in John Burdon-Sanderson's *Handbook of the Sphygmograph* with English captions. The flexible steel spring (fixed at the screw P) ends in a plate of ivory at its end (K), which rests upon the radial artery. Because the spring is flexible and elastic, the slight rise and fall of the radial pulse is transmitted to a pair of levers that multiply the movement of the artery and inscribe the pulse wave onto a sheet of glazed paper mounted on a moveable frame. John Burdon-Sanderson, *Handbook of the Sphygmograph: Being a Guide to Its Use in Clinical Research, to Which is Appended A Lecture Delivered at the Royal College of Physicians on the 29th of March 1867 on the Mode and Duration of the Contraction of the Heart in Health and Disease* (London: Robert Hardwicke, 1867), frontispiece.

As his biographer points out, Burdon-Sanderson had not merely fiddled with the sphygmograph, but combined clinical observations on patients with post-mortem examinations and physiological experiments on animals to advance his understanding of cardiac physiology. Burdon-Sanderson's own initial enthusiasm soon waned as he grew disillusioned with the instrument at the same time that his career moved in new directions. His private practice and self-identification as a clinician gave way to academic medicine when he was appointed professor of practical physiology and histology at University College London in 1874.[18] His career further

---

the Mode and Duration of the Contraction of the Heart in Health and Disease," 39; the quotation in the *Handbook* is on page 65.

[18] Romano, *Making Medicine Scientific*, 89–91.

advanced in 1895, when he was named Regius Professor of Medicine at Oxford, a post he held until 1904.

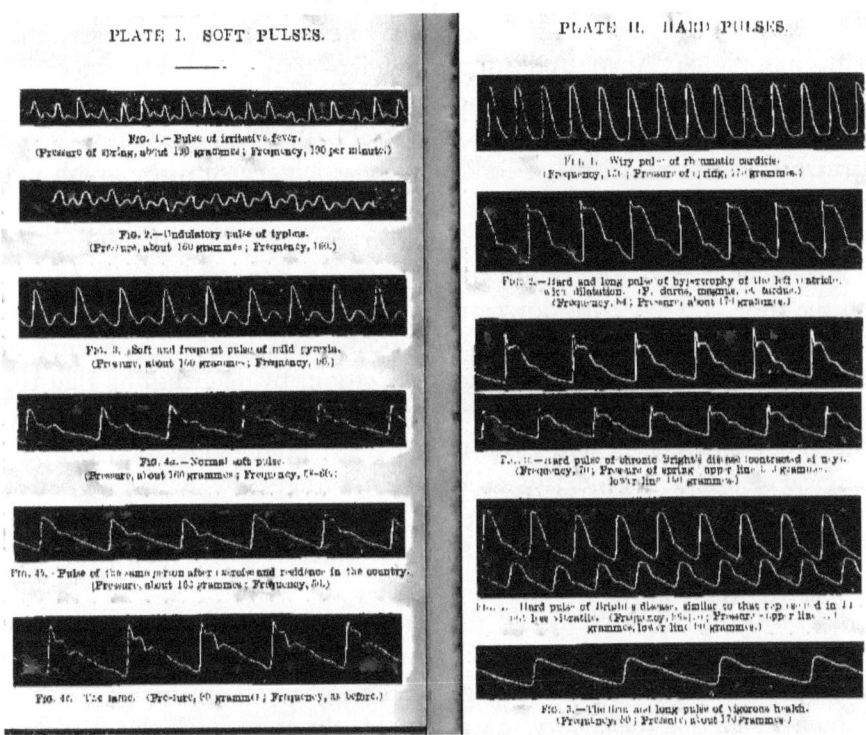

FIGURE 26: Burdon-Sanderson's examples of "hard" and "soft" pulses, a visual representation of the *pulsus durus* and *pulsus mollis* of classical pulse study. John Burdon-Sanderson, *Handbook of the Sphygmograph: Being a Guide to Its Use in Clinical Research, to Which is Appended A Lecture Delivered at the Royal College of Physicians on the 29th of March 1867 on the Mode and Duration of the Contraction of the Heart in Health and Disease* (London: Robert Hardwicke, 1867), between pages 32 and 33.

ANSTIE: SPHYGMOGRAPHIC CONSULTATION

Francis E. Anstie was an energetic young clinician and medical author/editor with broad-ranging interests in therapeutics, public welfare, nervous diseases, and the medical education of women. His tragic early death was due to rapidly progressive septicemia secondary to a cut received during the autopsy of a child who died in an institutional epidemic of peritonitis. Among those colleagues who attended him was Burdon-Sanderson.[19]

Physicians adept in the use of new technologies would grow increasingly important as consultants in all areas of medicine. A report from King's College Hospital in late 1865 or early 1866 demonstrated that sphygmographers Anstie and Burdon-Sanderson were already being called in as consultants. The consultation described in the report was related to localization of an aneurysm (a blood vessel ballooning or malformation; British spelling aneurism), a condition in which the sphygmograph was truly of practical use to the clinician.

The key to diagnosing and localizing an aneurysm—and determining if it was operable—was the asymmetry of the sphygmographic tracings taken on the right and left arms downstream from the vascular abnormality. In the reported case, a patient with a large post-traumatic thoracic aneurysm was examined by Anstie to help in localization. By determining that the radial pulse waves were equal bilaterally, Anstie was able to conclude that the aneurysm was located close to the heart (and inoperable with the surgical techinques of the day) rather than in a more distal branching artery leading to the arm. Burdon-Sanderson was also consulted (or perhaps he reviewed the tracings done by Anstie) and concurred. Autopsy confirmed their findings.

In a similar case published the same year, Anstie was able to show unequal pulses in the radial arteries in what proved to be a case of axillary artery aneurysm; unequal tracings in the right and left radial arteries demonstrated that the aneurysm was distal to the point at which the central artery branched off to the upper extremity.[20]

Burdon-Sanderson and others quickly recognized the particular value of the sphygmograph in locating such vascular malformations. Even as he cautioned against premature confidence in the device, he affirmed its clinical value in localizing aneurysms, declaring: "It is not likely that, with the one exception of certain aneurisms, the instrument will ever be of much use in the discovery of organic lesions."[21]

---

[19] "Francis Edmund Anstie" (obituary), *Lancet* 2 (1874): 433–34.

[20] "Report from King's College Hospital: Large Aneurismal Tumour in the Posterior Triangle, Diagnosed by the Aid of the Sphygmograph; Haemorrhage from Rupture; Death; Autopsy," *Lancet* 1 (1866): 65–66; "St. Mary's Hospital: Aneurism of the Axillary Artery: Examination by the Sphygmograph," *Lancet* 1 (1866): 176.

[21] Burdon-Sanderson, *Handbook*, 65.

THE SPHYGMOGRAPH AS A GUIDE TO THERAPY

Anstie described how he used the sphygmograph in clinical practice, championing its use in prognosis and in judging the effects of therapy:

> The value of being able to *mathematically estimate* the resistance of a pulse, wich we owe in the first instance to Dr. Sanderson, is very great. The practical instances to which it may be turned are very numerous, but I shall content myself with one which will not fail to impress the reader. If, on examining a patient with acute febrile symptoms (no matter what the cause), I find that the pressure which is best suited to bringing out the maximum pulse curve is very low (say 100 to 120 grammes), I am pretty certain that the case will require wine [a stimulant]. If on the other hand, I discover that the pulse requires 200 grammes power to elicit its maximum trace, then the case does not, at any rate as yet, require stimulation.[22]

Thus Anstie was particularly interested in using the sphygmograph for the practical purposes of guiding therapy and determining prognosis. The place of alcohol in medical therapy was controversial at the time. Anstie attempted to place medicinal alcohol, whether as a stimulant or "narcotic" (here used in the general sense of a sedative) on a more scientific basis by using sphygmographic tracings to demonstrate the clinical progress of a patient treated with alcohol.[23] From one point of view, Anstie was using anecdotal evidence from a highly idiosyncratic and unproven device to diagnose, or at least evaluate, vague febrile conditions as yet undefined by the emerging germ theory, in order to justify the prescription of useless and possibly dangerous therapy. But from the point of view of British medicine in the 1860s, he was applying a promising and innovative technology, stamped with the cachet of French science, to a group of illnesses defined by current nosologies, in order to select from among available therapeutic options.

---

[22] Francis E. Anstie, "On Certain Modifications of Marey's Sphygmograph," *Lancet* 1 (1868): 784; italics in original.

[23] Francis E. Anstie, "Lectures on the Prognosis and Therapy of Certain Acute Diseases, with Specific Reference to the Indications Afforded by the Graphic Study of the Pulse." *Lancet* 2 (1867): 385–87. Two lectures were published in five segments by the *Lancet*.

THE SPHYGMOGRAPH AND THE FEVER PULSE

A year earlier, Anstie had presented a series of lectures to the Royal College of Physicians in London on the subject of the sphygmograph. At that time, he emphasized the correlation between a specific abnormality in the shape of the downslope of the pulse wave with the condition of the febrile patient."[24] What Anstie termed "fever pulses" were important signs of a grave prognosis at a time when prognostication was a key function of the consulting physician and diseases such as typhoid ran rampant. The sphygmograph, so it seemed, could detect subtle changes in the rapid pulse of a feverish patient that were undectable by simple pulse palpation.

Anstie also took serial sphygmographic tracings in two apparent cases of cardiac disease with rapid pulse. He found that a sharp apex in the pulse curve was a "good augery," while a blunt apex in the pulse curve was "ill-omened."[25] Variations in the shape of successive pulse waves and undulation of the baseline also heralded a poor prognosis.[26] Such sphygmographic subtleties were impractical for the average clinician, even if he had the means, interest, and time to "fiddle" with the Marey sphygmograph as Burdon-Sanderson and Anstie had done. Anstie's observations would only have been of practical value to a small number of elite consultants.

TECHNICAL EXPERTISE AND A WARNING

Technical expertise and experience were important from the outset, thus helping to justify sphygmographic consultation. In a 1868 *Lancet* article (a year after Burdon-Sanderson's *Handbook of the Sphygmograph* appeared), entitled "On Certain Modifications of Marey's Sphygmograph," Anstie pointed out that Marey's original instrument required up to fifteen minutes for optimal adjustment before a good pulse recording (or, "not infrequently" any pulse recording at all) could be obtained. As described in Burdon-Sanderson's *Handbook* and (mentioned earlier) elastic bands were used to fix the hyperextended wrist to a pad, holding the wrist firmly in position (see Figure 23).

Anstie also elaborated on the value of a smoked glass/stylus recording system over a paper/ink recording system as described by

---

[24] Anstie "Lectures on the Prognosis and Therapy of Certain Acute Diseases," *Lancet* 2 (1867): 35–36 (Lecture i); quotation, 36.

[25] Ibid., 63–65.

[26] Ibid., 123–24.

Burdon-Sanderson: "Glass slides are blackened with the smoke of parafine; and the writing lever is armed with a needle point. . . . [T]he resulting traces are delicate and beautiful."[27] Slides were preserved by coating the tracing with photographic varnish. For Anstie, this modification of the Marey sphygmograph produced a tracing that was both scientific and aesthetic.

An important practical problem was the pressure which ought to be applied directly upon the artery. Generally, the examiner looked for the pressure that would result in the "most distinctly marked trace."[28] Anstie credited Burdon-Sanderson with originating the principle of "graduation of pressure on the tactile spring upon the artery."[29] In something of a precocious post-mortem, he concluded a lecture with a warning similar to that offered by Burdon-Sanderson:

> Used in conjunction with the strictest and most diligent observance of other means of clinical research, I believe that the instrument affords us an additional test of the progress of acute disease and the patient's chances of safety which is of very high value. But without this careful and constant reference to the other features of each case we have no warrant for reposing trust in the indications of the sphygmograph. And I am bound to insist strongly upon the paramount necessity for the observer to qualify himself for his task by acquiring a thorough familiarity with the manipulation of the instrument before he attempts to apply it to the investigation of disease. For this purpose he must examine great numbers of healthy pulses, and must satisfy himself, by repeated examinations of the pulses of particular persons, that he is able so to use the apparatus as to obtain uniform results in the same physiological conditions; otherwise he will inevitably obtain fallacious indications, which will disgust him with the instrument, and induce him to throw undeserved discredit on a mode of investigation which he has really never properly understood.[30]

---

[27] Anstie, "On Certain Modifications of Marey's Sphygmograph," 783–84.
[28] T. A. McBride, "The Utility of the Sphygmograph in Medicine," *Archives of Medicine* (New York) 1 (1879): 192.
[29] Anstie, "On Certain Modifications of Marey's Sphygmograph," 784.
[30] Anstie, "Lectures on the Prognosis and Therapy of Certain Acute Diseases," 124.

Both Burdon-Sanderson and Anstie, in spite of various technical limitations and an abundance of cautionary remarks, recognized the great contribution of the sphygmograph to medical progress—in effect, a paradigm change—as "instruments of precision" made their way into medical practice. The sphygmogram was indeed "a permanent record—as faithful as a photograph" and the pulse was truly *"armed with a pen."*

SPHYGMOSYSTOLE: GARROD AND SPHYGMOGRAPHIC TIME INTERVALS

Alfred Henry Garrod, the son and brother of prominent British physicians, was a young fellow of St. John's College (Cambridge) when he undertook detailed sphygmographic studies (with a modified Marey sphygmograph) of the pulse. His interest as an experimental physiologist was in the measurement and interpretation of time intervals within the cardiac/pulse cycle rather than in the shape of the pulse tracing.

Garrod's early paper, "On the Relative Duration of the Component Parts of the Radial Sphygmographic Trace in Health," was presented before the Royal Society of London in 1870. He wanted to understand how the relative durations of ventricular contraction (systole) and filling (diastole) were related to the heart rate. The duration of systole was taken to be the time (in fractions of a second) between the initial rise in the radial pulse trace as the ventricle pumped blood through the open aortic valve and the beginning of a secondary rise in the downward slope of the pulse marking the closure of the aortic valve. Diastole commenced with the closure of the aortic valve and ended with the opening of the aortic valve. He noted that an earlier investigator had attempted to measure these two intervals by timing heart sounds heard through the stethoscope, a very difficult (if not impossible) undertaking at the normal human heart rate.

Garrod took multiple pulse tracings at different heart rates and then graphed the ratios of systole to the whole pulse beat on the "y" axis vs. the pulse rate on the "x" axis. He derived a mathematical model for the inverse relationship between the ratio of systole to the duration of the whole pulse as the pulse rate increased; that is, systole occupied more of the cardiac cycle at slower pulse rates.[31]

---

[31] Alfred H. Garrod, "On the Relative Duration of the Component Parts of the Radial Sphygmographic Trace in Health," *Proceedings of the Royal Society of London* 18 (1869–70): 351–54.

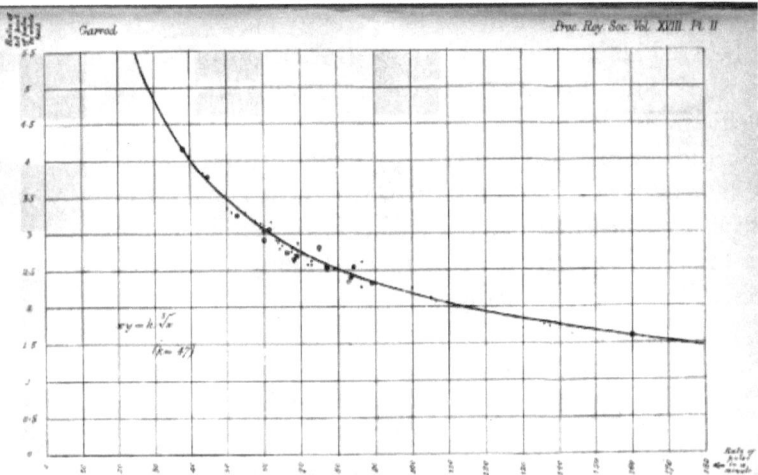

FIGURE 27: A. H. Garrod's graph showing decrease in ratio of systole to "whole beat" vs. heart rate. W. A. Forbes, "Biographical Notice," in *The Collected Scientific Papers of the late Henry Garrod, M.A., F.R.S.* (London: R. H. Porter, 1881): 17. Original in A. H. Garrod, "On the Relative Duration of the Component Parts of the Radial Sphygmographic Trace in Health," *Proceedings of the Royal Society of London* 18 (1869–70): plate between 352–53.

In 1871, Garrod studied the relation of the apex cardiograph (the pressure tracing taken with a sensor over the ventricular impulse against the chest wall) and the tracing taken at the radial pulse. He was interested in the exact relation between the contraction of the heart and the rise in the pulse at the wrist, an interval too short to be appreciated by comparing stethoscopic sounds over the heart to the palpable pulse at the wrist. He developed a complex apparatus to take simultaneous cardiac and radial artery tracings. Again, he derived mathematical formulae to define the "cardio-arterial intervals." In general, the cardio-arterial interval varied inversely with the pulse rate.[32]

In 1874, continuing with an paper entitled "On Some Points Connected with the Circulation of the Blood, Arrived At from a Study of the Sphygmograph-Trace," Garrod used the terms "sphygmosystole" to refer to the measured interval between the onset of systole and the closure of the aortic valve. He now elevated his previous work with pulse intervals to the status of a scientific "law" (i.e.: the length of cardiosystole is constant

---

[32] Alfred H. Garrod, "On the Mutual Relations of the Apex Cardiograph and the Radial Sphygmographic Trace," *Proceedings of the Royal Society of London* 19 (1870): 318–24.

for any given pulse rate and varies as the square root of the length of the pulse beat). The law held true for measurements of pulses in the carotid and posterior tibial (ankle) arteries, suggesting that it also held true for the aortic pulses.[33]

Garrod's work was limited to experimental physiology with no immediate clinical application. In an 1871 article in the *Journal of Anatomy and Physiology*, he explained the scientific impulse behind his emphasis on timed intervals (and their mathematical analysis) rather than the more subjective shape of the tracings:

> The Sphygmograph is a bad haemodynamometer [instrument to measure the blood pressure] at its best, and as such its employment will probably diminish. A glance at the work of Dr. Loraine [a Parisian investigator] will shew [sic] that numberless variations in the character of a tracing can be introduced by very small changes in the position, &c. [etc.] of the subject experimented on. But there is one part of the trace which is not affected in any way by these complications, and that is the relation borne by the *length* of the different portions of each beat to one another. Whether the arm is raised or lowered, whether the pressure is great or small, the interval between the systolic rise and the commencement of the diastolic rise does not vary in the least. These intervals cannot be correctly estimated except by the aid of the sphygmograph; and as the value of any method of investigation is greatest in that direction in which it is least infuenced by surrounding circumstances, it is, as it will be my endeavour to prove when considering the tracings themselves, that the measurement of these intervals that we must look [to] for the future value of the sphygmograph.[34]

Garrod would prove to be largely correct. Subtleties in the wave forms were frustratingly subjective and operator dependent, though, as we shall see, Frederick Akbar Mahomed, working in London in the 1870s would discover much about the blood pressure from the shape of the tracings.

---

[33] Alfred H. Garrod, "On Some Points Connected with the Circulation of the Blood, Arrived at from a Study of the Sphygmograph-Trace (abstract)," *Proceedings of the Royal Society of London* 22 (1873): 291–93; full paper *Proceedings of the Royal Society of London* 23 (1874): 140–51.

[34] Alfred H. Garrod, "On Sphygmography," *Journal of Anatomy and Physiology* 6 (1871–72): 404.

More detailed investigations of cardiac and pulse intervals would later be undertaken by an innovative American sphygmograph man named Alonzo Thrasher Keyt (see Chapter 5). Garrod's interest and expertise soon turned to comparative zoology; his promising career was cut short by his death in 1879 at age thirty-three from tuberculosis. In recent decades, precise numerical measurements have become integral components of electrocardiography, echocardiography, and cardiac catheterization

BROADBENT: THE SPHYGMOGRAPH AS TEACHING TOOL

In his classic 1890 book, *The Pulse* ("Illustrated with 59 Sphygmographic Tracings"), London clinician and medical school lecturer William Broadbent remarked of the sphygmograph: ". . . the application of the graphic method by means of the admirable sphygmograph invented by Marey led to a scientific study of the pulse and to a comprehension of its indications never before possible."[35] Broadbent emphasized the educational value of the sphygmograph in teaching medical students to examine and interpret the pulse; the sphygmograph "rediscovered for us the indications furnished by the pulse." He handed around pulse tracings for students to inspect and interpret, but he did not expect the students to become sphygmographers. Rather, his goals in exhibiting pulse tracings were to foster a better knowledge of cardiovascular physiology, prepare students to read and understand the evolving medical literature, and to better enable them to interpret pulse palpation with the examining finger at the bedside. This simple demonstration of the portability of the pulse tracing underscores the the power of the graphic method. But the sphygmograph, warned Broadbent, was not to be used recklessly:

> The sphygmograph is invaluable as an exact means of observation, and has been a great means of educating us how to feel and properly appreciate the pulse—has, in fact, as I said, rediscovered for us the indications furnished by the pulse. It will never come into use in general practice, for it demands not only

---

[35] William H. Broadbent, *The Pulse* (London: Cassell, 1890; Philadelphia: Lea Brothers, 1890), 15. The British and American editions of Broadbent's book, *The Pulse*, are identical; both are based on the Croonian Lectures delivered at the Royal College of Physicians in 1887 (information courtesy W. Bruce Fye); William H. Broadbent, "The Pulse: The Croonian Lecture Delivered to the Royal College of Physicians, 1887," *British Medical Journal* 1 (1887): 655–60.

time and care at each application, but also a careful preliminary training. It is an instrument of precision and requires a skilled workman.[36]

BEYOND LONDON: THE SPHYGMOGRAPH IN THE PROVINCES

In 1867, a promising young medical student made an important and valid observation using the sphygmograph. While still a student at Edinburgh, Thomas Lauder Brunton was impressed by early sphygmographic experiments conducted by Arthur Gamgee, one of the city's leading physicians. Brunton, while working on the wards at Edinburgh's Royal Infirmary, had seen that phlebotomy (therapeutic bloodletting) seemed to relieve and even prevent angina attacks (heart pain due to what is now known to be coronary artery disease). Aware that amyl nitrite dilated the blood vessels and reduced the tension in the arteries (without the need to open a vein with a lancet and bleed the patient), Brunton thought such a "medical phlebotomy" using inhaled amyl nitrite might be helpful in angina. Angina attacks were indeed aborted by the drug and the clinical course seemed to be reflected in serial sphygmographic tracings. Brunton wrote:

> From observations during the attack, and from an examination of numerous sphygmographic tracings taken while the patients were free from pain, while it was coming on, at its height, passing off under the influence of amyl, and again completely gone, I find that when the attack comes on gradually the pulse becomes smaller, and the arterial tension greater as the pain increases in severity. During the attack the breathing is quick, the pulse small and rapid, and the arterial tension high, owing, I believe, to contaction of the systemic capillaries. As the nitrite is inhaled the pulse becomes slower and fuller, the tension diminished, and the breathing less hurried. . . . not till the volume as well as tension of the pulse became normal, did I feel sure that the pain would not return.[37]

---

[36] William H. Broadbent, "The Pulse: Its Diagnostic, Prognostic, and Therapeutic Indications," *Lancet* 2 (1875): 549.

[37] T. Lauder Brunton, "On the Use of Amyl Nitrite in Angina Pectoris," *Lancet* 2, 97–98: 1867. For a detailed history of Brunton's work with amyl nitrite, see W. Bruce Fye, "T. Lauder Brunton and Amyl Nitrite: A Victorian Vasodilator," *Circulation* 74 (1986): 22–29.

Years later, Brunton recalled his youthful enthusiasm for the sphygmograph and his experiments with amyl nitrite, adding serial sphygmographic tracings to support his clinical observations:

> I was able to watch a patient at every hour of the day and night, and to observe every phase of the attack. By the aid of Marey's sphygmograph, I discovered that during the paroxysm [i.e., the painful anginal attack], the blood pressure rose and the pulse became quick . . . [T]he experiments of Marey and Chauveau enabled me to say, from the form of the tracing, what I could not have discoverd by the finger, that the arterioles were excessively contracted.[38]

Brunton's studies with the sphygmograph appeared in the *Lancet* in 1867, suggesting that Gamgee and Brunton were working with the sphygmograph independently of Burdon-Sanderson and his colleagues in London.[39]

Work with the sphygmograph was proceeding independently in Birmingham as well. In early 1866, Balthazar Foster, a young consultant and anatomy professor at Queen's College in Birmingham, published an article in the *British Medical Journal* describing his work with the sphygmograph as presented before the Midland Medical Society. Acknowledging his debt to Anstie for acquainting him with Marey's sphygmograph, Foster published several of his own tracings. He was clearly attempting to integrate Marey's sphygmograph into clinical practice just a year or two after Burdon-Sanderson and Anstie in London were conducting the earliest British studies with the sphygmograph.

Foster was particularly interested in the "senile pulse," examining octogenarians through the courtesy of the medical officer of the Birmingham workhouse, as well as various structural cardiac abnormalities identified in patients in several Birmingham hospitals. Of the "senile pulse" he wrote: "I allude to that *Senile Change in the Vessels* which gives to the finger placed over the radial [wrist] artery the

---

[38] T. Lauder Brunton, *Pharmacology and Therapeutics; or Medicine Past and Present* (London: Macmillan and Co., 1880), 139–40.

[39] Brunton became a leading expert in the application of physiologic principles to clinical pharmacology. He was the co-author, with Burdon-Sanderson and others of the *Handbook for the Physiology Laboratory*; Edward Klein, john Burdon-Sanderson, Michael Foster, T. Lauder Brunton, *Handbook for the Physiology Laboratory* (Philadelphia: Lindsay & Blakiston, 1873).

sensaton of resting on a hard inelastic tube." Such a pulse, often found at a "comparatively early period of life," was well recognized through autopsy studies to be associated with degenerative changes in the heart and hypertrophy (enlargement) of the left ventricle, the main pumping chamber of the heart. Modern terminology would label this premature atherosclerosis with ventricular hypertrophy and, in the late stages, cardiac decompensation.

Foster believed that the sphygmograph expanded the clinician's ability to study and characterize the "senile pulse." His article in the *British Medical Journal* (1866), included tracings he had taken in patients with a characteristic hard pulse detected by palpation:

> In the better understood diseases of the heart and great vessels, we can arrive at a diagnosis by the ordinary means employed [palpation of the pulse and cardiac impulse, percussion of the heart border, and auscultation with the stethoscope] the instrument of Marey can afford us useful confirmatory evidence, and in many it can perfect a diagnosis which percussion and auscultation have failed to complete. The pulse-trace alone often enables those skilled in its interpretation to foretell the sounds to be heard on auscultation; and in doubtful cases, by the information it yields, augments in no small degree the certainty of the diagnosis.[40]

Foster's lectures to the Midland Medical Society, "On the Use of the Sphygmograph in the Investigation of Disease," were published as a pamphlet in 1866 and also in the *British Medical Journal*. A chapter on sphygmography was included in a book published in England and Philadelphia 1874, in which Foster attempted to correlate a wide variety of valvular and other structural cardiac disorders with sphygmographic tracings and autopsy findings.[41]

---

[40] Balthazar W. Foster, "On the Use of the Sphygmograph in the Investigation of Disease," *British Medical Journal* 1 (1866): 275–78, 330–33; quotation 330.

[41] Balthazar W. Foster, *On the Use of the Sphygmograph in the Investigation of Disease* (London: John Churchill & Sons, 1866); Balthazar W. Foster, "Cases Illustrating the Use of the Sphygmograph and Cardiograph in the Study of Diseases of the Heart and Great Vessels," in *Clinical Medicine: Lectures and Essays* (London: J. and A. Churchill, 1874; Philadelphia, Lindsay and Blakiston, 1874), 267–330. As noted previously, the term cardiograph as used here refers to the application of the sphygmographic sensor to the chest over the apex of the heart, thus producing a tracing of the upward thrust of the contracting heart.

In a 1866 prize-winning essay on shock, Furneaux Jordan, a Birmingham colleague, invited Foster to assist in a study of surgical and trauma patients with the sphygmograph. Foster studied Jordan's patients pre- and post-operatively. He also took sphygmographic tracings of a patient under chloroform anesthesia during "operation of the saw" in the course of an amputation.[42]

"LONDON CALLING"— TAKING ON A PROVINCIAL UPSTART

A minor tiff over priority erupted in the *Lancet*. Upon receipt of Foster's handbook, a *Lancet* editorialist huffed, ". . . we are sorry we cannot speak with approbation." The editorial questioned Foster's right to publish a monograph on the sphygmograph and took him and his friends to task for claims of priority. The *Lancet* pointed out that the work of Anstie and Burdon-Sanderson in London was "in full progress at a time when Dr. Foster himself was probably unaware even of the existence of Marey's sphygmograph." Foster's pamphlet was little more than a *"réchauffé"* (rewarming) of Marey's published work.[43]

Foster replied testily to the *Lancet* that he had in fact acknowledged his gratitude to Anstie in his monograph and was happy to express his debt to Burdon-Sanderson. Furthermore, continued Foster, the true priority may have rested with Hughes Bennet, who had demonstrated a sphygmograph in Bath in September of 1864. Be that as it may, Foster denied that his own work was merely a copy of work done earlier by Marey. The contested pamphlet presented original tracings taken by himself as well as fully acknowledged copies of tracings by Marey. Marey had, in fact, corresponded with him, complimenting Foster and asking to use some of his tracings.

Foster may have been responding to a perceived slight by the London elite toward provincial physicians like himself. He ended his response by taking the high (and correct) scientific road: "I regret that you should call into question my right to repeat and extend M. Marey's researches. . . . Is it not true that the independent investigation of new facts by a number of observers is the legitimate and most fruitful method of promoting their application to the uses of our art?"[44]

---

[42] Furneaux Jordan, "On Shock after Surgical Operations and Injuries: The Sphymograph in Shock," *British Medical Journal* 1 (1867): 192–93.

[43] "The Sphygmograph in English Medical Practice" (editorial), *Lancet* 1 (1866): 579.

[44] Balthazar Foster, "The Sphygmograph in English Medical Practice" (letter), *Lancet* 1

The *British Medical Journal* was viewed as the voice of the provincial practitioner, while the *Lancet* was the voice of the London elite.[45] Anstie, who was on the editorial board of the *Lancet*, wrote a guardedly mollifying letter, proclaiming the sphygmograph "public property for several years." He rather tartly referred to his own paper of November 1865 in the *Lancet*, but concluded with the dignified (and patriotic) reflection that the "united efforts of numerous English sphygmographers now at work will render most important services to clinical research."[46]

Foster apparently enjoyed some positive reputation outside Birmingham. In 1866–67, the *Medical Record* (New York) published a reprint of a review from the August 1866 *Dublin Quarterly Journal of Medical Science* of Foster's handbook, *On the Use of the Sphygmograph in the Investigation of Disease*. The Dublin reviewer, noting the pioneering use of Marey's sphygmograph by Burdon-Sanderson and Anstie, considered Foster's work to be "the first publication likely to introduce [the sphygmograph] to British practitioners." (Foster's book credited Anstie with acquainting him with the instrument and being the first in Britain to make a presentation to a medical society, perhaps a response to Anstie's letter in the *Lancet* in November 1865.) The *Dublin Quarterly* reviewer predicted that as "the instrument comes into extensive use so many observations will be recorded that valuable information will be afforded in the diagnosis of all diseases in which examination of the pulse by the finger has hitherto been relied on." To underscore Foster's appeal to ordinary practitioners (outside the London elite), he was praised as "a practical physician and an industrious clinical teacher."[47]

BENJAMIN WARD RICHARDSON: THE SPHYGMOPHONE

Some sphygmographers, perhaps mindful of the stethoscope as an invaluable diagnostic aid, added sound to the workings of the

---

(1866): 634.
[45] Robert G. Frank, Jr., "The Telltale Heart: Physiological Instruments, Graphic Methods, and Clinical Hopes," in *The Investigative Enterprise*, ed. William Coleman and Fredrick L. Holmes (Berkeley: University of California Press, 1988), 219–20.
[46] Frances E. Anstie, "The Sphygmograph in English Medical Practice," *Lancet* 1 (1866): 671.
[47] "On the Use of the Sphygmograph in the Investigation of Disease, by B. W. Foster" (review), *Dublin Quarterly Journal of Medical Science* 42 (1866): 125–28; "New Instruments: The Sphygmograph," *Medical Record* (New York) 1 (1866–67): 580–81.

sphygmograph. In 1879, Benjamin Ward Richardson, a leading London physician, sanitarian, and pharmacologist, was fiddling with an audiometer when it occurred to him that he might get a secondary or telephonic sound from the movements of the pulse at the wrist." By attaching wires and microphones to a Pond sphygmograph (see Chapter 6), Richardson was able to transmit the scratchings of the recording stylus to a telephone. The transmitted sounds were rather telegraphic, each pulse wave giving two long and one short sounds, the whole resembling the words "bother it." Richardson thought the device might be useful in teaching. The Richardson "sphygmophone" seems to have been stillborn in his laboratory. However, Richardson did modify the British Dudgeon sphygmograph; Richardson's Standard Sphygmograph was included in an American instrument catalog ca. 1893.[48]

A year later, American inventor W. H. H. Barton patented a sphygmophone that appears to have converted pulse motion into an audible signal.[49] Nothing further is known of the inventor or his sphygmophone. Presumably, the sphygmophone was intended to emit a sound with each pulse beat, an innovation echoed by the ubiquitous beeping pulse monitors in today's intensive care units.

THE SPHYGMOGRAPH AS SPHYGMOMANOMETER: BLOOD PRESSURE MEASUREMENT

An intriguing application of sphygmography was its projected role in determining the pressure within the arteries. Physicians had long characterized the palpable pulse as "hard" or "soft." Until the mid-nineteenth century, the pulse associated with what we now call hypertension would have been described as the *pulsus magnus durus et tardus*. At first glance, it would seem that the pressure exerted on the artery by the sensor of the

---

[48] Benjamin Ward Richardson, "Note on the Invention of a Method for Making the Movements of the Pulse Audible by the Telephone. The Sphygmophone," *Proceedings of the Royal Society of London* 29 (1879): 70; Benjamin Ward Richardson, "A Standard Sphygmograph," in *Aloe's Illustrated and Priced Catalogue of Superior Surgical Instruments, Physician's Supplies and Hospital Furnishings*, 6th ed. (St. Louis: A. S. Aloe Co., ca. 1893), 351, 354–55.

[49] Barton, W. H. H., "Sphygmophone, U.S. Patent No. 232,105, 14 September 1880," www.google.com/patents/US232105 (accessed 2 February 2017). Only the drawing can be viewed at the website; the exact working and purpose of Barton's sphygmophone are unknown. Barton of Brockton, MA, appears to have patented a number of devices including a thermostat and furnace damper.

sphygmograph should be a measure of arterial pressure. However, the pressure exerted on the artery by the sphygmograph—typically adjusted by the operator to produce the best possible waveform—was a function of the instrument and the anatomy of the patient's wrist, as well as the properties of the arterial wall. Intuitively, one might also suppose that the height of the wave produced by the sphygmograph would correlate with blood pressure, but this too was a function of the state of the arterial wall, the anatomy of the wrist, and the performance of the springs and levers in the instrument itself.

The systolic blood pressure as measured by modern sphygmomanometers (blood pressure devices) is determined by the pressure necessary to *obliterate* the arterial pulse—such a pressure would produce no wave on a sphygmograph—rather than the pressure required to produce a distinct wave on the sphygmograph. Interestingly, it was Vierordt, inventor of the earliest sphygmograph, who enunciated the principle of determining the blood pressure in 1855, declaring that the systolic blood pressure was equal to the counterpressure sufficient to obliterate the arterial pulsations.[50]

Ever the innovator, Marey built an imaginative device for measuring the pressure, applying Vierordt's principle of vascular occlusion. He filled a glass box with water and placed the subject's forearm in the box. The pressure in the box could be increased or decreased by means of a leveling bulb. The box was connected to a shallow cup or drum with a thin elastic membrane (a tambour or "lever drum" similar to that used by Marey to record cardiac pulsations), which carried a writing lever to record pulse waves on a kymograph, thus producing a sphygmogram or pulse tracing. As the operator increased the pressure in the closed box (indicated by a mercury manometer), "a moment comes," wrote Marey, "when the pulsations [of the artery] cease." The pressure necessary to obliterate the pulse was taken as the [systolic] blood pressure.[51] Although it bore the hallmark of Marey's ingenuity, the instrument was clumsy and impractical. The fact that the entire forearm with its cushion of soft tissues was being compressed, rather than the artery alone, was bound to produce erroneous readings.[52]

---

[50] Ralph Major, "The History of Taking the Blood Pressure," *Annals of Medical History* n.s. 2 (1930): 51–52.

[51] Étienne-Jules Marey, *Physiologie expérimentale: Travaux du laboratoire de M. Marey* (Paris: G. Masson, 1876), 2:317–18.

[52] Major, "History of Taking the Blood Pressure," 52; Eion O'Brien and Desmond Fitzgerald, "The History of Indirect Blood Pressure Measurement," in *Handbook of Hypertension*, ed. E. O'Brien and K. O'Malley (Amsterdam: Elsevier Science Publishers, 1991): 14:10.

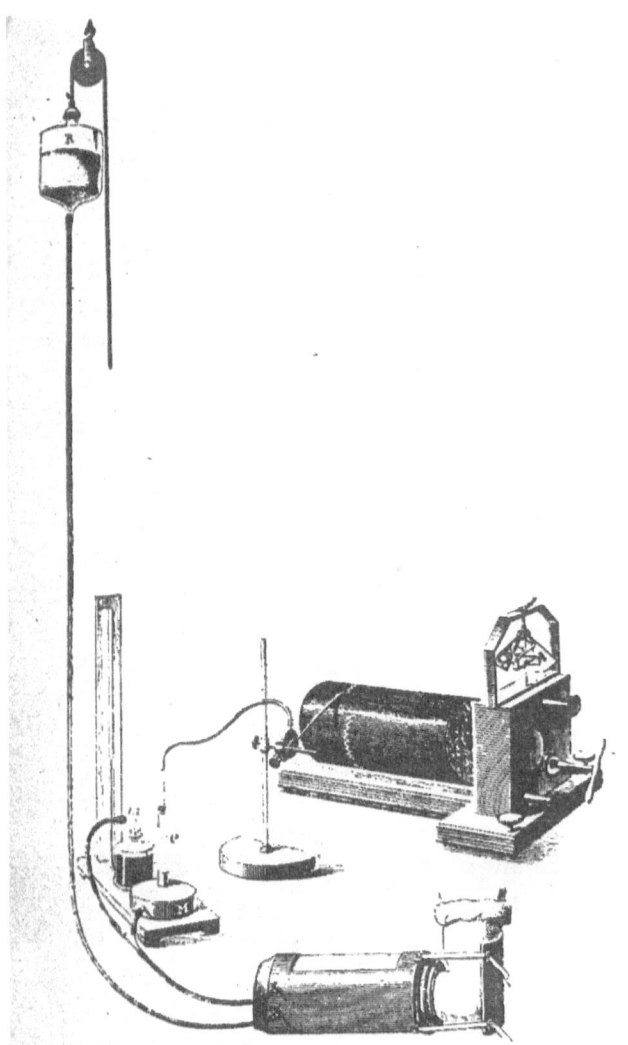

FIGURE 28: Marey's hydraulic blood pressure device, incorporating pulse tracings and the concept of pulse obliteration as the systolic pressure. Étienne-Jules Marey, *Physiologie expérimentale: Travaux du laboratoire de M. Marey* (Paris: G. Masson, 1876), 317.

The numerical determination of blood pressure would prove to be beyond the capabilities of the sphygmograph and similar instruments. Burdon-Sanderson, in *A Handbook for the Physiological Laboratory*, commented pessimistically in 1873, "We have already seen that the sphygmograph is of no use as a gauge of arterial pressure," although one could follow trends in pressure by serial determinations and get a general qualitative notion of the arterial pressure.[53]

MAHOMED: THE FORGOTTEN MASTER OF BLOOD PRESSURE MEASUREMENT

The late-nineteenth-century master of the sphygmograph with respect to arterial tension—and the man who first elucidated primary hypertension (i.e. high blood pressure *not* seconday to kidney disease or any other organ dysfunction) and its harmful effect on the organs of the body—was Frederick Akbar Mahomed of Guy's Hospital in London. While still a medical student, Mahomed, the grandson of an immigrant Indian military surgeon and operator of medicinal baths in London, modified Marey's device, winning the Pupils' Physical Society Prize of 1870 for his unpublished essay, "On The Sphygmograph." Mahomed's introduction to his unpublished essay suggests that the staff at Guy's Hospital had already given up on the sphygmograph, so recently introduced from France: "Mr. President and Gentlemen; In bringing under your notice this evening the Sphygmograph, some apology is necessary; for I am aware that it is an instrument which has already been condemned in this hospital, and having been put to the test, has been cast aside as useless."[54]

As his detailed investigations into chronic kidney disease (then known as Bright's disease) progressed through the 1870s, Mahomed emphasized that sphygmographic pulse study had a critical role to play in clinical medicine. In Mahomed's hands, pulse study, refocused on arterial tension, would prove to be revolutionary. Building on Burdon-Sanderson's

---

[53] Edward Klein, John Burdon-Sanderson, Michael Foster, and T. Lauder Brunton, *A Handbook for the Physiology Laboratory* (London, J. and A. Churchill; Philadelphia: Lindsay & Blakiston, 1873), 229. Burdon-Sanderson wrote the section on cardiovascular physiology, "Blood Circulation, Respiration, and Animal Heat." The *Handbook*, a model of its kind, received lavish praise from Henry P. Bowditch, professor of physiology at Harvard. Without specifically mentioning the sphygmograph, Bowditch cites Burdon-Sanderson's "important experiments which have thrown so much light on the functions of the nervous system in regulating the movements of the heart, and the resistance offered by the arteries to the flow of blood." Henry P. Bowditch (as H. P. B.), "Bibliographic Notice of *Handbook for the Physiological Laboratory*." *Boston Medical and Surgical Journal* 89 (1873): 360–61.

[54] J. Stuart Cameron and Jackie Hicks, "Frederick Akbar Mahomed and His Role in the Description of Hypertension at Guy's Hospital," *Kidney International* 49 (1996): 1492. The first page of Mahomed's handwritten essay, "On the Sphygmograph," is reproduced by Cameron and Hicks as an illustration.

modification of the Marey sphygmograph, Mahomed (and the jeweler who suggested the adjustment and assembled the instrument) added a screw that allowed him to measure the pressure needed to occlude the radial artery in precise troy weights. He evolved a system for using the shape of the pulse wave forms to qualitatively identify high arterial tension (high blood pressure) and low arterial tension. He could not, however, assign a number in units such as millimeters of mercury to his findings.

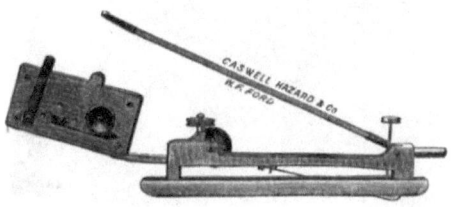

FIGURE 29: Mahomed's modification of the Marey sphygmograph, allowing measurement of the precise pressure applied to the artery. T. A. McBride, "The Utility of the Sphygmograph in Medicine," *Archives of Medicine* 1 (1879), 185.

In a comprehensive 1879 article entitled "The Utility of the Sphygmograph" for the *Archives of Medicine* (New York), gifted young New York consultant Thomas A. McBride reviewed Mahomed's methods for the benefit of an American audience. He was very familiar with Mahomed's work and described his improvements on the basic Marey model:

> The great advantage of this [Mahomed's] instrument is that the amount of pressure employed can be estimated quite accurately. The amount of pressure used [to apply the sensor firmly to the artery at the wrist] is registered upon a dial, and the pressure is applied to the spring which rests upon the artery by means of an eccentric. It is necessary in using the Marey or Mahomed to place the forearm upon a padded splint and the instrument is then applied to the forearm and fastened to the splint by tapes or elastic bands.[55]

As was well known to all sphygmographers, the sphygmographic pulse wave had several components reflecting the opening and closing of the aortic valve and the expansion and relaxation of the arteries as the left ventricle pumped blood into the aorta and through the arterial system of

---

[55] McBride, "Utility of the Sphygmograph," 186–89.

the body. Each component was subject to variation by a range of conditions affecting the circulation.

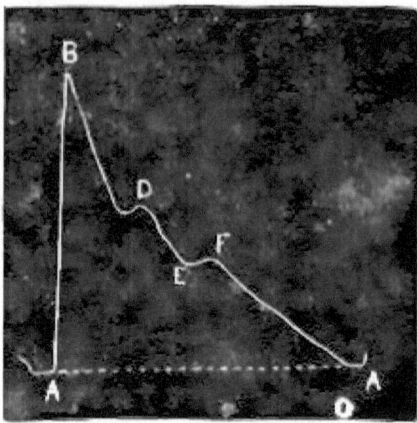

FIGURE 30: Components of the pulse wave as recorded by the sphygmograph: AB: upstroke or percussion wave; D: the tidal wave; E: aortic or dicrotic notch; F: dicrotic wave; AA: the respiratory or base line. T. A. McBride, "The Utility of the Sphygmograph in Medicine," *Archives of Medicine* 1 (1879), 187.

There was some confusion regarding the mechanism of the various components of the normal pulse wave as visualized with the sphygmograph. McBride attributes much of the currently correct explanation to the work of Mahomed. In this scheme, the wave of a single pulse beat consists of three components; the following schema uses the notation of McBride:

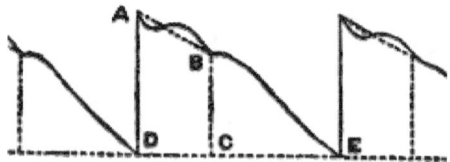

FIGURE 31: Mahomed's two methods for identifying a high pressure pulse. If any part of the curve extended above a line drawn from the apex of the upstroke to the bottom of the notch preceding the dicrotic wave (line AB), then the pulse was a high pressure pulse. Also, the higher the notch above the baseline (line BC), the higher the blood pressure. Frederick Akbar Mahomed, "Some of the Clinical Aspects of Chronic Bright's Disease," *Guy's Hospital Reports* 24 (3rd ser.) (1879): 371.

1. percussion wave: the sudden upstroke as the aortic valve opens and the artery is filled with blood; the momentum of the lever arm of the sphygmograph causes the lever to overshoot the true height of the pulse wave (B in Figure 30)
2. tidal wave: the true maximal influx of blood into the artery, seen as a dip and second peak following the maximal point of the percussion wave (D in Figure 30)
3. dicrotic wave: a notch in the downward arm of the arterial wave due to closure of the aortic valve followed by a sudden bump or dicrotic wave (E and F in Figure 30)[56]

Mahomed's method of identifying elevated blood pressure—a "high-tension pulse"— from sphygmographic tracings was relatively objective and straightforward:

> A line must be drawn from the apex of the upstroke to the bottom of the notch preceding the dicrotic wave [AB in Mahomed's diagram, Figure 31]. No part of the tracing should rise above this line; if it does, then the pulse is one of high pressure. The height of this notch is another good gauge of pressure; the higher it is from the base line of the tracing the higher is the pressure; the nearer it approaches the line the lower is the pressure [BC in Mahomed's diagram].[57]

Mahomed used his modified sphygmograph as a research instrument to study the form and pressure of the pulse in hundreds of patients with a wide variety of diseases, most importantly chronic kidney disease (then known as Bright's disease). The relation between kidney disease and pathological changes in the blood vessels at autopsy was already widely recognized. The pathophysiology was generally thought to follow a path from diseased kidneys to high arterial tension. In Mahomed's words (1879): "Thus, the sequence is supposed to be, first, the kidney; second, retained effete material [in this case, retained nitrogenous cell waste] in the blood; third, impeded circulation; fourth, the cardio-vascular changes characteristic of Bright's disease." By relying on "morbid anatomy" (autopsy studies), Mahomed believed that "functional" disorders such as abnormalities of the pulse (and particularly high arterial tension) were being ignored.

---

[56] Ibid., 190–91.
[57] Frederick Akbar Mahomed, "Some of the Clinical Aspects of Chronic Bright's Disease," *Guy's Hospital Reports* 24 (1879): 370–71.

Mahomed's systematic sphygmographic study of the pressure in the arteries yielded profound insight into human disease, challenging the conventional wisdom that diseased kidneys invariably *caused* high arterial tension diseased arteries. By the late 1870s, Mahomed's correlation of clinical disease and his meticulous acquisition and analysis of sphygmographic tracings led him to conclude that high arterial pressure often *preceded*, and indeed caused, some forms of kidney disease as well as cardiac disease and cerebrovascular disease (then often referred to as "apoplexy").[58] Mahomed was the first to define what we now call essential hypertension, a universally acknowledged—and now aggressively treated—risk factor (to use a modern term) for progressive end-organ damage in middle age.

Mahomed, who promised much for the future of cardiovascular physiology and diagnosis, drifted into other areas of medical inquiry; he died in 1884 at age thirty-five of typhoid fever. He was attended in his final illness by his mentor and colleague William Broadbent, who later published important works on the pulse and the use of the sphygmograph.

A 1996 biographical study by nephrologists J. Stewart Cameron and Jackie Hicks of Guy's and St. Thomas' Hospital (London) provides insight into the rapid eclipse of Mahomed's reputation. His identification of essential hypertension based on his meticulous work with the sphygmograph was forgotten; credit went to the later work of an investigator (Thomas Clifford Allbutt, see below) armed with an early sphygmomanometer (blood pressure cuff). The difficulties of applying the sphygmograph and interpreting its complex waves played a key role in relegating Mahomed to undeserved obscurity.[59]

Broadbent, who was Mahomed's friend and colleague and himself a respected British authority on cardiology, devoted a chapter of his 1890 monograph on the pulse to the problem of the high tension pulse. Again, it must be stressed that the pressure applied to the artery was not the blood pressure; in fact, as Broadbent pointed out in 1875 (and all experienced sphygmographers knew): "The value of its [the sphygmograph's] revelations depends entirely on the intelligence which is brought to bear on its employment. . . . Completely different tracings may be obtained from the same pulse by variations in the pressure employed." As noted earlier, the ideal pressure to be applied to the artery when recording a sphygmogram was that which, by trial and error, produced the best pulse tracing.[60]

---

[58] Ibid., 364–68.
[59] Cameron and Hicks, "Frederick Akbar Mahomed," 1503.
[60] Broadbent, "The Pulse: Its Diagnostic, Prognostic, and Therapeutic Indications," 549; Broadbent, "The Pulse: The Croonian Lecture," 655–60.

As Mahomed had shown two decades earlier earlier, the high tension pulse was a harbinger—indeed, often the cause—of a shortened life: "It points out tendencies which later result in serious illness or fatal disease, and its recognition often directs us to measures by which ailments may be relieved, and enables us to foresee and sometimes to avert premature death." Broadbent characterized the high tension pulse wave as having "an upstroke with a faint inclination forwards, a round or flat summit and a gradual decline without a dicrotic notch or wave."[61] Such subjective descriptions continued to underscore the inutility of the sphygmograph for practical blood pressure determination. Compared to these purely subjective and vague observations, the sphygmomanometer (modern blood pressure apparatus), with its numerical readout in millimeters of mercury, would, at the turn of the twentieth century, offer obvious advantages in precision, standardization, and practical utility.

Mahomed's unsigned memorialist (probably Broadbent) in the *Lancet*, remarked that Mahomed's "fervent advocacy did much to re-establish the sphygmograph in clinical estimation," while gently suggesting that operator subjectivity and skill was difficult to ignore:

> It was a common saying that no one but Mahomed could interpret all the teachings of the sphygmograph, and it may be that this study of its records led him to place too strong a reliance upon the faithfulness of a mechanical contrivance, without due allowance for its necessary imperfections.[62]

STEELL: PURSUING THE HIGH TENSION PULSE

Reliance on the shape of the sphygmographic curve limited the qualitative determination of high arterial pressure to a few highly motivated clinicians. Graham Steell of Manchester published his short monograph, *The Use of the Sphygmograph in Clinical Medicine*, in 1899, dedicating it to the memory of "the late lamented Dr. F. A. Mahomed" and his "eloquent advocacy" of the unfairly neglected sphygmograph, often seen as a "mere toy of faddists." Steell returned to the synedoche of the "physician's finger" to describe traditional pulse study:

---

[61] Broadbent, *The Pulse*, 147–49.
[62] "Frederick A. Mahomed" (obituary), *Lancet* 2 (1884): 973.

> Again, we are told that the physician's "finger" should be educated, and instrumental aid eschewed. My answer is that as an educator of the "finger" ["finger" standing, of course, for the cerebral center that receives the impressions conveyed by the finger] the sphygmograph is *facile princeps* [easily the best]. This fact alone should render the instrument at least deserving of respect. To those who would trust the "finger" absolutely, I might say that I believe the most cultured "finger" will occasionally err without an appeal to instrumental aid.[63]

Steell suggested that the degree of applied pressure on the artery "will usually be found to be considerable in high tension pulses and small in low tension pulses." In fact, Steell's description of the "high tension pulse" was so highly subjective as to discourage all but the most dedicated investigators and practitioners. The challenge of diagnosing the high-tension pulse was made more difficult by the uncertainties about a normal pulse tracing. Steell observed:

> It is difficult to define the characters of a normal pulse-tracing, inasmuch as there are physiological differences in the pulses of different individuals. One man has normally a fairly high-tension pulse, another, equally healthy, a fairly low-tension pulse, and the pulse of the same man at different times and under the influence of temporary circumstances may vary as greatly in its character.[64]

Steell devoted very little of his monograph to the high tension pulse, focusing mainly on diseases of the heart valves and disturbances in cardiac rhythm. Of the high-tension pulse, he describes pertinent characteristics of several illustrative tracings: "well-developed" tidal wave, sustained or prolonged tidal wave, aortic notch located high above respiratory line, no exaggeration of the dicrotic notch. Low-tension pulses were characterized by the reverse or absence of these features.[65] All these highly subjective subtleties would become evaluable only *after* the novice had mastered the pesky intricacies of the sphygmograph.

---

[63] Graham Steell, *The Use of the Sphygmograph in Clinical Medicine* (Manchester: Sherratt & Hughes, 1899), 5.

[64] Ibid., 6.

[65] Ibid., 6–9. Steell's name remains in cardiology textbooks today in association with a characteristic heart murmur.

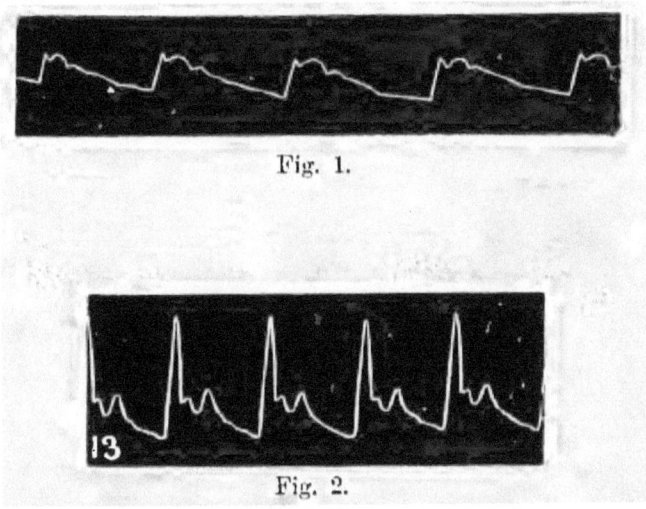

FIGURE 32: Examples from Graham Steell (1899) of a high tension/pressure pulse (top tracing) and low tension/pressure pulse (bottom tracing) emphasizing the "well-developed" or "sustained" tidal wave in the high pressure pulse and the "absent" or "ill developed" tidal wave in the lower pressure pulse. The tidal wave is the peak immediately following the high and sharp primary or percussion wave. Graham Steell, *The Use of the Sphygmograph in Clinical Medicine* (Manchester: Sherratt & Hughes, 1899), 7.

VON BASCH: FIRST GLIMPSE OF THE HOLY GRAIL OF HYPERTENSION

In the early 1880s, Samuel Siegfried Ritter von Basch, working in Vienna, was able to quantitate systolic pressure in millimeters of mercury (mm Hg) using a rubber bulb (pelotte) filled with mercury. The bulb was pressed against the radial artery and the mercury transmitted the impulse to a calibrated manometer. A cradle was later added to steady the subject's wrist. Von Basch was able to record systolic pressures (the applied pressure at which the pulse was obliterated), reporting a range of 110 to 160 mm Hg. He went on to develop several other models of his sphygmomanometer and introduced an aneroid gauge in place of the mercury manometer. Other Europeans modified the von Basch device, most notably Pierre Carl Edouard Potain of Paris, who subsituted an air-filled pelotte to compress the artery in his 1889 sphygmomanometer. With the introduction of the now-familiar occlusive arm cuff by Italian Scipione Riva-Rocci in the mid-1890s, the modern era of sphygmomanometry began.[66]

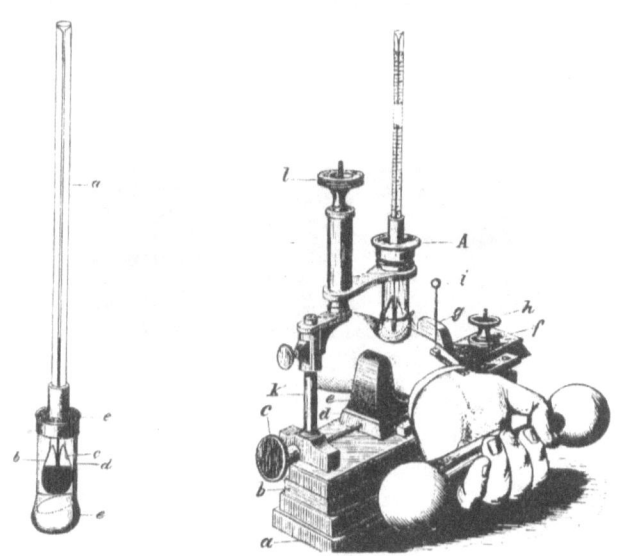

FIGURE 33: Von Basch's sphygmomanometer, an early device to determining the blood pressure in millimeters of mercury. The mercury-filled bulb (pelotte) was pressed against the radial artery and the pulsations transmitted to the calibrated glass monometer. Basch later added a frame to restrain the wrist during measurement of the blood pressure. Reproduced in N. H. Naqvi and M. D. Blaufox, *Blood Pressure Measurement: An Illustrated History* (New York: Parthenon, 1998), 58; original in von Basch articles ca. 1880.

ALLBUTT: HYPERPIESIA—ESSENTIAL HYPERTENSION

In 1892, encouraged by hindsight and familiar with early models of blood pressure devices, T. Clifford Allbutt, Regius Professor of Medicine at Cambridge, reflected with some disdain on what was sometimes referred to as the "personal equation" in sphygmography:

> Some of the earlier workers with the instrument [he mentions Burdon-Sanderson and Mahomed] . . . published excellent

---

[66] N. H. Naqvi and M. D. Blaufox, *Blood Pressure Measurement: An Illustrated History* (New York: Parthenon Publishing Group, 1998), 57–59, 67–68.

curves; then unfortunately books and papers [by others] . . . were furnished with tracings, some new, many of them hackneyed clichés, not a few of which were unskilful merely as tracings; while many other showed a want of appreciation of the limits and capacities of the sphygmograph itself. Too often the observer had taken pains to read into its records what the instrument was incapable of describing; or had interpreted as physiological, features due only to its mishandling, its defaults, or its inertia. There is no such thing as "the normal pulse tracing" a good tracing implies not only a sensitive make of instrument, but also a sensitive manipulator. Many an amorphous tracing betrays to the reader that the instrument had not followed the artery; some of its finer waves were beyond the capacity of the instrument used, or of any instrument; or again beyond the user's dexterity. So we are treated to rows of comparatively structureless bumps.[67]

Allbutt had begun his own pulse and cardiac investigations with the sphygmograph:

> Until his sphygmomanometer was introduced by von Basch in 1887, my own work . . . was done entirely with Marey's sphygmograph and cardiograph. Invaluable as were the records of the sphygmograph in revealing the form and rhythm of the pulse, yet, after may attempts to adapt it to even approximate recording of blood pressures, we had to admit that for this purpose another kind of instrument would be required.[68]

Allbutt then turned to the von Basch and Potain devices until they were eclipsed by the arm cuff instruments. He was not satisfied with the Riva-Rocci prototype of the modern sphygomanometer and went on to use several other early models to measure blood pressure as accurately as possible.[69] In 1896, Allbutt coined the term "hyperpiesia" (*piesia*, Latin for pressure) for hypertension and eclipsed Mahomed as the "discoverer" of essential hypertension. "Today," conclude Cameron and Hicks in their biographical portrait of Mahomed, "Allbutt rightly is given credit for

---

[67] T. Clifford Allbutt, Diseases of the Arteries Including Angina Pectoris (London: Macmillan and Co., 1915), 58.
[68] Ibid., 57.
[69] Ibid., 84–85.

placing hypertension firmly center stage in human disease, but at the expense of occluding Mahomed's contribution in his writings."[70]

PICTURING CARDIAC ARRHYTHMIAS

Later in the century, physicians began to use the sphygmograph to study "ominous pulse irregularities"—the first efforts to clarify the vast and complex study of cardiac arrhythmias. Earlier physicians had remarked that the pulse was irregular but attempted no analysis. In 1879, a review article by McBride in the New York based *Archives of Medicine* mentioned the utility of the sphygmograph in counting extremely rapid pulses (he recorded a pulse as fast as 165 beats per minute; the currently accepted normal range is 60 to 100 per minute) and observed that in some conditions, "certain irregularities of the pulse-beat are observed, and these have often a certain rhythmical character, which is sometimes impossible to appreciate by touch. The sphygmograph, however, inscribes the beats in legible characters."[71]

In 1899, Steell devoted a chapter in his book, *Use of the Sphygmograph in Clinical Medicine*, to the application of the instrument to pulse irregularities. He described bigeminal and trigeminal pulses (two or three regular beats followed by an apparent "skip" or pause), as well as the chaotically disordered "*delirium cordis*" (the irregular pulse usually associated with atrial fibrillation and now characterized as "irregularly irregular" to distinguish it from patterned irregularities): "individual curves of most different type and magnitude being huddled together in the wildest disorder." He also observed that some apparently healthy individuals have "habitually irregular pulses." One particularly interesting series of tracings showed the highly irregular pulse associated with alcoholic heart disease (cardiomyopathy, referring to degeneration of the heart muscle), followed by a spontaneous reversion to a regular rate and rhythm and a subsequent episode of a regular but very rapid rate of 160 beats per minute (tachycardia).[72] Such arryhthmias would be more accurately characterized with the introduction of the electrocardiograph at the turn of the twentieth century.

---

[70] Cameron and Hicks, "Frederick Akbar Mahomed," 1503; Naqvi and Blaufox, *Blood Pressure Measurement*, 57–59.

[71] McBride, "Utility of the Sphygmograph," 193.

[72] Steell, *Use of the Sphygmograph*, 43–57, tracings from pages 52 and 53.

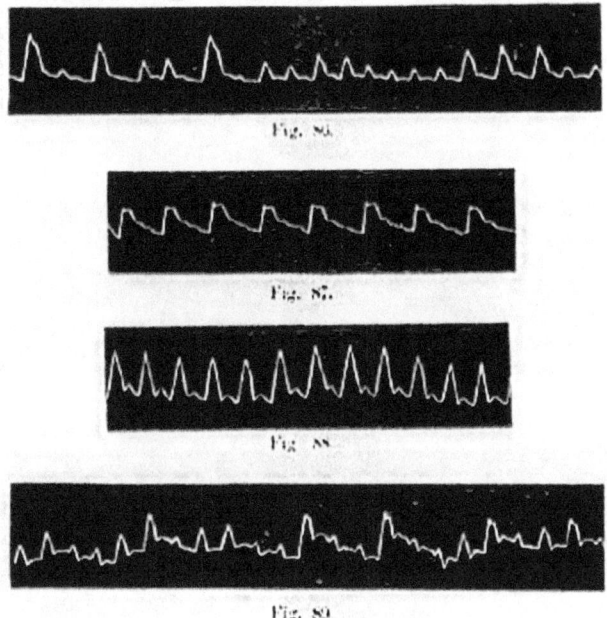

FIGURE 34: Serial tracings from a case of alcoholic cardiomyopathy (heart muscle deterioration) showing an irregularly irregular pulse probably atrial fibrillation (then called *delirium cordis*), followed by two tracings of a regular heart rate, the first showing high tension and the second showing low tension. The fourth tracing shows an irregularly irregular pulse in a patient with kidney disease. Graham Steell, *The Use of the Sphygmograph in Clinical Medicine* (Manchester: Sherratt & Hughes, 1899), 53.

MACKENZIE: THE POLYGRAPH

The confusion about arrhythmias in the decades prior to the introduction of the electrocardiograph was partly resolved by the brilliant investigations of James Mackenzie—"pioneer in the graphic study of cardiac arrhythmias," a graduate of Edinburgh, the leading British clinical cardiologist of his day, and the author of a "sterling" book on the pulse. He began his work with the sphygmograph while still in general practice, studying the irregular rhythms associated with heart failure in pregnant women. Surprisingly, Mackenzie, a native Scot, was not a consultant associated with a prestigious hospital during two and half decades of work with the sphygmograph and later the polygraph. In the introduction to his important work, *The Study of the Pulse* (1902), he commented that his research, often interrupted, was conducted and the book written "amid the distractions of the life of a busy general practitioner." After thirty years as a general practitioner in Lancashire, Mackenzie came to London as a consultant in 1907.[73]

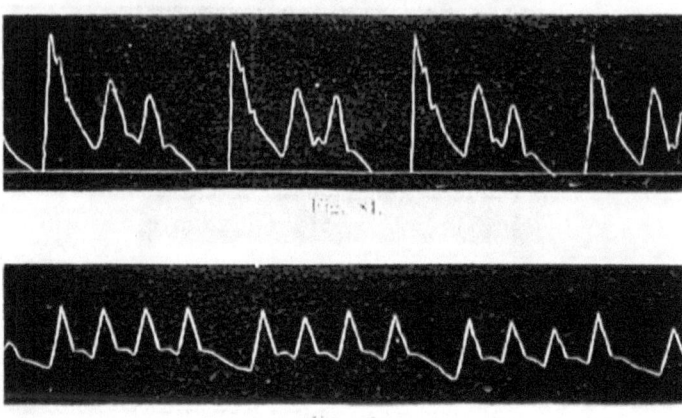

FIGURE 35: Patterned pulse irregularity (regularly irregular), showing three regular beats followed by a dropped beat (trigeminy) and four regular beats followed by a dropped beat (85). More precise characterization of such pulses would be possible with the electrocardiogram introduced some years later. Graham Steell, *The Use of the Sphygmograph in Clinical Medicine* (Manchester: Sherratt & Hughes, 1899), 52.

Mackenzie wrote in 1902: "It is now the fashion to decry the value of the sphygmograph. . . . In my opinion the instrument has never yet had a fair chance. It was expected to give information of a kind that it was incapable of displaying." In fact, Mackenzie, far from relegating the sphygmograph to the physiology laboratory, set out to demonstrate the usefulness of the instrument in general practice.[74]

Mackenzie's seminal contribution was his study of the venous pulse waves in the neck (a window into the function of the right side of the heart) simultaneously with the standard sphygmographic arterial waves (an indication of left-sided cardiac function). He designed two

---

[73] Fielding H. Garrison, *An Introduction to the History of Medicine*, 4th ed. (Philadelphia: W.B. Saunders, 1929), 687–88; James Mackenzie, *The Study of the Pulse: Arterial Venous and Hepatic, and of the Movements of the Heart*, (Edinburgh and London: Young J. Pentland, 1902), x.

[74] Mackenzie, *Study of the Pulse*, ix.

instruments to expand the reach of the sphygmograph, which could only record arterial and cardiac (more specifically left ventricular) waves: the polygraph and the "clinical polygraph." An existing instrument (Knoll's polygraph)—a device for recording multiple physiological events simultaneously— proved to be "elaborate and bulky" as well as "unwieldy."[75] In the early 1890s, Mackenzie designed his more convenient clinical polygraph, which incorporated a Dudgeon-style sphymgograph (see Chapter 7) along with a small cup-shaped sensor for recording the pulsations of the veins in the neck (pulsations over the liver similarly reflected right heart function).

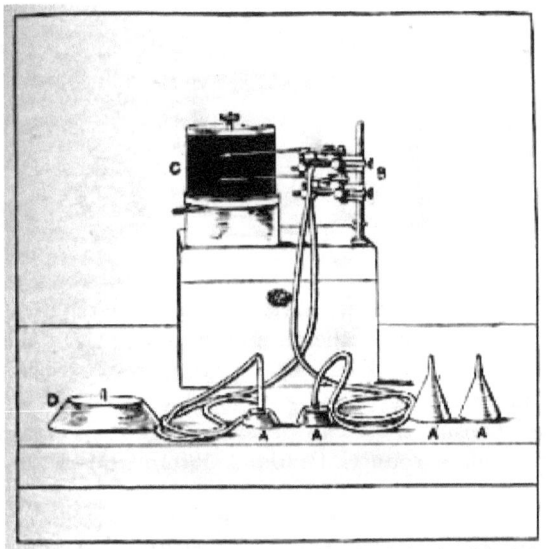

FIGURE 36: Knoll's polygraph used by Mackenzie. Several "receivers" allow simultaneous recordings of arterial, cardiac, and venous pulses. The sensor (D) at left is used to record liver pulsations, a reflection of venous blood return to the heart. James Mackenzie, *The Study of the Pulse: Arterial Venous and Hepatic, and of the Movements of the Heart*, (Edinburgh and London: Young J. Pentland, 1902), 9.

The receiver transmitted pulsations via a "tambour" (a drumhead-shaped apparatus such as that used by Marey to transmit movements to a recording device) to a recording stylus. Most importantly, the pulsations

---

[75] Ibid., 9–10.

of the artery (or cardiac apex) as detected by the sphygmograph could be recorded *simultaneously* with the venous pulsations (in the liver or neck veins), allowing Mackenzie to correlate events in the left side of the heart with events in the right side of the heart. The instrument was still fussy and somewhat idiosyncratic, but it opened up entirely new insights into the the cardiac cycle and the intricacies of the circulation.[76]

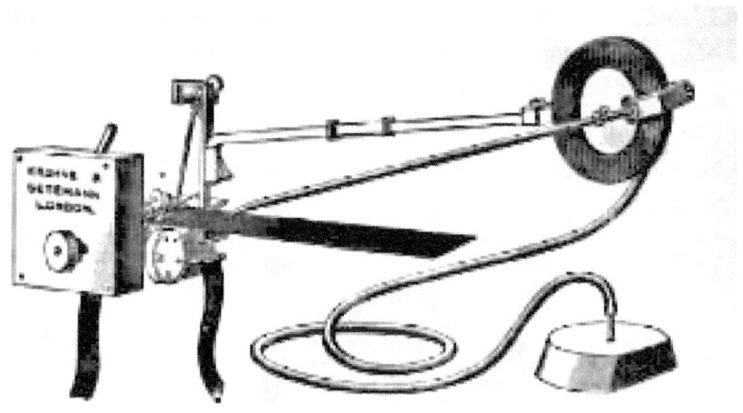

FIGURE 37: The portable Mackenzie clinical polygraph, which permitted multiple simultaneous tracings of the carotid artery, cardiac impulse, radial pulse, and venous pulses (jugular or liver). The sphygmograph at the left is a British Dudgeon model rather than a Marey type sphygmograph. James Mackenzie, *The Study of the Pulse: Arterial Venous and Hepatic, and of the Movements of the Heart*, (Edinburgh and London: Young J. Pentland, 1902), 10, 185.

The clinical polygraph led Mackenzie to a unique understanding of the previously obscure origin of cardiac arrhythmias and the nature of heart block (failures in the normal pacemaking functions of the heart), as well as a better understanding of the common clinical condition of heart failure. His 1902 book, *The Study of the Pulse*, and the 1919 *The Future of Medicine*, detail these important investigations with many illustrative paired recordings. His careful analysis of the venous pulse in the neck, with its multiple waves (atrial or "a" wave, ventricular or "v" wave, and carotid or "c" wave —visible to the acute observer as the "dancing" venous pulses in the neck)—not only guided the interpretation of his paired recordings, but also taught clinicians how to glean valuable information from a careful

---

[76] Ibid., 9–15.

bedside visual examination of the neck veins.⁷⁷ Though often neglected today, the astute clinician can still glean useful information from a visual examination of neck veins.

The neglect of cardiac arrhythmias by nineteenth-century sphygmographers was largely due to the brief duration of the recording made by available sphygmographs—often no more than a dozen beats. Mackenzie recognized, as had others before him, that the study of cardiac arrhythmias required tracings of longer duration. To overcome the problem of a flat recording surface limited to a few inches (and therefore a few pulse cycles), he devised his "ink polygraph" in 1906, in which a roll of recording paper allowed tracings of over an hour.⁷⁸

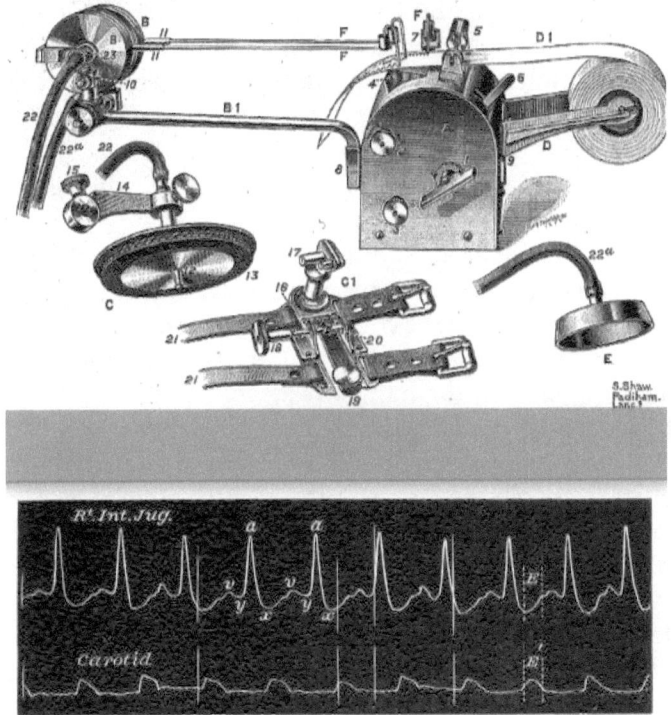

FIGURE 38: Mackenzie's ink polygraph, which enabled him to record long tracings vital to the elucidation of cardiac arrhythmias (the portable sphygmographs using smoked glass or paper mounted on a frame generally

---

⁷⁷ Ibid., chapters 16 to 31; James Mackenzie, *The Future of Medicine* (London: Oxford University Press, 1919), 82–100.

⁷⁸ Alex Mair, *Sir James Mackenzie, M.D., 1853–1925: General Practitioner* (Edinburgh: Churchill Livingstone, 1973), 92–95; Mackenzie, *Future of Medicine*, 91–94.

recorded about 10 seconds of pulse beats). Note the long roll of recording paper at the top right and the paired recording pens at the end of twin levers F. Wellcome Images, Wikimedia Commons, https://commons.wikimedia.org/wiki/File:The_Ink_polygraph_Wellcome_L0004447.jpg (accessed 14 January 2017). Simultaneous tracings of the jugular (venous) and radial (arterial) pulses correlating right and left heart activity. James Mackenzie, *The Study of the Pulse: Arterial Venous and Hepatic, and of the Movements of the Heart*, (Edinburgh and London: Young J. Pentland, 1902), 185.

WITHERING, MACKENZIE, AND FOXGLOVE

Among the uses to which Mackenzie profitably applied his polygraph was the study of the action of digitalis (derived from foxglove) upon the heart. Introduced in the late-eighteenth century by the observant William Withering of Birmingham, digitalis had been used, overused, and misused for more than a century to treat congestive heart failure and atrial fibrillation, along with a host of other cardiac as well as non-cardiac conditions. Withering himself had discovered its value in congestive heart failure and its ability to slow the heart rate, a potentially dangerous side effect (Chapter 1).

Mackenzie contributed significantly to the understanding of the complex actions of digitalis in various forms of heart disease, although much work remained to be done in the course of the twentieth century. Mackenzie wrote, "By the use of this instrument [i.e., the Mackenzie polygraph] the action of digitalis on the human heart was studied for the first time with accuracy, and its methods of use intelligently described."[79] Although much of Mackenzie's work would be corrected and revised by others using newer medical technologies, he made a key contribution to modern clinical pharmacology and cardiology. "None of these shortcomings," writes a modern historian of Withering and digitalis, "should hide the fact that it was through the agency of Mackenzie that the modern use of digitalis in treating fast atrial fibrillation was established."[80]

It is important to stress that the polygraph, as applied by Mackenzie and those who used the instrument over the next two decades, was not a mere extension of work done with the sphygmograph. Early sphygmograph men sought insights into "the state of the circulation," a broad and poorly defined concept. Mahomed and Mackenzie asked narrower and more specific questions. They were rewarded with valuable insights into

---

[79] Mackenzie, *Future of Medicine*, 88–89.

[80] J. K. Aronson, *An Account of the Foxglove and Its Medical Uses, 1785-1985* (London: Oxford University Press, 1985), 327–30.

cardiovascular physiology. In Mackenzie's hands, the sphygmograph/polygraph revolutionized clinical medicine and ushered in modern clinical cardiology.

MACKENZIE: TOO MUCH TECHNOLOGY?

Early sphygmographers, following the lead of Burdon-Sanderson, warned against overdependence on the sphygmograph because its messages were confusing and inconclusive. Later, Mackenzie cautioned against a similar overreliance on the polygraph, not because its messages were confusing and inconclusive, but because it dulled the senses of the physician and threatened to replace clinical judgment. At the end of his career, having retired to his native Scotland, Mackenzie, a clinician first and foremost, reflected on the place of the polygraph in British medical practice. "This instrument," wrote Mackenzie, "is useful mainly in research work. For routine practice no instrument is necessary, and as soon as I had found out the knowledge it could convey, I set about discovering means by which the information could be obtained by the unaided senses."[81]

As the sphygmograph educated the palpating finger of the clinician at the bedside, the venous pulse wave recorder educated the eye. Once Mackenzie had used his polygraph to "decode" the venous pulse, any well-instructed clinician could learn to interpret the venous pulsations in the neck by intelligent and informed observation. (In fact, "reading" the venous pulse in the neck, especially in the presence of a rapid pulse, is far from simple; today, few physicians claim much skill in this area of physical diagnosis.) Too much technology, warned Mackenzie, can lead the clinician astray and even cause harm to the patient: "In the employment of laboratory methods [including diagnostic instruments], so much attention is given to the results of the instrument that the patient is often ignored." His words, written in 1919, continue to resonate a century later.

Returning to the very foundations of clinical cardiology, Mackenzie placed the practitioner and the patient—the finger on the pulse—at the center of medical practice: "The *tactus eruditus* [learned touch of the physician's finger on the pulse] is no fanciful idea, but a factor of importance in the perfecting of that necessary instrument to clinical medicine—the trained physician."[82]

---

[81] Mackenzie, *Future of Medicine*, 94–95.
[82] Ibid., 183, 185.

Within Mackenzie's lifetime, it would become clear that instruments such as the electrocardiograph, x-ray machine, and the sphygmomanometer could yield information that no amount of clinical sophistication could elicit by physical examination. The paradigmatic problem in the twentieth century is not the reliance on technology as Mackenzie saw it, but rather the shift of emphasis from the traditional balanced triad of physician, patient, and disease toward a tetrad in which technology, in an almost deterministic fashion, seems to define the disease and dictate the actions of the physician and the responses of the patient.

Chapter 4

"Sphygmographic Hieroglyphics": The Amateur Science of Edgar Holden

Physiological research in America had its intellectual and methodological origins in the academic centers, research institutes, and great hospitals of Europe. But the project, amorphous and halting in the ante-bellum years, had a distinctly American trajectory. Also important was an American tradition of amateur research—that is, research conducted in private settings, supported by private funds, and undertaken in private time stolen from medical practice.

The systematic gastric physiology experiments of army surgeon William Beaumont (1825–1833) and the far more slapdash trials of etherization by a pair of New England dentists (mid-1840s) were distinctly American ventures and models for future amateur medical scientific research. Between 1825 and 1833, Beaumont conducted elegant experiments in digestion. It is difficult to imagine a more quintessentially American researcher than the apprentice-trained Beaumont, a military surgeon's mate during the War of 1812 and a failed grocer/druggist, who spent his productive years as an army surgeon at remote frontier posts in Michigan and Missouri.

His experimental subject, Alexis St. Martin, was a hardy voyageur with a fortuitous (for Beaumont) gastrocutaneous fistula caused by a gunshot wound, through which Beaumont could sample gastric juices. What is less well known is that Beaumont tried mightily to interest Americans in his book, *Experiments and Observations on the Gastric Juice and the Physiology of Digestion* (1833). Given the state of American medicine in the 1830s, his failure was inevitable. Europeans, however, responded enthusiastically with publications by and about Beaumont in British and Continental journals.[1] Although Beaumont was not part of the broader institutional growth of American physiology that began in the late 1850s, he was a prime example of a Yankee who was ingenious, resourceful, shamelessly self-promoting, and not at all intimidated by the mystique of European medical institutions. Four decades later, innovative Americans did indeed exemplify the amateur science of men like Beaumont in their novel experiments with the sphygmograph.

Edgar Holden, a young Newark practitioner, was among the country's first students of the sphygmograph and the first to use a modified Marey sphygmograph to conduct laboratory and clinical research. Holden exemplified the amateur science that constituted American medical research in the nineteenth century. Not only was he outside the European sphere, but he was also outside the new American scientific elite. Within a matter of a few years in the 1870s, Holden embraced the European literature on the sphygmograph, conducted novel physiologic and pharmacologic experiments with his own modification of the Marey instrument, won a major prize for his work, published an impressive monograph, and ultimately became disillusioned with the once-promising new technology. Holden, America's first "sphygmograph man," offered an explicit, albeit minor and little-heeded, challenge to the self-confident European hegemony in scientific medicine.

PHYSIOLOGICAL RESEARCH IN AMERICA: THE EUROPEAN CONNECTION:

Between 1815 and the 1850s, at least one thousand Americans studied or observed, for varying periods of time, medical practice and research in Paris.[2] The attraction and influence of Parisian physiologist Claude Bernard—and of Paris as a destination for American medical graduates —was beginning to fade by the 1860s. In 1869, American Henry Bowditch, the future Harvard physiologist and reformer of education in the basic medical sciences, found Bernard's laboratory poorly equipped and

---

[1] Estelle Brodman, "William Beaumont and the Transfer of Biomedical Information," *Federation Proceedings* (Federation of the American Societies of Experimental Biology) 44 (1985): 9–17.

[2] John Harley Warner, *Against the Spirit of System: The French Impulse in Nineteenth-Century American Medicine* (Princeton: Princeton University Press, 1998), 3.

lacking in facilities for the instruction of students. He wrote to his mentor, European trained anatomist and physiologist Jeffries Wyman, "The want of a good laboratory for practical instruction in physiology is seriously felt in Paris. The Frenchmen acknowledge the great advantage the Germans have over them in this respect."[3]

In the field of physiology, the dominant influence on American students after the Civil War was the German system of laboratory research and teaching epitomized by Carl Ludwig in Liepzig. Bowditch continued his studies under Ludwig, an inspiring role model and the undisputed leader in experimental physiology in the 1860s and 1870s.[4] Ludwig's physiology laboratory became the training ground for young men from abroad, nurturing them in the unfamiliar process of scientific research and encouraging mutual support—"a little world unto itself." In Ludwig's laboratory, workers were regularly exposed to new instruments such as the sphygmograph and learned where to seek out the best makers and suppliers.[5]

It is estimated that some fifteen thousand Americans studied in Germany, Austria, or Switzerland in the four decades after 1870. Many of these already held American degrees and sought post-graduate training abroad. Most were attracted to clinical rather than laboratory courses of study, but it seems likely that all became attuned to some degree to the important role of the laboratory in medical education and the rising importance of the laboratory as a source of authority in medicine.

Among those who pursued laboratory study were men like William Welch and other future founders of academic medicine and the basic sciences in United States medical colleges.[6] These men returned to the United States with what historian of American medical education Kenneth Ludmerer terms a "new world view ... intellectually and temperamentally at odds with ... the elite, French-trained physicians of the older generation."[7]

---

[3] Letter from Bowditch to Jeffries Wyman, 1869; cited in W. Bruce Fye, *Development of American Physiology: Scientific Medicine in the Nineteenth Century* (Baltimore: Johns Hopkins University Press, 1987), 96; 255, footnote 16.

[4] Ibid., 307.

[5] Robert G. Frank Jr., "American Physiologists in German Laboratories, 1865–1914," in *Physiology in the American Context, 1850–1940*, ed. Gerald L. Geison (Bethesda: American Physiological Society, 1987), 35–36, 39. Fye, *Development of American Physiology*, 102.

[6] Thomas Neville Bonner, *American Doctors and German Universities: A Chapter in International Intellectual Relations, 1870-1914* (Lincoln, NE: University of Nebraska Press, 1953), 23–24.

[7] Kenneth M. Ludmerer, *Learning to Heal: The Development of American Medical Education* (Baltimore: Johns Hopkins University Press, 1985), 35.

American physicians challenged French empiricism and the cachet of experience by promoting the authority of the laboratory and enthusiastically embracing new technologies.

At mid-century, the medical research environment in America was but dimly discernable. The relation of early American physiologists to nascent academic, scientific, and medical institutions was tenuous. Both John Call Dalton, professor of physiology at the Columbia College of Physicians and Surgeons, and Bowditch at Harvard Medical School self-consciously sought to insert their European training in physiology into an academic setting that was yet to coalesce.[8] At mid-century, gifted university administrators, generous philanthropists, and forward-looking physicians had not yet embarked on what would prove to be a revolutionary movement to amalgamate research programs, medical schools, and hospitals into a system of medical education that would surpass European systems in the wake of World War I. In 1910, the Flexner report (*Medical Education in the United States and Canada: A Report to the Carnegie Foundation for the Advancement of Teaching*) codified and publicized this maturing process.

RESEARCH IN THE AMERICAN MEDICAL COLLEGE

For ante-bellum American physicians, research was not a component of medical education; most instructors and students considered research irrelevant to the practical medical needs of a growing nation. Dalton, who was appointed professor of physiology at New York's College of Physicians and Surgeons in 1855, had been inspired by the lectures and demonstrations by Bernard in Paris. In a memorial address for Dalton, S. Weir Mitchell, a Philadelphia medical graduate who briefly studied physiology in France in the early 1850s, captured with a simile the essence of the typical pre-Dalton physiology lecture: "A physiological lecture was in that day a more or less well stated resume of the best foreign books, without experiments or striking illustrations. It was like hearing about a foreign land into which we were forbidden to enter."[9]

---

[8] See especially Fye, *Development of American Physiology*: Chapter 1, "John Call Dalton, Jr.: Pioneer Vivisector and America's 'First Professional Physiologist,'" 15–53 and Chapter 3, "Henry P. Bowditch: The Prototypical Full-Time Physiologist and Educational Reformer," 92–128.

[9] S. Weir Mitchell, "Memoir of John Call Dalton, 1825–1889: Read before the National Academy, April 16, 1890," *Biographical Memoirs of the National Academy of Sciences* 3

Even under Dalton's enlightened mid-century approach to teaching physiology, students at Columbia would not have access to modest laboratory facilities until the late 1870s. Participation in research by students and hands-on experience in the physiology laboratory was not possible without major endowments, a process which began in the 1880s. Students did, however, witness vivisection demonstrations conducted before the class by Dalton.[10] Research oriented physiology instructors such as Dalton were paid to teach. Dalton conducted his own productive physiological research privately, at his personal expense, although he was granted the use of a small room at the College.[11]

PRIVATE RESEARCHERS OUTSIDE ESTABLISHED MEDICAL COLLEGES

Men outside academic settings also conducted private research in physiology. Mitchell in Philadelphia, for example, taught at a private extramural medical school and later established his own laboratory at the Philadelphia School of Anatomy in the mid-1850s.[12] Although forced to support his family by wearying medical practice, Mitchell had the advantage of an established institutional structure in Philadelphia and the support of like-minded colleagues in institutions such as the Academy of Natural Sciences of Philadelphia and the Philadelphia Biological Society.

Like his friend Mitchell, William Hammond, a graduate of New York's University Medical College (1848) with post-graduate work at the Pennsylvania Medical College in Philadelphia, enjoyed a supportive environment that was academic in its outlook, if not as prestigious and institutionalized as that in major European cities. Hammond was an army surgeon and avid amateur physiologist who had conducted private physiological research while serving at remote military posts. Like Mitchell, he was active in the scientific societies of Philadelphia in the late 1850s. Hammond's hopes for the professorship of anatomy and physiology at the University of Maryland evaporated in 1859, and he resumed his military

---

(1890): 179.

[10] Fye, *Development of American Physiology*, 47, 112–4; Sandra W. Moss, *Edgar Holden, M.D., of Newark, New Jersey: Provincial Physician on a National Stage* (Xlibris, 2014), 61–63.

[11] Fye, *Development of American Physiology*, 5, 28–29.

[12] Ibid., 57–58.

career.[13] As discussed in a later chapter, Hammond is known to have bought a sphygmograph in Paris in 1865, returning with it to the United States in 1866.[14]

"YANKEE INGENUITY" AND THE AMERICAN SPHYGMOGRAPH MEN

In contrast to Hammond and Mitchell, there is a sense of "Yankee ingenuity" about the technical and scientific endeavors of Holden and two other American sphygmograph men who lacked the collegial advantages of major cities such as Philadelphia. (see Chapters 5 and 6)

Knowledge of the sphygmograph entered American consciousness through European journals and monographs. A report in the *Medical Record* (New York) for 1866–67, under the heading "New Instruments," quoted portions of an article about M(onsieur) Marey's "contrivance" (i.e., the sphygmograph) from the *Dublin Quarterly Journal of Medicine*.[15] The instrument itself entered the country in the hands of returning American medical graduates, traveling friends of curious American practitioners, and quite likely through orders submitted to European instrument makers.

While most interested Americans were content to use such imported instruments (and imported guidelines for interpretation), a handful of Americans considered themselves equal to the task of improving upon European designs and methods. It is these latter innovators who are referred to here as the "American sphygmograph men." Users of instruments purchased through instrument supply houses are referred to simply as sphygmographers. Unlike many of their contemporaries who would later play key roles in founding and developing the medical sciences in America, none of the three American sphygmograph men whose work is described in this and the following two chapters studied formally or systematically in Europe and indeed there is no evidence that any of them visited Germany

---

[13] Bonnie E. Blustein, *Preserve Your Love for Science: Life of William A. Hammond, American Neurologist* (Cambridge, MA: Cambridge University Press, 1991), 38–50. Hammond was Surgeon General at the outset of the Civil War and suffered through a vindictive court-martial in 1864. He later had a distinguished career as a neurologist in New York.

[14] William A. Hammond, "The Sphygmograph as an Instrument of Precision (With Apologies to Dr. Leonhardt)," *New York Medical Journal* 58 (1893): 588.

[15] "New Instruments: The Sphygmograph," *Medical Record* (New York) 1 (1866–1867): 580–81.

or the leading European sphygmograph men in France or Britain. Thus, they had no opportunity to benefit from the well-equipped laboratories of Europe, where they would have encountered sophisticated apparatus and training in laboratory techniques.

THE SOUND AND LIGHT SHOW OF J. B. UPHAM OF BOSTON

The sphygmograph touched the United States lightly in the 1860s and 1870s. An unnamed contributor to the *Boston Medical and Surgical Journal* declared in 1867: "Like the laryngoscope, it is comparatively of recent origin, and can hardly as yet be said to have been introduced to any considerable extent (in this country at all events) into practical use by the profession."[16]

The sphygmograph may have been introduced in America as early as 1865. J. B. Upham of Boston, visiting physician to Boston City Hospital, first exhibited a Marey sphygmograph to the Boston Society for Medical Improvement in December of that year. Upham described the instrument and its application to the "diagnosis of obscure diseases affecting the arterial system, illustrating the point by reference to a series of original observations in his practice at the City Hospital." At subsequent meetings between 1866 and 1867, Upham showed original tracings taken from patients with a wide variety of cardiac and non-cardiac disorders, and, in some cases, verified his findings at autopsy. Among his cardiovascular cases were thoracic aortic aneurysms and abnormalities of the aortic and mitral valves. Like many sphygmographers, he took pulse tracings in febrile illnesses such as typhoid, typhus, and pneumonia, seeking characteristic pulses to aid in diagnosis. An observer remarked in the *Boston Medical and Surgical Journal* that Upham's sphygmograms, "by their manifest and marked variation from the healthy pulse-form, and from each other, show the exceeding delicacy of the instrument, and its power, with patient manipulation, to do all that Marey and his zealous co-workers have claimed for it."[17]

---

[16] "Some Further Improvements in Medical Science," *Boston Medical and Surgical Journal* 76 (1867): 359.

[17] Ibid., 359.

Upham seems to have been something of a showman. At an 1869 meeting of the American Association for the Advancement of Science in Salem, Upham produced a cardiac light show. It is not clear how the sphygmograph was involved in the chain of "translations" from the heartbeats of patients (in Boston) through telegraph wires to an audience some miles distant in Salem, but a report of this demonstration, entitled "Sphygmography by Telegraph," in the *British Medical Journal* suggests that the actual wavy sphygmogram patterns were transmitted. However, given the technology of the day, the transmission was limited to a visible pulse "flash."[18] The audience was impressed and the demonstration reached beyond the medical literature to be reported in *Scientific American*:

> At the conclusion of his lecture [on the action of the heart], Dr. Upham gave some remarkable experiments. The beatings of the hearts of several of the physicians and patients of the City Hospital, in Boston, were automatically transmitted by telegraph from the hospital to the hall in Salem [about fourteen miles distant]. By means of the magnesium light these pulsations were made to manifest themselves to the sight by the vibration of a beam of light on the wall of the darkened room [in Salem]. A regular pulse of 60 per minute was first sent. Then was transmitted the healthy pulse of an excited person, regular, but having a rapidity of 90 per minute. But the most interesting cases were those of a patient suffering from pneumonia, whose pulsations numbered 118 per minute, and that of another afflicted with organic disease of the heart. The irregularity of the beats in this latter case was vividly impressed on the mind by the sounds of the instrument. Prof. Farmer, the well-known electrician, assisted by a skillful operator from Boston, had charge of the electical arrangements in Salem. Dr. Knight was in charge at the hospital in Boston. The Franklin Telegraph, too, gave the free use of their lines for the experiments, which were successful to a degree even surpassing the anticipations of Dr. Upham.[19]

Clearly, Upham was pushing the concept of "translation" to the limits of available technology, both through the recording of sphygmographic waves and their graphic presentation, to an audience remote in time and

---

[18] "Sphygmography by Telegraph," *British Medical Journal* 2 (1869): 355–56.
[19] "The Science Association," *Scientific American* n.s. 21 (1869): 162.

place from the patient and through projection of real time and visual pulse transmission to a distant audience (as described in the *Scientific American* report). His experiments in this latter direction presage our modern beeping cardiac monitors with readouts of pulse waves and an instantly calculated pulse rate.

EARLY AMERICAN EXPERIENCE WITH THE SPHYGMOGRAPH

A few forward looking and intellectually curious physicians acquired sphygmographs by the late 1860s and used them in a variety of settings. An early application of the sphygmograph to medical teaching in America was announced in 1868 at the meeting of the Middlesex South District Medical Society (Massachusetts) in October 1868. Jeffries Wyman, professor of anatomy at Harvard College, "exhibited a model of a sphygmograph, modified for the lecture room by a combination of levers, which greatly increases the sweep of the index."[20] Wyman's use of a wide-swinging amplified recording arm indicates his interest in using the sphygmograph to teach cardiac physiology; it is unlikely that he was attempting to teach students how to use the device in their future practices.

In 1868, Samuel B. Ward of New York read a paper before the New York Medical Journal Association about his experience with "Marey's Improved Sphygmograph." His published address featured several original tracings, including a tracing of his own arteries, and several tracings credited to Marey. Ward was impressed by the work of a physician in Dublin who had made over three thousand tracings and claimed to have identified the sphygmographic signs of convalescence in typhus.[21]

By 1869, and probably some years earlier, Dalton at the College of Physicians and Surgeons was using a sphygmograph. In an article on the circulation published by the popular magazine *The Galaxy*, Dalton invoked a comparison to the microscope, a medical device with which he was intimately familiar:

> An instrument has been contrived within a few years, by which some of these peculiarities of the pulse may be indicated with

---

[20] Charles E. Vaughan, "Middlesex South District Medical Society, October 14, 1868," *Boston Medical and Surgical Journal* 79 (1869): 233.

[21] Samuel B. Ward, "The Sphygmograph, and Some of Its Uses," *Medical Record* (New York) 3 (1868–69): 385–89.

rather more delicacy than it is possible to perceive them by the finger, and by which they may, at the same time, be registered for future examination. . . . The index [the inscribing arm] is thus made to oscillate upon its hinge with a movement which translates, as it were, and at the same time magnifies the peculiarities of the arterial pulsations. It serves in this way as a kind of microscope, to make minute variations in the size of the artery readily appreciable by the eye.

In language aimed at a general audience, Dalton proceeded to describe the sphygmograph (probably a Marey instrument). He used a modified Ludwig kymograph to record the pulse tracing. This gave him a thirty-second tracing (about forty heartbeats) rather than the six or so seconds that the portable Marey sphygmograph recorded on a short strip of smoked glass or paper.

Now for the registering apparatus. At the other end of the brass frame is a cylinder about two inches in diameter, which is made to revolve, at will, by clockwork, finishing one complete revolution in exactly thirty seconds. Upon this cylinder is fastened a paper or cardboard of the proper width, with its surface covered by a coating of lampblack. Everything being in readiness, the apparatus fastened in its place, and the clockwork wound up, the operator sets it in motion by touching a small knob on the top of the cylinder. As the cylinder revolves, the point of the index, pressing gently against its sides, traces on the blackened surface of the paper a white line, whose curves and oscillations faithfully portray every peculiarity of the arterial pulsation. The revolution of the cylinder completed, the paper is removed, and this becomes a permanent register, not only of the exact number of pulsations during an interval of thirty seconds, but also of their extent, their regularity, and various other qualities.[22]

In all likelihood, Dalton recorded animal pulses in his laboratory, as he was not a clinician with access to patients; or perhaps he recruited student volunteers. Dalton's article in *The Galaxy* was quite possibly the first instance in which the *méthode graphique* was laid before a wide non-medical audience in the United States.

---

[22] John Call Dalton, "How the Blood Circulates," *The Galaxy* 8 (1869): 673–74.

By 1870, a sphygmograph, probably the Marey model, was in use at the Pennsylvania Hospital in Philadelphia. Jacob Mendes DaCosta, a leading diagnostician, used the sphygmograph to study a cardiac patient with an alarming reaction to chloral hydrate, a newly introduced sedative. DaCosta used serial sphygmographic tracings (reproduced in his published article) to determine when the patient could safely receive a second dose of the drug. [23]

In the 1873 edition of his comprehensive textbook of medicine, distinguished American professor and diagnostician Austin Flint Sr. gave a lengthy discussion of Marey's sphygmograph, describing it as "an instrument ingeniously contrived to represent to the eye the movements of the pulse." Stopping short of recommending its use in clinical practice, Flint concluded, "The sphygmograph has undoubtedly enlarged our resources for obtaining data for diagnosis and prognosis."[24]

It seems evident, then, that some American physicians—the intellectual elites with an interest in physiology in major cities such as New York, Philadelphia, and Boston—enthusiastically embraced the sphygmograph and the graphic method, at least for a short time. Like the early British sphygmographers, they sought to inform their colleagues of the new technology and struggled to define its place in medical practice.

EDGAR HOLDEN: FIRST AMERICAN SPHYGMOGRAPH MAN

The balance of the present chapter concerns Edgar Holden of Newark, New Jersey, America's first sphygmograph man and the first American to conduct systematic research with the sphygmograph. Holden's encounter with the sphygmograph illustrates the amateur and isolated nature of medical research in America and the reliance of intellectually active American physicians on British and European authority in medical science. Holden's initial enthusiasm, intense experimentation (including pharmacologic trials), and ultimate disillusionment mirror the experience of Burdon-Sanderson and his contemporaries in Britain. Holden was

---

[23] Jacob M. DaCosta, "Clinical Notes on Chloral," *American Journal of the Medical Sciences* 59 (1870): 364.

[24] Austin Flint, Sr., *A Treatise on the Principles and Practice of Medicine; Designed for the Use of Practitioners and Students of Medicine*, 4th ed. (Philadelphia: Henry C. Lea, 1873), 114–17.

familiar with the work of Burdon-Sanderson and, quite likely, other British and Continental sphygmograph men.

In 1874, Holden published a lengthy monograph on the study of the pulse by means of his modified Marey sphygmograph. Although his investigations earned him a modest place—little more than a footnote—in medical history, his engagement with an instrument associated with the European academic elite marks him as an outstanding private researcher in post-bellum America. The nature of his experiments with the sphygmograph reveal much about Holden as a student of technology and, briefly, a physiologist. While he may not have articulated philosophical reflections on space and time, Holden grasped the possibilities of graphic representation of the pulse, anticipating that such "pulse writing" could impact diagnosis, prognosis, and therapy.

NEWARK: THE MEDICAL LANDSCAPE AT MID-CENTURY

In order to place Holden's research with the sphygmograph in perspective, it is helpful to begin with a brief description of medical practice and the post-Civil War research environment in New Jersey, and particularly Newark and surrounding Essex County. Medical historians, most notably Stephen Wickes, a nineteenth-century practitioner, and David Cowen, a modern historian, have written invaluable histories of medicine within the state.[25] However, regional and national historians of medicine have tended to ignore New Jersey, leaving the impression that there was nothing of importance between the Hudson River in the northeast and the Delaware River in the southwest.[26] Holden spent his distinguished and multifaceted career in this heretofore unremarked medical community.

---

[25] David L. Cowen, *Medicine and Health in New Jersey: A History* (Princeton: D. Van Nostrand, 1964); Cowen's scholarly history of New Jersey medicine, published in 1964, remains the best single volume work on the subject. Practitioner Stephen Wickes assembled and edited the records of the Medical Society of New Jersey from 1766 to 1858. In addition, he wrote an early history of New Jersey medicine. Stephen Wickes, *History of Medicine in New Jersey, and of Its Medical Men, From the Settlement of the Province to A.D. 1800* (Newark: Martin L. Dennis, 1879). See also Karen Reeds, *A State of Health: New Jersey's Medical Heritage* (New Brunswick, NJ: Rutgers University Press, 2001).

[26] New Jersey physicians are remembered, if at all, for forming the first colonial medical society (1766). A well-organized narrative history of the first two centuries of the Medical Society of New Jersey, based on published transactions and journals, is *The Healing Art*. Fred B. Rogers and A. Reasoner Sayre. *The Healing Art: A History of the*

"Sphygmographic Hieroglyphics": The Amateur Science of Edgar Holden

New Jersey's Essex County and its largest city, Newark, kept an eye turned to New York in all matters, medical and otherwise. Essex County, a growing urban industrial center with a rapidly expanding population, was home to a mature medical community with capable and relatively well-educated practitioners. Nevertheless, the absence of a medical school condemned Essex County (and New Jersey) to a provincial status in American medicine until the mid-twentieth century. For the intellectually curious practitioner, often a man with some European experience, medical authority originated in Britain and the Continent, and, increasingly, in New York and Philadelphia.[27] New Jersey was, with few exceptions, an importer of medical knowledge and medical trainees.

Many Essex County men received their diplomas from the College of Physicians and Surgeons in New York. A few studied at prestigious medical centers in Edinburgh, Paris, and later Germany. For example, Abraham Coles of Newark, a graduate of Jefferson Medical College in Philadelphia, traveled to Europe and "being in Paris during the bloody revolution of June, 1848, improved the frequent opportunities which he had, in hospitals and elsewhere, to add to his store of experience as a surgeon."[28] Edward Ill, son of a German immigrant physician, apprenticed in Newark with his father and graduated from the College of Physicians and Surgeons in 1875. After two years at medical schools in Germany and Austria he returned to Newark and became a well-regarded consultant in surgery, obstetrics, and gynecology.[29]

The post-bellum years were a time of renewed optimism in medicine. Surgery and its newly-emerging subspecialties were making steady gains. Although the new scientific medicine had yet to produce great advances in medical therapeutics, physicians were increasingly confident that the laboratories and great teaching hospitals of Europe would not fail them. The historian of the Essex District Medical Society, an older man in failing

---

Medical Society of New Jersey (Trenton: Medical Society of New Jersey, 1966).

[27] The early history of the Essex District Medical Society was published in 1867 by an older physician with deep roots in the medical community; J. Henry Clark, "The First Fifty Years of the District Medical Society of Essex County," *Transactions of the Medical Society of New Jersey* (1867): 77–181. A brief biography of Clark appears in William H. Shaw, comp., "The Medical Profession of Essex County," in *History of Essex and Hudson Counties, New Jersey* (Philadelphia: Everts & Peck, 1884), 311–12.

[28] Shaw, "Medical Profession of Essex County," 332. For a biography of Abraham Coles, see Fred B. Rogers, *Help Bringers: Versatile Physicians of New Jersey* (New York: Vantage Press, 1960), 72–80.

[29] Shaw, "Medical Profession of Essex County," 345; "Dr. Edward J. Ill (obituary)," *Journal of the Medical Society of New Jersey* 39 (1942): 402.

health, spoke in 1867 of a "golden age [of medicine] . . . all about us . . . in this day of wonderful expansion."[30]

EMBRACING THE NEW "INSTRUMENTS OF PRECISION"

In general, American physicians, while ever mindful of the art of medicine with its comfortable historical references, were proud of the technological progress represented by the accelerating parade of "scopes" for revealing and "graphs" for reading the hidden body. Carleton Chapman's *Order Out of Chaos: John Shaw Billings and America's Coming of Age* focuses on a physician whose professional life extended from the Civil War to the early twentieth century. Billings enjoyed a decent American medical education, found himself tested by the Civil War, and went on to become an authority on diverse medical endeavors that he helped define. Billing's multiple arenas included medical architecture, public health, medical education, and the methods of the medical archivist. His stage was national and his innovations were of lasting importance.[31] In 1881, Billings, as driving force behind the monumental *Index-Catalogue of the Library of the Surgeon-General's Office*, addressed an international medical congress on "Our Medical Literature," a subject on which he was uniquely qualified to comment. Billings welcomed the infusions of the physical sciences into medicine, especially in "increasing the delicacy and accuracy of measurements. . . . of expressing manifestations of force in terms of another force, or of dimension in space or time." He named the galvanometer, microscope, thermometer, and sphygmograph as prime contributors to the goal of establishing a permanent, objective medical record.[32]

In the decades that followed, New Jersey physicians, too, increasingly embraced new diagnostic technologies and were proud to list the many new "meters" and "scopes" that had become available. In 1883, John Snowden of Camden County, the outgoing president of the Medical Society of New Jersey, spoke on "The Advances Made in Medicine by Physical Diagnosis." Auscultation with the stethoscope remained the foundation

---

[30] Clark, "First Fifty Years," 178.
[31] Carleton B. Chapman, *Order Out of Chaos: John Shaw Billings and America's Coming of Age* (Boston: Boston Medical Library, 1994). The *Index Catalogue*, a landmark in medical information retrieval, was published volume by volume between 1880 and 1895.
[32] John S. Billings, "An Address on Our Medical Literature," *British Medical Journal* 2 (1881): 262–68.

of cardiopulmonary diagnosis. Snowden asked rhetorically, "How helpless would the diagnostician be without them?" By 1883, the thermometer was "recognized as an indispensable mechanical aid in the diagnosis of disease." Snowden went on to mention Hutchinson's spirometer (volume of inspired and expired air, see Chapter 1), the pneumatometer (force of inspiration and expiration), the phonometer (variant of percussion using a tuning fork), the stethometer (chest wall excursion), and the cyrtometer (dimensions of the chest). For cardiovascular diagnosis, he named the pulsuhr ("tension, fulness [sic] and volume of the pulse"), and the cardiometer (distance of the cardiac apex from the midline, an indication of heart size). Snowden then listed the various scopes and related diagnostic armamentarium: laryngoscope, rhinoscope, otoscope, acoumeter (a primitive audiometer), ophthalmoscope, radiometer or photometer (visual acuity), meatoscope (urethral examination), endoscope (specifically, the cystoscope to examine the bladder), *speculum vaginae* (vaginal speculum) and anal speculum. With improvements in illumination technology, instruments such as the esophagoscope and the gastroscope were entering practice. The "enteroscope," an early sigmoidoscope, had to date proved a failure. Neurologists employed the aesthesiometer to detect sensory impairment. The microscope had already proven its value in pathological diagnosis.

Snowden did not neglect his fellow New Jerseyan, Edgar Holden, loyally proclaiming the Holden sphygmograph, with which Snowden himself probably had little if any experience, "the most perfect instrument." He marveled at the rapidity with which such technology had been introduced. From this somewhat tedious catalogue of instruments, it is evident that the very promise of medical technology had enormous appeal to New Jersey physicians. For Snowden, who was sixty years old and nearing the end of his career, technology seemed to promise a magical future. He concluded his address with a hopeful vision: "Judging from the past, what must be the capacity of our noble profession a century hence, for the investigation and cure of disease?"[33]

IN THE SHADOW OF NEW YORK: DISPENSARIES AND HOSPITALS

Newark lagged far behind New York and Philadelphia in its medical institutions. Dispensaries and hospitals, which served as sites of informal

---

[33] John W. Snowden, "The Advances Made in Medicine by Physical Diagnosis," *Transactions of the Medical Society of New Jersey* (1883): 56–78 passim.

postgraduate education and embryonic specialization, came late to the area despite a rapidly growing immigrant and native-born population. New York, Philadelphia, Boston, and Baltimore had opened dispensaries by 1800. The Newark City Dispensary, staffed for limited hours by volunteer community physicians, opened in 1857.[34]

By mid-century, most large American cities found it necessary and desirable to build hospitals. Inspired by a sense of stewardship, prominent citizens saw the hospital as a place to care for the "deserving" sick poor, often recent immigrants who could not be expected to recover their health in squalid urban dwellings. In cities such as Boston, hospitals became a locus of prestigious volunteer practice for elite private physicians. Religious and ethnic groups founded hospitals for the care of their co-religionists or fellow immigrants. Physicians and their private patients increasingly saw well-equipped hospitals as symbols of medical progress and superior medical care.[35]

Newark's first hospital was a Civil War military hospital, opened in a converted warehouse near the Passaic River in 1862.[36] In 1863, a committee of the Medical Society huffed, "It is a shame to the State that, notwithstanding its wealth and resources, and its *needs*, it has not a [civilian] hospital within its borders."[37] In Newark, the almshouse bore the brunt of the municipal burden for chronic institutional care. In 1868, the dangerously overcrowded almshouse, with its population of sick poor

---

[34] Charles E. Rosenberg, "Social Class and Medical Care in Nineteenth-Century America: The Rise and Fall of the Dispensary," *Journal of the History of Medicine and Allied Sciences* 29 (1974): 33. The first dispensary was founded in Philadelphia in 1786, New York in 1791, Boston in 1796, and Baltimore in 1800. Newark Dispensary notice in *Newark Daily Advertiser*, 21 December 1857. Medical articles in the *Newark Daily Advertiser* extracted under the direction of Samuel Berg, a New Jersey physician. Berg's extracts, typed verbatim from the newspaper, are the only record of this publication known to exist. Samuel Berg, comp., *Medical Practice and Hospital Development in Newark, N.J., 1850–1887 as Reported in* Newark Daily Advertiser (ca. 1940), New Jersey Room, Newark Public Library.

[35] Morris J. Vogel, *The Invention of the Modern Hospital: Boston 1870-1930* (Chicago: University of Chicago Press, 1980), 2–3, 10–12, 97–110.

[36] The history of the Ward Hospital is taken in part from a series of articles written by a Newark physician who had worked at the hospital since its inception. The articles were unsigned. "History of the 'Ward' U.S.A. General Hospital," *Ward Hospital Bulletin*, 15 June 1865–10 August 1865. *The Ward Hospital Bulletin* published seven issues between June 1865 (two months after Appomattox) and August, 1865. For a modern history of the Ward Hospital, see Sandra W. Moss, "Newark's Civil War Hospital," *New Jersey Heritage Magazine* 2 (2004): 18–28.

[37] Stephen Wickes, Thos. Ryerson, and R. M. Cooper, "Report of the Standing Committee," *Transactions of the Medical Society of New Jersey* (1863): 35–36. I am indebted to Cowen, *Medicine and Health*, for drawing my attention to this report.

"huddled together in the rooms and halls," expanded to house three hundred residents.[38] Religious and ethnic groups were meeting some of the city's needs for hospital beds. In the late 1860s, St. Michael's Hospital (Catholic) and St. Barnabas Hospital (Episcopalian) opened in converted residences. The cohesive German-American community opened the Newark German Hospital in late 1870.[39] Finally, in September 1882, a twenty-five bed municipal hospital designed to "accommodate patients who can not be accommodated in the other hospitals" (i.e., the indigent poor) was opened in Newark in a new wing attached to, but administered separately from, the city almshouse.[40]

MEDICAL SCHOOLS IN NEW JERSEY, OR THE LACK THEREOF

Medical schools were far from prestigious institutions in nineteenth-century America. But by the turn of the twentieth century, research-minded physicians, as well as leading clinicians, would begin to coalesce around the better medical schools. In symbiotic relationships with major teaching hospitals and enlightened universities, American medical schools emerged from trade school status to respected institutions for education, research, and patient care.

Despite its venerable medical society (founded in 1766) and relatively well-trained graduates of schools such as the College of Physicians and Surgeons in New York, New Jersey had no medical school. There was, indeed, a puzzling lack of concern among physicians on this score, despite the fact that medical life in the shadows of New York City and Philadelphia occasionally rankled. By 1886, there were eight medical schools in New York City (regular. eclectic, and homeopathic) and four additional regular schools in upstate New York. Philadelphia had four regular schools and a homeopathic school by 1886. At that date, New Jersey claimed only two medical colleges, both "extinct": Livingston University in Haddonfield, a diploma mill, and the Hygeio-Therapeutic College in Bergen Heights. The Council on Medical Education and Hospital of the American Medical

---

[38] "The Newark City Almshouse—Description of the New Building," *Newark Daily Advertiser*, 15 July 1868.

[39] John T. Cunningham, *Clara Maass: A Nurse, A Hospital, A Spirit* (Cedar Grove, NJ: Rae Publishing, 1968), 15–24.

[40] "The Opening of the New City Hospital," *Newark Daily Advertiser*, 12 August 1882, 5 September 1882.

Association used the terms "fraudulent" and "charter revoked" for both these "schools," and added "mongrel institution" for the latter. By 1891, two additional equally unsavory schools, one "disreputable" and the other "fraudulent," had their charters revoked.[41] After the turn of the twentieth century, the top ranks of American medical schools would become centers for the promulgation of new medical knowledge generated in laboratories and at the bedside. New Jersey would not fully participate in this venture until the latter half of the twentieth century.

MEDICAL RESEARCH IN NEW JERSEY

For many American practitioners, medical research was characterized by such pursuits as the correlation of climatological and environmental observations with local patterns of illness. Though pedestrian and unoriginal, these activities satisfied the scientific curiosity of the more thoughtful physicians, fit in well with prevailing etiological theories, and helped organize the confusing array of diseases and symptoms that characterized general practice prior to the Civil War. In time, of course, the definition of what counted as scientific research would evolve.[42] In keeping with this view of scientific medicine, Essex County physicians avidly published details of the medical topography and climatology of their towns. Stephen Wickes studied the medical topography of Orange (near Newark in Essex County) in 1859, extolling the general healthfulness of the area.[43] The genre seemed inexhaustible; in 1887, the *Transactions of the Medical Society of New Jersey* published a tedious 160 page article, replete

---

[41] *Medical and Surgical Directory of the Unites States* (Detroit: R. L. Polk, 1886), 110–13, 116–17; Council on Medical Education and Hospitals (American Medical Association), *Medical Colleges of the United States and of Foreign Countries* (American Medical Association, 1918, reprinted from *American Medical Directory*, 6th ed., 1918), 12.

[42] For a study of New Jersey climatological research, see Sandra W. Moss, "The Doctor as Weatherman: Medical Topography in Nineteenth-Century New Jersey," *Journal of the Rutgers University Libraries* 62 (2006): 59–74. Medical historian Owsei Temkin suggested that what was "scientific" to a general practitioner would not be seen as "scientific" by a German-trained laboratory physiologist. What counts as "scientific medicine" changes not only with time, but also with the sensibilities and perceptions of the individual physician. Gerald L. Geison, "Divided We Stand: Physiologists and Clinicians in the American Context," in *The Therapeutic Revolution: Essays in the Social History of American Medicine*, ed. Morris J. Vogel and Charles E. Rosenberg (Philadelphia: University of Pennsylvania Press, 1979), 82.

[43] Stephen Wickes, "Medical Topography of Orange, N.J.," *Transactions of the Medical Society of New Jersey* (1859): 78–82.

with tables, on the year-by-year history of "The Climatology and Diseases of Essex County."⁴⁴

Nourishing a spirit of scientific inquiry was not the mandate of mid-century proprietary American medical schools.⁴⁵ Medical schools in America existed to turn out practitioners for a frontier nation. The American Medical Association lamented in 1858 that existing didactic physiology lecture courses in American schools, "so beautiful, so important," were beyond the comprehension of generally ill-prepared students.⁴⁶ Despite the qualms and anxieties of distinguished professors such as Oliver Wendell Holmes of Harvard, who cautioned students to steer clear of "dig[ging] in far-off fields for the hidden waters of alien sciences," forward-thinking physicians were acutely uncomfortable with the state of medical science in America.⁴⁷

Despite the absence of medical schools and teaching hospitals within the state, leading New Jersey physicians began to see themselves as participants in, or at least beneficiaries of, a new scientific medicine. In 1888, Ezra Mundy Hunt, a Middlesex county physician active in national and state public health circles, commented in response to a provocation: "There is no medical wilderness between New York and Philadelphia."⁴⁸ Was New Jersey a medical wilderness? The intellectual and research activities of New Jersey practitioners (all researchers were first and foremost practitioners) provide some answers to this question and frame the sphygmographic research efforts of Edgar Holden.

---

44 [Stephen Wickes?], "The Climatology and Diseases of Essex County," *Transactions of the Medical Society of New Jersey* (1887): 71–230. Sphygmograph researcher Edgar Holden supplied some of the data used in the preparation of this lengthy article, 230. The author of the unsigned article is most likely Stephen Wickes of Orange.

45 William G. Rothstein, *American Physicians in the 19th Century: From Sects to Science* (Baltimore: Johns Hopkins University Press, 1972), 102–4.

46 William Henry Anderson, "Report of the Committee on Education," *Transactions of the American Medical Association* 9 (1856): 559–60.

47 Charles R. Bardeen, "Oliver Wendell Holmes," in *A Cyclopedia of American Medical Biography*, ed. Howard A. Kelly (Philadelphia: W. B. Saunders, 1912), 1:420. Holmes also warned students not to be diverted by the "muddy sewer of politics" or the "enchanted streams of literature."

48 Ezra Mundy Hunt, "Origin of Disease and Micro-organisms as Related Thereto," *Transactions of the Medical Society of New Jersey* (1888): 110–12. Although unattributed by Hunt, the deprecating remarks were probably in response to comments made by Dowling Benjamin of Camden to the effect that there were only two physicians in New Jersey who accepted the germ theory in 1867. See Dowling Benjamin, "The Present Position of Antiseptic Practice," *Transactions of the Medical Society of New Jersey* (1887): 253.

NEW JERSEY'S CONTRIBUTIONS TO THE MEDICAL LITERATURE

New Jersey's medical literature remained strictly provincial. Joseph Parrish, a Philadelphian who practiced briefly in Burlington County, published *The New Jersey Medical Reporter* from 1847 until 1864, when it was reborn in Philadelphia as the far more prestigious *Medical and Surgical Reporter*. *The Country Practitioner* was edited and published in tiny Beverly, New Jersey, between 1879 and 1881 by Ellis P. Townsend, an ambitious local physician. Abstracts from other journals far outnumbered the modest original contributions. The editor saw his reader, the "country practitioner," as isolated from "the fraternity," a self reliant man, "fighting his way alone through emergencies that would cause some of the great medical luminaries to stagger in their traces." *The Country Practitioner* ceased publication when the editor moved to Camden, New Jersey and then on to Montana.[49]

The state's sole medical publication after 1859 was the annual *Transactions of the Medical Society of New Jersey*, a collection of unedited essays and case reports submitted through the county medical societies, as well as the transcripts of presidential addresses and other society business. "Reports of District Societies," the structural backbone of the *Transactions*, focused on medical conditions as encountered and managed by the physicians of each county. The emphasis in these reports was on personal experience and, by extension, personal authority. Scientific medicine was promoted in occasional articles by specialists such as A. Mead Edwards of Newark, whose expertise and skill were evident in "The Microscope in Gynecology."[50]

MEDICAL RESEARCH IN NEW JERSEY AT MID-CENTURY

A general idea of the state of medical research in the purported medical wilderness of New Jersey can be gained by scanning the *Transactions of the Medical Society of New Jersey* for evidence of original research.[51] The

---

[49] Ellis P. Townsend, "To Medical Practitioners," *The Country Practitioner* 1 (1879): 1–3; Sandra W. Moss, *The Country Practitioner: Ellis P. Townsend's Brave Little Medical Journal* (Xlibris, 2011).

[50] A. Mead Edwards, "The Microscope in Gynecology," *Transactions of the Medical Society of New Jersey* (1875): 140–60.

[51] I am indebted to David Cowen, who previously surveyed the *Transactions of the Medical Society of New Jersey* for citation of many worthy publications. See Cowen, *Medicine and Health*, 56–59.

autopsy was a circumscribed form of research which demonstrated a spirit of inquiry. Practicing physicians performed their own autopsies, usually with a few medical colleagues to share the educational experience. In 1867, a doctor from rural Burlington County enjoined New Jersey's country physician to make more frequent "*post mortem* examinations for the correction of diagnosis, and justification, or not, of the practice pursued."[52]

One popular form of research was the gathering of responses to vexing medical questions by means of "circular letters." In 1874, for example, members of the various county medical societies were asked by the state organization about their use of chloral hydrate and their personal experience with hypodermic medications.[53] Such "collective investigation" did not challenge the status of the experienced practitioner as the legitimate source of medical authority.[54]

Trials of novel therapies, successful and otherwise, were an accepted form of clinical investigation. William Pierson Jr. of Orange attended a distressing case of rabies in a child. In desperation, he and a consultant resolved to try "electro-magnetism," a therapy one of them had merely read about.[55] C. C. Vanderbeck of Monmouth County was induced to try ergot for headache: "Having noticed in one of our late medical journals, the use of ergot in headache, I was induced to experiment with this article of the materia medica, in the very distressing affection, cephalgia."[56]

A handful of papers gave evidence of thoughtful systematic research. In a study of creosote as a therapeutic agent in the treatment of "phthisis pneumonalis" (pulmonary tuberculosis), pediatrician William Watson reported his experience with the drug in fifty successive unselected patients at St. Francis Hospital in Jersey City. He concluded that creosote was no cure, "yet it will benefit all."[57]

---

[52] J. P. Coleman, "Reports of District Societies (Burlington County)," *Transactions of the Medical Society of New Jersey* (1867): 226.

[53] Frank Wilmarth, "Reports of District Societies: Essex County," *Transactions of the Medical Society of New Jersey* (1874), 133–35.

[54] Harry M. Marks, *The Progress of Experiment: Science and Therapeutic Reform in the United States: 1900–1990* (Cambridge: Cambridge University Press, 1997), 43–44.

[55] William Pierson, Jr., "Case of Hydrophobia," *Transactions of the Medical Society of New Jersey* (1864): 100–1; current was applied for half an hour "without producing the least abatement of the symptoms or any apparent effect upon the child." Those who have not seen a child die of hydrophobia might criticize Pierson for turning to such a seemingly foolish therapy. However, neurophysiology and galvanic currents were current topics of research, and many distinguished practitioners used electric current in their therapeutic regimens.

[56] C. C. Vanderbeck, "The Use of Ergot in Headache," *Transactions of the Medical Society of New Jersey* (1873): 194–95. Vanderbeck presented two cases, and noted that patients were requesting "headache drops" of him. Ergot preparations continue to be used for migraine headaches today.

[57] William P. Watson, "The Value of Creosote in Fifty Cases of Disease of the Air

Two occupational health studies impress the modern reader as examples of first-class clinical research. Forgotten by historians of industrial health is an 1860 investigation by Dr. Addison Freeman of Orange entitled "Mercurial Disease Among Hatters." Freeman reported that "during the winter of 1858–9 and following spring there prevailed quite extensively among the hatters of Orange, Newark, Bloomfield and Millburn [all in Essex County] a disease showing all the characteristics of Mercurial Salivation and Stomatitis." He conducted a thorough study of the hatmaking process, pinpointing the high risk among hat finishers who were exposed to mercury used in a manufacturing step called carating. Freeman tested for mercury in the fabric, and advised changes in processing and ventilation.[58]

Jonathan Stevenson of Camden took advantage of his position as examining surgeon for Civil War draftees to evaluate the health of young men in six southern New Jersey counties. Finding that many draftees were glassblowers in regional industries, he measured chest expansion and developed a summary profile of their health. He found them to be of "slight physical development," perhaps due to their employment in adolescence. He concluded that the "continued and violent exercise of their lungs" as glassblowers contributed to emphysema and cardiac hypertrophy.[59]

In 1878, Alexander Dougherty of Newark, intrigued by apparently mild cases of diabetes, asked directors of institutions such as the New Jersey State Lunatic Asylum and the New Jersey Soldier's Home for "their kind cooperation to ascertain what amount of glycosuria [sugar in the urine] there might be among the [asymptomatic] patients under their charge." Dougherty concluded that "a slight glycosuria is very common, and very commonly overlooked, because not at all suspected; belonging to the border land between a state of health, and one of disease."[60] For a busy practitioner, this was indeed a careful and useful clinical study.

Passages," *Transactions of the Medical Society of New Jersey* (1889): 117–42.

[58] J. Addison Freeman, "Mercurial Disease among Hatters," *Transactions of the Medical Society of New Jersey* (1860), 61–64. For the history of mercury toxicity in the New Jersey hatting industry, see Helen Sheehan and Richard Wedeen, "Hatters' Shakes," in *Toxic Circles: Environmental Hazards from the Workplace into the Community*, ed. Helen Sheehan and Richard Wedeen (New Brunswick, NJ: Rutgers University Press, 1993), 26–54. Addison's promising career was cut short by his death from pneumonia at age thirty-one during service in the medical corps during the Civil War.

[59] Jonathan R. Stevenson, "Vital Statistics," *Transactions of the Medical Society of New Jersey* (1864): 145–53.

[60] Alexander M. Dougherty, "Observations on Glycosuria, Historical and Clinical," *Transactions of the Medical Society of New Jersey* (1878): 116–17. In today's diagnostic terminology, some of these patients would probably be classified as mild cases of non-insulin-dependent or adult onset diabetics; others would have impaired glucose

One New Jersey physician, perhaps overestimating his own sophistication as a researcher, set up a laboratory at Orange Memorial Hospital in East Orange for "diagnostic and pathological research."[61] Joseph Stickler was one of the first American physicians to travel to Berlin to assess Koch's much-heralded (and soon discredited) tuberculin treatment for tuberculosis. Stickler's New Jersey memorialist recalled that "he brought the experienced thus gained to bear upon his service in the phthisis [tuberculosis] wards of the [Orange] hospital. It will be remembered by the members of this society, how disappointed the Doctor was at the results of his numerous experiments in this direction."[62] Using methods learned in European laboratories, Stickler conducted unsuccessful and dangerous experiments in children in an effort to produce immunity to scarlet fever.[63] A colleague recalled: "Dr. Stickler was a fearless investigator in several lines of pathological research" and a "scientific physician." Stickler's slight (posthumous) national reputation rested not on his research findings, but on harsh criticism in the antivivisectionist press.[64]

A MEDICAL BACKWATER?

The first glimmer of quality domestic medical research was becoming evident at mid-century in the pages of American medical journals.[65] An informal review of leading American journals of the day suggests that contributions to the medical literature, even at the rudimentary level of the case report, were confined to a mere handful of New Jersey physicians.

---

tolerance, a pre-diabetic state.
[61] "Joseph William Stickler" (obituary), *Transactions of the Medical Society of New Jersey* (1899): 286–88.
[62] Ibid., 287. Koch developed his tuberculin treatment in 1890; several subjects died following the treatment and it fell into disrepute.
[63] Joseph W. Stickler, "Foot and Mouth Disease as It Affects Man and Animals, and Its Relation to Human Scarlatina as a Prophylactic," *Boston Medical and Surgical Journal* 117 (1887): 607–9; Joseph W. Stickler, "Scarlet Fever Reproduced by Inoculation; Some Important Points Deducted Therefrom," *Transactions of the Medical Society of New Jersey* (1897): 201–12. Ethics in experimentation were presumed to reside within the well-trained physician, polished by experience and moral authority. Superintendents of orphanages routinely gave consent for experiments on children in their charge. Susan E. Lederer, *Subjected to Science: Human Experimentation in America before the Second World War* (Baltimore, Johns Hopkins University Press, 1995), 15–16, 73–100.
[64] "Joseph William Stickler" (obituary), 287; Lederer, *Subjected to Science*, 76, 93.
[65] W. Bruce Fye, "The Literature of American Internal Medicine: A Historical View," *Annals of Internal Medicine* 106 (1987), 451–60.

Of the published notes or articles originating in New Jersey, most were of negligible quality and importance. The names of Jersey practitioners were rarely if ever found on the title pages of medical textbooks.

Thus, New Jersey at mid-century was something of a medical backwater—an importer rather than an exporter of medical knowledge, sparsely represented in America's developing medical literature. Not surprisingly, the state suffered from a medical brain drain, as men who sought academic and professional advancement went to New York or Philadelphia. For example, Edward Gamaliel Janeway of New Brunswick took the road to New York and academic distinction. A brilliant diagnostician, Janeway was professor of medical practice at Bellevue Hospital Medical College and served as commissioner of health for New York in the late 1870s.[66] Joseph Pancoast, born in Burlington County, studied medicine in Philadelphia, where he became a leading professor of surgery and a widely acclaimed innovator and author.[67]

This, then, was the medical community that Edgar Holden, the first of America's sphygmograph men, joined at the close of the Civil War. Holden would practice in Newark until his death in 1909. With respect to competence, intelligence, and personal excellence, his New Jersey colleagues represented a spectrum similar to that in any practice environment outside of the best academic centers of the day.

RENAISSANCE MAN OF NEWARK MEDICINE— THE EARLY YEARS

Holden's half-century medical career stood in sharp contrast to the careers of European academics, hospital men, consultants, and researchers like Marey, Burdon-Sanderson, Mahomed, and Mackenzie. For his time and place, Holden was something of a renaissance man. Although never counted among the ranks of the American medical elite, Holden transcended the provinciality of late-nineteenth-century Newark. His early and brief engagement with the sphygmograph is best seen in the context of a varied and productive medical life.[68]

---

[66] Fielding H. Garrison, *An Introduction to the History of Medicine*, 4th ed. (Philadelphia: W. B. Saunders, 1929), 633.

[67] "Pancoast, Joseph," in *Appleton's Cyclopaedia of American Biography*, eds. Grant Wilson and John Fiske (New York: D. Appleton, 1888): 4:641–42.

[68] For a detailed biography of Holden, see Moss, *Edgar Holden*.

Born in 1838 into a manufacturing family with deep roots in colonial Massachusetts, Holden came to Newark in 1852.[69] There is no evidence that he contemplated a career in medicine prior to entering Princeton in 1856. His academic record was undistinguished, and his standings in chemistry and anatomy were below average. Despite his mediocre grades, Princeton offered Holden a superior pre-medical education at a time when most medical schools required only a high school diploma or the loosely construed "equivalent."[70]

Like many aspiring physicians from northern New Jersey, Holden enrolled at the College of Physicians and Surgeons in New York in 1859. By the dismal standard of mid-nineteenth-century American medical education, this was an outstanding school.[71] The faculty of prominent medical practitioners sought to make courses as "demonstrative and practical as possible."[72] Among the instructors was young physiologist John Call Dalton.[73] Eager to distinguish Physicians and Surgeons from barebones proprietary schools, the 1859 catalogue promised that "Professor Dalton will teach Physiology as a science of observation and experiment."[74] A privately conducted survey of New York medical colleges

---

[69] Family history, courtesy Joan Smith, Westfield, N.J., a great granddaughter by Holden's first marriage, and William Birdsall, Chatham, N.J., a great grandson by Holden's second marriage. Family records of W. Birdsall suggest that Asa Holden may have worked as a shipbuilder and foundryman.

[70] Registrar's Grade Books, AC #116, 1802-1906, Box 11 (1853 Oct–1863 Jun), Seeley G. Mudd Manuscript Library, Princeton University. Each record lists course grade and rank. On the diploma or "equivalent," see Robert P. Hudson, "Abraham Flexner in Perspective: American Medical Education, 1865–1910," *Bulletin of the History of Medicine* 46 (1972): 546. 545–48. A survey of 222 New Jersey and Pennsylvania physicians, completed in 1882, found that 178 had no college training, although date of graduation was not considered; C. McIntire Jr., *The Percentage of College-Bred Men in the Medical Profession* (Philadelphia: American Academy of Medicine, 1883): 3–6; cited in Hudson, "Abraham Flexner," 547.

[71] In many schools, there was a serious disjunction between catalogue descriptions and the actual medical school experience. Historian Gert Brieger concluded that "the catalog promises seem to have been fulfilled at Physicians and Surgeons." Gert Brieger, Editor's note preceding *"Annual Catalogue of the College of Physicians and Surgeons, in the City of New York, 1849-50,"* in *Medical America in the Nineteenth Century: Readings from the Literature* (Baltimore: Johns Hopkins University Press, 1972), 37–38.

[72] Ibid., 38–42.

[73] For a biography of Dalton and an analysis of his critical role in American physiology, see Fye, *Development of American Physiology*, 15–53.

[74] College of Physicians and Surgeons in the City of New York, *Catalogue of the Officers of the University and of the College and Annual Announcement of Lectures; Fifty-Third Session, 1859–60* (New York: Baker and Godwin, 1859), 8–9. Copies held at Archives and Special Collections, Augustus C. Long Health Sciences Library, Columbia University,

in 1858 concluded: "Probably a more full and perfect course of instruction in physiology is here [Physicians and Surgeons] given than in any other institution in this country."[75] A biographer remarked of Dalton: "By the experimental method he brought [medical students] face to face with the facts of physiology so that the science became something more than a résumé of the best foreign textbooks."[76] Holden's interest in cardiovascular physiology was most likely stimulated by Dalton.

Upon graduation, he took up a post as assistant physician at King's County Hospital in Flatbush (Brooklyn), an institution managed by the Superintendents of the Poor.[77] The average daily census was about 340 patients with some 2300 admissions annually, so he would have seen a wide range of cases.[78] Although not a requirement for practice, ambitious young medical graduates considered it important to their future career prospects in cities such as New York to spend some time as a house physician in a hospital or dispensary.[79]

IRONCLAD SURGEON

Holden's future career plans were likely focused on New York, but the Civil War intervened and he joined the naval medical service in late

---

New York.

[75] J. C. B[artlett], "The Profession in New York: Impressions of a Visitor," *Boston Medical and Surgical Journal* 58 (1858): 301.

[76] Howard A. Kelly and Walter L. Burrage, *American Medical Biographies* (Baltimore: Norman, Remington Co., 1920), 278.

[77] "Death Comes to Dr. Holden" (obituary), *Newark Evening News*, 19 July 1909. Holden's obituary in the *Transactions of the Thirty-First Annual Meeting of the American Laryngological Association* (1909): 393–95 states that he was an "interne" at the hospital; J. E. N., "Dr. Edgar Holden" (obituary), *Transactions of the American Larnygological Association* (1909): 393. However, the word "intern" did not appear until the Civil War. Hudson, "Abraham Flexner," 553, footnote 45. Confirmation of Holden's appointment as resident physician: Thomas Turner, "Annual Report of the Resident Physician of Kings County Hospital," in *Annual Report of the Superintendents of the Poor of Kings County, for the Year Ending July 31, 1861* (Brooklyn, Daily Eagle Print, 1861), 49; reference courtesy Jack Termine, Archives and Special Collections, SUNY Downstate Medical Center.

[78] L. B. Proctor, "History of the Superintendents of the Poor for the County of Kings," in *The Civil, Political, Professional Record of the County of Kings and the City of Brooklyn N.Y. from 1683 to 1884*, ed. Henry R. Stiles New York: W. W. Munsel and Co., 1884), 1:483–84.

[79] Rosenberg, "Social Class and Medical Care," 40–41.

1861.⁸⁰ In four years as a naval medical officer, he logged sixteen months of active sea duty and participated as surgeon in three major naval battles (Hampton Roads aboard the *Minnesota*, Charleston Harbor aboard the monitor *Passaic*, and the epic battle of Albemarle Sound between the CSS *Albemarle* and the USS *Sassacus*)."⁸¹ Holden's lifelong commitment to publication in medical journals began in 1866 with an article in the *American Journal of the Medical Sciences*, entitled "An Inquiry into the Causes of Certain Diseases on Ships of War." Included among the maladies was "ironclad fever," a fatal encephalitis-like illness that afflicted sailors on the early ironclads, possibly caused by subacute carbon monoxide poisoning.⁸² Following his discharge from the navy in 1864, Holden took up a part-time post in Newark's Ward Army Hospital, serving until the hospital was decommissioned in September 1865.⁸³

NEWARK PRACTITIONER

Holden emerged from the war a self-confident and experienced clinician. His multifaceted career embodied many of the dominant themes of postbellum American medicine: medical research and technology, specialization, hospital practice, and public health. His mastery of insurance medicine, epidemiology, laryngology, and cardiopulmonary medicine were evidence of an extraordinary intellect. Certainly nothing in his formal training had prepared him for such breadth of achievement. In obituaries and biographies, he was cited as "a prominent physician of Newark," "one of the leading medical men in New Jersey," "an acknowledged authority in the department of otolaryngology," "a highly cultured and trained man in the learned profession he adorned [and] also an executive of marked and successful administrative ability," and "one of the leading specialists of his day."⁸⁴

---

[80] Holden signed up for the navy at the Brooklyn Navy Yard according to his second wife's Declaration for Widow's Pension, 1909; family records, W. Birdsall.

[81] *Register of the Commissioned, Warrant, and Volunteer Officers of the Navy of the United States to January 1, 1862 (1863, 1864, 1865)* (Washington: Government Printing Office, 1862–1865). For a summary of Holden's military service, see also Clark, "First Fifty Years," 165–67 and Moss, *Edgar Holden*, 81–145; Edgar Holden, "The First Cruise of the 'Monitor' *Passaic*," *Harper's Monthly Magazine* 27 (October 1863), 577–95. The *Passaic* came close to sinking in the same storm that claimed the *Monitor*.

[82] Edgar Holden, "An Inquiry into the Causes of Certain Diseases on Ships of War," *American Journal of the Medical Sciences* 51 (1866): 75–84.

[83] Moss, *Edgar Holden*, 123–24.

[84] J. E. N., "Dr. Edgar Holden" (obituary), 393–95; "Death Comes to Dr. Holden" (obituary), *Newark Evening News*, 19 July 1909; "Holden" (obituary), *Journal of the*

Holden maintained a private practice in Newark between 1865 and 1891.[85] Although he began as a general practitioner, in later years he became identified as a medical consultant and a specialist in laryngology. He directed the throat and chest clinic at St. Michael's Hospital, visited patients at home or in consultation at two local hospitals, performed general surgery including chest and abdominal operations, and tinkered with new medical devices including three instruments designed to detect lung disease.[86] Laryngology was tailor-made for Holden, a forward-looking physician with surgical skills and a fondness for modifying and inventing medical hardware. He was an early member of the American Laryngological Association (founded 1879) and served as vice-president in 1889.[87]

An early interest in cardiac disease was evidenced by an 1867 article in the *American Journal of the Medical Sciences*, a prominent Philadelphia publication. Combining over thirteen hundred "selected and insured lives" from the files of the Mutual Benefit Live Insurance Company, four hundred from "books of county physicians," and three hundred from his general practice in the community, Holden studied the effect of familial disorders on subsequent organic cardiac and brain disorders. Although his study was amorphous and his methods incapable of yielding meaningful data, the work was nevertheless an ambitious undertaking for a young man in practice for little more than two years.[88]

Medical Society of New Jersey 6 (1909): 137–38; "Edgar Holden, M.D." (obituary). *Journal of the American Medical Association* 53 (1909): 474; "Holden, Edgar." *National Cyclopaedia of American Biography* (New York: James T. White, 1916), 15:91–92; "Dr. Edgar Holden (obituary)," *New Jersey Historical Society Proceedings*, n.s. 1 (1916): 106–7; "Holden, Edgar, M.D.," *Biographical Encyclopaedia of New Jersey of the Nineteenth Century* (Philadelphia: Galaxy Publishing: 1877), 284; "Holden, Edgar," in *Cyclopedia of New Jersey Biography* (New York; American Historical Society, 1923) 330–31; "In Memoriam, Edgar Holden," *Circular No. 13, Military Order of the Loyal Legion of the United States* (New York: Military Order of the Loyal Legion of the United States, 1909), pamphlet in the collection of great grandson W. Birdsall.

[85] Samuel W. Butler, *Medical Register of the United States* (Philadelphia: Office of the *Medical and Surgical Reporter*, 1874), 452; A. E. M. Purdy, comp., *The Medical Register of New York, New Jersey, and Connecticut for the Year Commencing June 1, 1875* (New York: G. P. Putnam's Sons, 1875), 158.

[86] Holden's name first appeared on the list of consulting physicians at St. Barnabas in 1874, although he may have been on the staff for some time. A. E. M. Purdy, comp., *Medical Register of New York, New Jersey and Connecticut for the Year Commencing June 1, 1874* (New York: William Wood, 1874), 141; Moss, *Edgar Holden*, 437–46.

[87] J. E. N., "Dr. Edgar Holden," 394.

[88] Edgar Holden, "On the Influence of Antecedent Disorders upon Organic Affections of the Heart and Brain," *American Journal of the Medical Sciences* 54 (1867): 54–67.

"THE REPROACH OF OUR PROFESSION"

Holden gained a reputation in New Jersey not as a sphygmograph man, but as something of an expert in tuberculosis, a disease of epidemiological importance and a centerpiece of rapidly evolving medical research. He was swept up in the transformation of tuberculosis from a hereditary and constitutional disease that claimed the lives of the best and brightest to "a contagion, something unclean . . . a blot on society, the symbol of all that was rotten in the industrial world."[89] In 1891, he addressed the Medical Society of New Jersey on the mechanism of the spread of tuberculosis: "One-fifth of the human family still succumb in grim dispair [sic] to the greatest scourge of our race." For Holden, tuberculosis remained "the *ignis fatuus* [will o' the wisp] of scientific study of all ages." As for the impotence of physicians in halting the disease, Holden reflected that it was "still, as for countless generations, the reproach of our profession."[90]

"BETTER THAN THE SYSTEM"

When compared to the meager output of most New Jersey physicians, the body of Holden's published work—over forty articles in addition to two book-length works—was truly astonishing, not only in quantity, but in relative quality. Between 1866 and 1897, he published regularly in the leading regional medical journals and national specialty journals of the day.[91] His publications extended well beyond his sphygmographic studies to include tuberculosis, insurance medicine, laryngology, and wide-ranging case reports drawn from general and specialty practice.

William Welch, a leader in American medical education reform, recalled that the nineteenth-century "system was about as bad as it could be." But, continued Welch, there were inspiring teachers, including such men as Dalton, Holden's physiology professor at the College of Physicians and Surgeons. Because of such gifted teachers, outstanding young

---

[89] René Dubos and Jean Dubos, *The White Plague: Tuberculosis, Man and Society* (Boston, Little, Brown & Co., 1952; reprint, New Brunswick, NJ: Rutgers University Press, 1987), 66. Pagination unchanged in reprint edition.

[90] Edgar Holden, "Tuberculosis—The Potential Factors in its Spread—Whether Hereditary Capacity, Inherited Bacilli or Transmission from the Lower Animals," *Transactions of the Medical Society of New Jersey* (1891): 83–107; quotation, 83. Koch identified the tubercle bacillus in 1882. The medical world was still reeling from the recent failure of Robert Koch's "tuberculin," widely and prematurely proclaimed as a cure.

[91] See the list of publications by Holden identified to date in Moss, *Edgar Holden*, 529–33.

physicians transcended their formal education. "The results," said Welch, in an oft-cited comment, "were better than the system."[92]

In a career spent outside the academic orbit of the relatively progressive medical schools, maturing teaching hospitals, and nascent research laboratories of the metropolis, Holden exemplified individual excellence far beyond that promised by his ante-bellum training and the provincial medical establishment of Essex County. He assiduously cultivated a familiarity with advances in European and American medicine. He made himself an expert in the field of sphygmography at a time when only a handful of academic physicians in England and on the Continent were exploring the mysteries of the recorded pulse wave.

HOLDEN'S EARLY WORK WITH THE SPHYGMOGRAPH

The origin of Holden's interest in the sphygmograph in the late 1860s is unclear. Holden may have been present at the meeting of the New York Medical Journal Association in 1868 when Samuel Ward described his work with the Marey sphygmograph.[93] There is no evidence, as noted earlier, that Holden traveled in Europe or England prior to 1870. If he owned a Marey sphygmograph, a point which is not clear in his writings, it would have been ordered from abroad or perhaps brought back by an acquaintance at his request.

With some steady income from the Mutual Benefit Life Insurance Company, Holden may have decided to seize the moment for research while he was still building a practice and had a few spare hours. Perhaps, at that particular point in his life, he was mulling over the idea of a New York hospital appointment or academic career, although there is no evidence that he attempted to establish any ties with New York medical schools.

Holden was at work on the sphygmograph by about 1868. At some point, he had delivered an early paper on the subject at a meeting of the

---

[92] William Henry Welch, "Medical Education in the United States: The Harvey Lecture" (1916), in *Papers and Addresses* by William Henry Welch (Baltimore: Johns Hopkins University Press, 1920), 3:120–21. Welch used the same phrasing nine years earlier in "Some of the Conditions Which Have Influenced the Development of American Medicine, Especially During the Past Century," *Bulletin of the Johns Hopkins Hospital* 19 (1908): 34; reprinted in *Papers and Addresses*, 289. Welch may have first used the phrase, "the results were better than the system" in an address on the occasion of the centennial of the College of Physicians and Surgeons in 1907.

[93] Ward, "Sphygmograph and Some of Its Uses," 385–89.

New York Journal Association (probably Holden's reference to the Medical Journal Association of New York).[94] In an 1871 article for the *Transactions of the Medical Society of New Jersey*, Holden remarked that it had been nearly three years since his modification of the Marey sphygmograph had been "laid before the profession" in the *Medical Record*, a New York journal. It is evident from this brief article that he was familiar with the Continental and British literature. In addition to Marey, he cited Vierordt, Anstie, and Burdon-Sanderson and was familiar with the "simple column of mercury" typical of the Hérisson sphygmoscope.[95]

Holden traveled to France and Italy with his wife in 1870, probably seeking sanatorium care for what appears to have been her advanced and ultimately fatal tubercular condition. He visited a number of European "hospitals and institutions of learning," but there is no mention of a course of study or of any personal interaction with a European sphygmographer.[96] Had Holden visited Marey's laboratory, he would almost certainly have mentioned the fact. While he might have visited some research institutions in France, Holden undertook no systematic physiologic training in Europe.

EARLY MODIFICATIONS OF THE MAREY SPHYGMOGRAPH

The originality of Holden's thinking is evident in his 1870–71 article, "The Availability of the Sphygmograph, with Description of a New Instrument," in which he introduced his earliest efforts at modifying the Marey sphygmograph. His design incorporated a wooden body with a steel spring and tracer. It was built to Holden's specifications by the respected George Tiemann surgical instrument company in New York. One unique feature was a "strap for binding to the wrist or leg." Holden seems to have anticipated recording a pulse in the lower extremity (most likely the popliteal pulse behind the knee); however there is no evidence that Holden used this early model to record lower extremity pulses.[97]

---

[94] Edgar Holden, "Introductory Note," in *The Sphygmograph: Its Physiological and Pathological Indications; The Essay to Which Was Awarded the Stevens Triennial Prize, by the College of Physicians and Surgeons, New York, April, 1873* (Philadelphia: Lindsay & Blakiston, 1874), 9.

[95] Holden, *The Sphygmograph*, 17, 18, 27, 29; Edgar Holden, "The Availability of the Sphygmograph, with Description of a New Instrument," *Medical Record* (New York) 5 (1870–71): 9–10.

[96] Shaw, "Medical Profession of Essex County," 322.

[97] Holden, "Availability of the Sphygmograph," 9–10. The article was "referred for

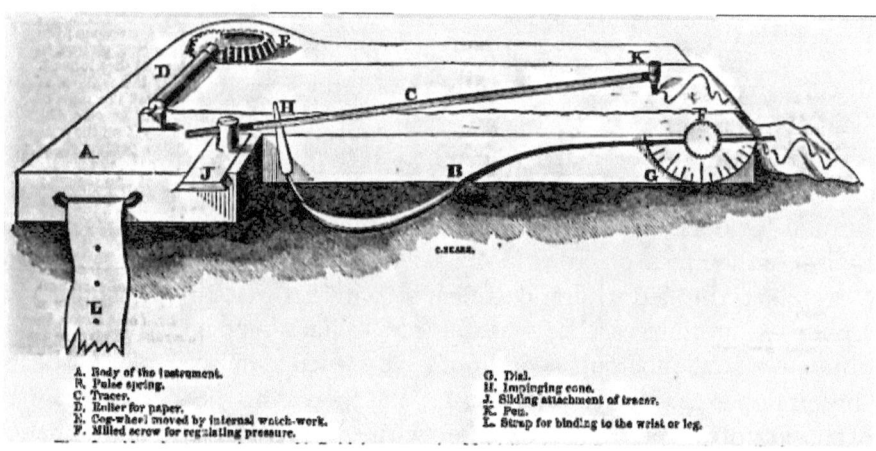

FIGURE 39: Early Holden sphygmograph based on the Marey sphygmograph with innovations in the pulse spring, pressure measurement, and tracer design. The instrument was manufactured to Holden's specifications by the George Tiemann company in New York. Note that the strap ("L") is labeled "strap for binding to the wrist or leg." Edgar Holden, "The Availability of the Sphygmograph, with Description of a New Instrument," *Medical Record* (New York) 5 (1870–71): 9.

In the dawning age of electricity, he thought first of applying an electric current and galvanometer to the sphygmograph. Although it is unclear how much experience he brought to the electrical project or whether he consulted someone with experience in a field such as telegraphy, Holden tried several modifications with different currents and metals. He was disappointed to discover that that "the instant of generation of the current commences a tracing which is incapable of noting the fine shades of the cardiac and arterial impulse." He soon abandoned experiments with electrical current.[98] It is intriguing to consider the help Holden might have obtained from Thomas Edison, who spent much of his career in New Jersey, had the sphygmographic project been started a few years later.[99]

---

publication" by the Essex County Medical Society. The George Tiemann company of New York, founded in 1826, manufactured an extensive range of medical devices, both diagnostic and therapeutic.

[98] Ibid., 9.

[99] In 1871, Edison was just beginning to set up a production shop in Newark for telegraph equipment. There is no known correspondence between the lesser and greater inventor. Matthew Josephson, *Edison: A Biography* (New York: John Wiley, 1992; New York: McGraw Hill, 1959), 84. A computerized search of the Edison papers at Rutgers

"Sphygmographic Hieroglyphics":
The Amateur Science of Edgar Holden

FURTHER DEVELOPMENT OF THE HOLDEN SPHYGMOGRAPH

Holden anticipated that his innovations would solve some of the problems of the original Marey sphygmograph and its British modifications: "Despairing of any success in the direction taken by the eminent observers of England and the continent, after their but partial success, it occurred to me that a new principle of construction might accomplish better results."[100] Accordingly, he adapted an ordinary watchwork to propel the paper, altered the writing tip to deliver ink, and redesigned the pulse spring system. As he emphasized in a long paper read before the Medical Society of New Jersey in 1871, there were no confining wrist straps in his later models as in the Marey and Burdon-Sanderson sphygmographs; Holden's instrument was simply pressed down upon the artery by the pressure of the examiner's hand on a metal bar atop the sphygmograph.

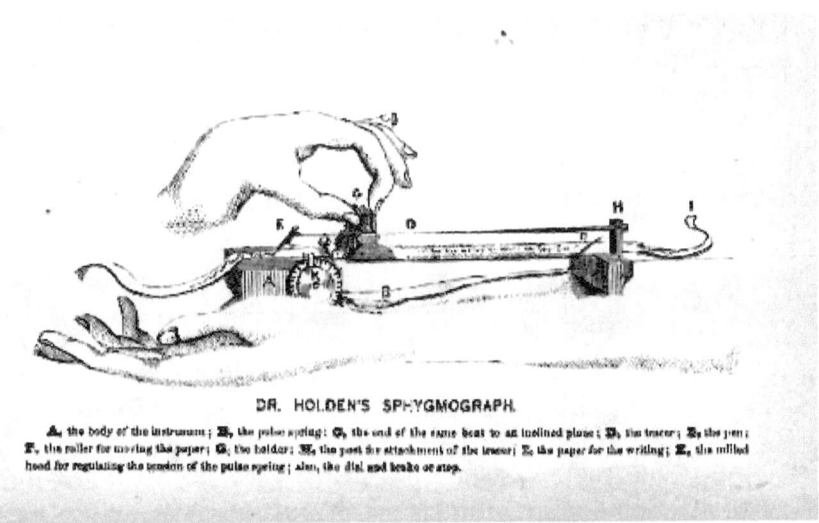

FIGURE 40: The redesigned Holden sphygmograph with basic parts clearly labeled. Note the absence of restraining bands and the "holder" for pressing down upon the artery. Edgar Holden, *The Sphygmograph: Its Physiological and Pathological Indications -- The Essay to Which was Awarded the Stevens Triennial Prize, by the College of Physicians and Surgeons, New York, April, 1873* (Philadelphia: Lindsay & Blakiston, 1874), frontispiece.

University failed to reveal any correspondence with Holden; courtesy Paul Israel, Thomas A. Edison Papers, Rutgers University.

[100] Holden, *The Sphygmograph*, 18-29.

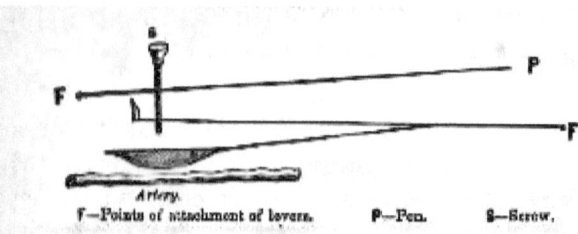

FIGURE 41: Schematic detail of the sensing and recording levers of the Holden sphymograph. Edgar Holden, *The Sphygmograph: Its Physiological and Pathological Indications -- The Essay to Which was Awarded the Stevens Triennial Prize, by the College of Physicians and Surgeons, New York, April, 1873* (Philadelphia: Lindsay & Blakiston, 1874), 19.

With his modified sphygmograph, Holden could take a tracing in one to three minutes, the observations not "marred by the fears of the patient, or the difficulties usually experienced in maintaining perfect quiet." It was this model that would appear in instrument catalogues as the "Holden sphygmograph."[101] Over the next two or three years, Holden perfected his sphygmograph and conducted exhaustive studies, both on his own constructed models of the cardiovascular system and on human subjects, including human volunteers, patients—and himself.

HOLDEN'S ARTIFICIAL HEART AND CIRCULATORY SYSTEM

Holden's long paper, "Circulatory Physiology and the Sphygmograph," was published in the *Transactions of the Medical Society of New Jersey* in 1871. As would be his lifelong practice, Holden familiarized himself with the relevant European literature. He took note early in his article of the "abstruse speculations heretofore indulged in by the eminent

---

[101] Edgar Holden, "Circulatory Physiology and the Sphygmograph," *Transactions of the Medical Society of New Jersey* (1871): 49; also published as a monograph: *The Sphygmograph and the Physiology of the Circulation: A Monograph Read Before the Medical Society of New Jersey, Upon Investigations Made Preparatory to a Larger Work on the Practical Value of the Sphygmograph.* New York: William Wood, 1871. *The American Armamentarium Chirurgicum*, published by the Tiemann Company, includes the Holden sphygmograph in its ca. 1879 catalog; George Tiemann & Co., *The American Armamentarium Chirurgicum* (New York: George Tiemann & Co., ca. 1879), I:87.

gentlemen whose names have become familiar."[102] The article was generously illustrated with tracings from patients with a variety of cardiac abnormalities. One tracing by Burdon-Sanderson was reproduced to illustrate a particular point.[103]

Both Marey and Burdon-Sanderson conducted experiments with artificial tubing serving as models for the arterial system. In 1867, Burdon-Sanderson commented on his as yet incomplete research in the "velocity of the transmission of vibrations, and to the production of successive movements identical to those of the pulse, in elastic tubes containing liquids."[104] Holden too experimented with artificial systems, building several novel pieces of apparatus, including an artificial heart and "capillary apparatus" made of rubber. Holden's artificial heart, was built to approximate the size of the human heart, but consisted of only one atrium and one ventricle (an approximation of the left side of the heart, which pumps blood into the aorta and the arteries of the body as detected by the sphygmograph; the right atrium and right ventricle pump blood into the pulmonary circulation and its action is not detected by the sphygmograph). Model valves were constructed of thin rubber (aortic) and leather (mitral) and were adjustable to approximate various forms of valvular disease.

Holden also constructed a large-scale sphygmograph, two feet in length, to inscribe tracings from his artificial heart. A simple mechanical "vascular system" consisted of rubber hosing connected to a steam engine. The distention of the hose as fluid passed along its length was recorded by means of a lightweight wooden lever six feet long, one end of which rested lightly upon the hose. The distal end of the lever recorded tracings of "pulse" waves up to six inches high for analysis.[105]

Unfortunately, there were no published illustrations of either the Holden artificial heart or the large scale sphygmograph; the instruments themselves and any original drawings have not survived. However, the article was generously illustrated with tracings from the artificial heart and vessels. Holden produced tracings from different sized "arteries" (tubes)

---

[102] Holden, "Circulatory Physiology and the Sphygmograph," 47.

[103] Ibid., 62.

[104] John Burdon-Sanderson, *Handbook of the Sphygmograph: Being a Guide to Its Use in Clinical Research, to Which is Appended A Lecture Delivered at the Royal College of Physicians on the 29th of March 1867 on the Mode and Duration of the Contraction of the Heart in Health and Disease* (London: Robert Hardwicke, 1867), vi; Ètienne Jules Marey, *La circulation du sang a l'état physiologique et dans les maladies* (Paris: G. Masson, 1881), 162–75.

[105] Holden, "Circulatory Physiology and the Sphygmograph," 47–53.

receiving "blood" (probably water, possibly alcohol) from the artificial heart—an approximation of the human pulse wave in health and disease. Part of this work was quite original, particularly in its use of the large inscribing lever. Holden confessed that some of the tracings were "very perplexing."[106]

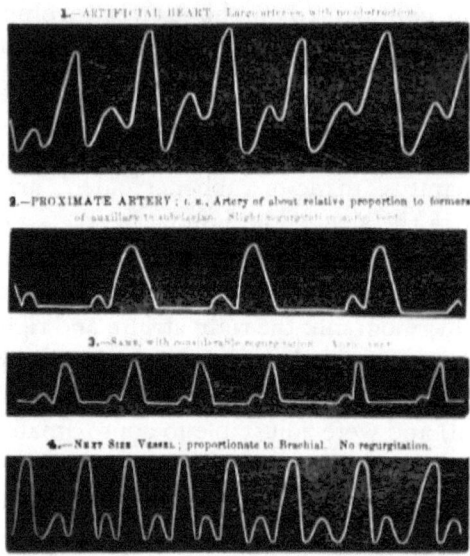

FIGURE 42: Holden sphygmograms of "pulses" in the artificial blood vessels connected to the Holden artificial heart recorded on his large scale sphygmograph. Holden experimented with various leaky valve modes and arterial configurations. Edgar Holden, "Circulatory Physiology and the Sphygmograph," *Transactions of the Medical Society of New Jersey* (1871): 51.

In his 1871 article, Holden urged patience. He warned, as he would a number of times, about the dangers of overreliance on the sphygmograph in making a diagnosis: "Now, so far as specific diagnosis goes, the science we are considering being in its infancy, is therefore far from perfect; thus tracings *apparently* similar result from very diverse sources, and our knowledge is at present too limited to enable us to read the hieroglyphics at first sight, always correctly."[107]

---

[106] Ibid., 51.
[107] Ibid., 66.

That the sphygmograph failed in making exact diagnoses was seen by Holden as a serious flaw. But in modern medical practice, many sophisticated tests—when combined with clinical acumen—are valued as supportive or confirmatory; others may help to rule out a diagnosis. Like successful twentieth-century technologies such as x-rays and electrocardiograms—and many that fell by the wayside—interpretation is always evolving, often requiring many decades as knowledge expands and technology is refined. Holden understood that the application of novel technology to clinical medicine was a work in progress:

> In concluding for the present [1871], however, permit me to express an opinion at variance with the fears of some who have found difficulties in the practical application of sphygmography, remarking that we should not allow our rules for interpretation to be too hastily formed, insasmuch as hitherto the expense and complex nature of the insturment used, the experience requisite to acquire dexterity, the difficulty of successful application, and the loss of valuable time in each case, have limited the number of workers and their observations.[108]

INSURANCE COMPANY MEDICAL DIRECTOR: DETERMINING SOUNDNESS

For forty years, Holden was president of the medical board of Newark's prestigious Mutual Benefit Life Insurance Company.[109] Mutual Benefit, founded in Newark in 1845, was the first life insurance company in New Jersey and the fourth in the nation. During the nineteenth century, Mutual Benefit was a successful, well-managed, and innovative company. In addition to a steady part-time income, his position with the company gained Holden access to health statistics and data that he incorporated into his broad array of published articles. Insurance medicine was an important, if circumscribed, subspecialty, requiring familiarity with the latest diagnostic technologies and such emerging fields as occupational health. As director, it was his job to establish criteria for insuring applicants, protect the assets

---

[108] Ibid., 67.

[109] Mildred F. Stone, *Since 1845: A History of the Mutual Benefit Life Insurance Company* (New Brunswick, Rutgers University Press, 1957), 95. Another reference gives 1865 as the date when Holden became a medical advisor at Mutual Benefit and 1869 as the date when he became president of the Board of Advisors: "Holden, Edgar, M.D.," in *Biographical Encyclopaedia of New Jersey*: 284.

of the company by rejecting bad "risks," keep the scattered field force of private physicians up to current standards of medical diagnosis, and apply evolving actuarial principles and data. In 1897, Holden was president of the Association of Life Insurance Medical Directors.[110] In the course of his duties at Mutual Benefit, Holden prepared a detailed and original analysis of the health of Newark. The *Mortality and Sanitary Record of Newark, N.J.*, graced by lavish colored graphs, tables, and maps, was published in 1880 and still remains of use to historians of public health.[111]

As an insurance company medial director, Holden was naturally intrigued by anything that might aid in determining prospects for longevity among applicants; like Burdon-Sanderson, he held out early hopes that the sphygmograph might prove to be a guide to "soundness."

> It is at once evident, that could we satisfactorily determine the variations compatible with health, the Sphygmographic record of an applicant for life insurance would be the safest record he could present as a test of his condition; and this single feature could hardly fail to be of great pecuniary value in a country where the assurane of life is almost universal. Those who know and lament the multitude of recklessly-made or ignorantly or fraudulently-made certificates of soundness, are aware that hundreds of thousands of dollars are annually sacrificed that might be saved by some such means.[112]

THE STEVENS TRIENNIAL PRIZE

In 1869–1870, the College of Physicians and Surgeons of New York stepped into the unsettled world of sphygmography. The Stevens

---

[110] Holden's presidential address was published in the journal of the organization. Edgar Holden, "The Factors Which Govern the Acceptance of Risks after Middle Life," *Medical Examiner New York* 7 (1897): 143–45.

[111] Edgar Holden, *Mortality and Sanitary Record of Newark, N.J.* (Newark: Mutual Benefit Life Insurance Company, 1880); also full text online at https://rucore.libraries.rutgers.edu/rutgers-lib/47899/ (accessed 28 February 2017). In his 1988 book, *Newark: The Nation's Unhealthiest City, 1832–1895*, Stuart Galishoff credits Holden's monograph with "la[ying] bare Newark's poor health record," in addition to giving "an important boost" to the cause of sewer construction; Stuart Galishoff, *Newark: The Nation's Unhealthiest City, 1832–1895* (New Brunswick, NJ: Rutgers University Press, 1988), 98, 122.

[112] Holden, *The Sphygmograph*, 86–87.

Triennial Prize, established by Alexander H. Stevens, the late president of the college (1841–1855), was "open for universal competition," offering a generous award of $200 for the best medical essay on an announced topic. The prize commission included the president of the college, the professor of physiology (John Call Dalton, Holden's former medical school professor), and the president of the alumni association. In 1869, essays on "The Sphygmograph: Its Physiological and Pathological Indications" were invited. Other topics for the competition included "The Use of the Thermometer in the Study of Disease" and "The Pathology, Symptoms and Treatment of Convulsive Affections."[113] The fact that the sphygmograph was the subject of a prize essay suggests that physiologically oriented American physicians were familiar with the instrument, or at least the current European literature on the subject. As noted above, Dalton was quite familiar with the sphygmograph, at least in laboratory applications, prior to 1869, and may have suggested the topic to his fellow prize commission members.

In all likelihood, the Stevens Triennial Prize competition was an unexpected opportunity that fell neatly into Holden's lap. Perhaps he saw the prestigious award as an ideal vehicle for putting his name before the medical profession. Holden may have discussed his work informally with Dalton, his former professor. Dalton was familiar with Marey's cardiovascular research and was particularly interested in Marey's experiments devoted to the propulsion of waves through elastic tubing. Dalton was using a sphygmograph (proabably an imported Marey model) by 1869.[114] Holden gathered some four to six years of sphygmographic work into a long essay and submitted it to the prize committee, probably in late 1872 or early 1873. At the spring 1873 commencement ceremonies at the College of Physicians and Surgeons, Holden was named the winner for his essay on the sphygmograph.

---

[113] John Shrady, comp., *Medical Register, New York and Vicinity, 1868* (New York: Baker and Godwin, 1868), 220. John Shrady comp., *Medical Register, New York and Vicinity, 1869–70* (New York: J. M. Bradstreet, 1869), 188–89. A. E. M. Purdy, comp., *The Medical Register of New York and Vicinity for the Year Commencing June 1, 1871* (New York: William Wood & Co., 1871), 234–35. The chronology of prize topics is somewhat confused, as there seems to have a substitution of the convulsion essay for the thermometer essay.

[114] John Call Dalton, *A Treatise on Human Physiology Designed for the Use of Students and Practitioners of Medicine*, 4th rev. ed. (Philadelphia: Henry C. Lea, 1867), 268–70; Dalton, "How the Blood Circulates," 667–77.

THE PUBLICATION OF *THE SPHYGMOGRAPH* (1874)

Holden published the prize-winning essay in 1874 as a book entitled *The Sphygmograph: Its Physiological and Pathological Indications; The Essay to Which Was Awarded the Stevens Triennial Prize, by the College of Physicians and Surgeons, New York, April, 1873*. Some modifications to the essay were made, "only as regards a certain diffusedness both of tracing and subject matter."[115]

The frontispiece featured paired images of "Prof. Marey's sphygmograph" and "Dr. Holden's sphygmograph." The drawing of the Holden sphygmograph applied to a patient's arm—without straps—demonstrated its apparent ease of use. There were detailed magnified drawings of specific features of the instrument, most notably the improved curving sensor that rested upon the artery.[116] In all, Holden illustrated his monograph with close to three hundred pulse tracings. In the closing line of his book, he reiterated that the tracings had been exhaustively reproduced, so that "the student desirous of forming his own conclusions may do so."[117] The book remains today in archival collections, an important work in the literature of sphygmography and one of two known American works on the subject.[118]

The clearly written essay, illustrated with hundreds of pulse tracings, was indeed impressive, demonstrating detailed knowledge of the European literature, cutting edge technology modified to his own specifications, evidence of serious private research, self-experimentation, experience with hundreds of patients, and great hopes for the future. Holden displayed his familiarity with Marey's work and the recent British literature by Burdon-Sanderson, Anstie, and others. His goal was to produce an affordable yet accurate sphygmograph, capable of distinguishing organic (structural) from functional heart disease.

---

[115] Holden, *The Sphygmograph*, 10.

[116] Ibid., frontispiece, 20, 23, 24, 25.

[117] Ibid., 163.

[118] Holden's monograph, *The Sphygmograph* was recently purchased by Special Collections at the University of Medicine and Dentistry in New Jersey for $1500. There are copies at the College of Physicians in Philadelphia and at the New York Academy of Medicine. The full text of the book is now available online: https://archive.org/stream/sphygmographitsp00hold#page/n13/mode/2up. An inexpensive "classic reprint" edition appeared in 2016. A second American monograph about the sphygmograph was published posthumously and consists of compilations of published articles by Alonzo T. Keyt of Cincinnati. Keyt and his work are discussed in Chapter 5.

"Sphygmographic Hieroglyphics":
The Amateur Science of Edgar Holden

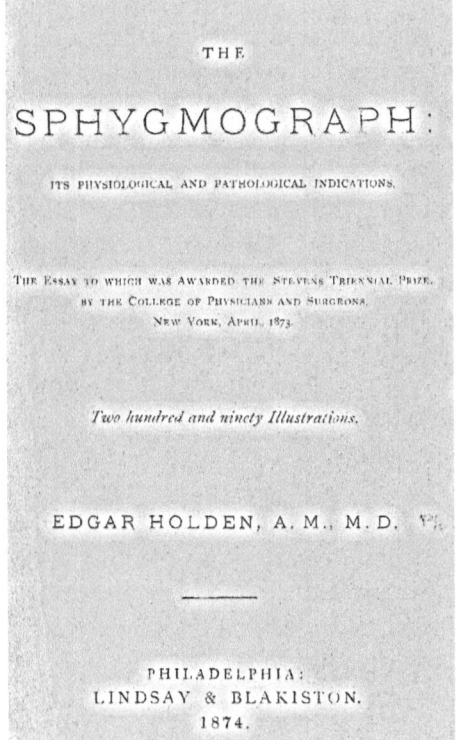

FIGURE 43: Holden's monograph, published in 1874, was based on his prize-winning work for which he was awarded the Steven's Triennial Prize by the College of Physicians and Surgeons in New York. Note the faint pencilled-in "PhD" after Holden's name; this copy of the monograph is in the possession of Holden's great-grandson, William Birdsall, of Chatham, New Jersey. Holden or his devoted wife probably added the "PhD" upon his receipt of the honorary degree from Princeton University in 1874.

THE SPHYGMOGRAPH: ITS PHYSIOLOGICAL AND PATHOLOGICAL INDICATIONS

Holden's monograph was divided into three parts, the first dealing with the basic operation of the sphygmograph and the interpretations of the sphygmogram, the second with tracings in various disease states, and the third with a series of experiments in which the sphygmograph was used to monitor the effects of drugs. Although he buried the statement deep in his first chapter, Holden had a fairly accurate view of the state of the art of sphygmography. The fundamental purpose of his study, he wrote, was not merely to build a better instrument, but to create an instrument capable of determining "whether there is any deep meaning in the blood current of the accessible arteries, of value in Physiology, Pathology or Therapeutics, which can be accurately ascertained and recorded" with a sphygmograph.[119]

In describing his own modified instrument, Holden demonstrated an understanding of mechanics and mechanical engineering, along with a good measure of ingenuity. Although there is no evidence that his modifications were ever incorporated by other designers or investigators, Holden noted that his sphygmograph was in good working order after several thousand tracings, and "could be duplicated by the maker at a cost of about one-third that of the imported instruments."[120] The Holden sphygmograph was capable of taking a reading in thirty seconds to two minutes and was not strapped to the patient's arm, thus obviating "nervous excitement due to the simple act of examination."[121] Regarding the wrist straps used by Marey and Burdon-Sanderson, Holden was mindful that the "difficulty of adjustment to the artery, even under favorable circumstances, is considerable; and when the patient is nervous and excited or frenzied by delirium, the tracing obtained after a prolonged trial cannot be accepted as the correct index of the pulsating wave."[122]

"SPHYGMOGRAPHIC HIEROGLYPHICS"

Holden began his monograph by summarizing the history of taking the pulse and the current status of sphygmology (pulse study). Echoing British authorities such as Broadbent, Holden asserted that the sphygmograph was not a substitute for the physician's art: "Every skillful, ambitious physician realizes in daily life that the *tactus eruditus* is to-day as valuable an acquirement as in the days of Galen."[123] Holden was not, of course, advocating a return to the "diffuse nomenclature" of the past or "the mysterious element so familiar to the student of ancient medicine," but rather a modern approach to pulse study. While not going so far as to endorse the "whimsical oddities" of the complex Chinese system of pulse study, in which a vast range of internal

---

[119] Holden, *The Sphygmograph*, 22–23.

[120] Ibid., 28 (footnote); the "maker" of the sphygmograph (to Holden's specifications) used in at least some of the experiments and cited here by Holden was Otto & Reynders, New York.

[121] Ibid., 29.

[122] Ibid., 20–21. For Burdon-Sanderson's instrument, see figure 23.

[123] Ibid., 30.

pathology was identified and localized by study of the pulse ("an extreme tax upon credulity"), Holden concluded that in the Chinese system "there was more of good sense than we are first inclined to believe."[124]

In a chapter entitled "The Translations of Tracings," Holden revealed his fondness for the expression "sphygmographic hieroglyphics." However, the more profound meaning of "translation" in the sense of "translation of physiological actions into the language of machines" may have been familiar concepts to him.[125] Holden explained the components of the normal pulse wave, identifying, as had others with some variations, the phases of the pulse wave: i. the shock wave or primary ascent; ii. the true systolic wave or wave of filling of the vessel with blood; iii. the diastolic collapse or descending wave; and iv. the wave of diastolic expansion or recurrent wave or wave of dicrotism.[126]

The first section of the book ended with a detailed discussion of the effect of various disease states, including hysteria, on the pulse wave. Holden devoted considerable attention to the "dicrotous wave," a much contested and poorly understood dip in the downstroke of the dominant contractile pulse wave. He related the dicrotic wave to the state of the capillary circulation and predicted that it "may be of value as a ground for prognosis when occurring during the progress of any wasting disease."[127] The relevant point here is that Holden sought physiological explanations for puzzling pulse wave contours.

THE UTILITY OF "SPHYGMOGRAPHIC HIEROGLYPHICS"

In the second section of the book, Holden focused on the utility of the sphygmograph. Apparently familiar with recent concepts of vascular degeneration, he quoted without attribution the observation that "the earliest beginnings of what may be called degenerative disease consist in structural alteration of the minutest arteries."[128] Holden anticipated, perhaps drawing

---

[124] Ibid., 32–33.

[125] "The Translation of Physiological Actions into the Language of Machines" is a chapter title in Stanley Joel Reiser, *Medicine and the Reign of Technology* (Cambridge: Cambridge University Press, 1978), 91–121.

[126] Holden, *The Sphygmograph*, 38–44.

[127] Ibid., 54–63; quotation, 62. Holden's wide knowledge of the medical literature was evidenced by his citation of an essay by M. Voisin in the *Biennial Retrospect of the Sydenham Society, 1867–8*, in which dicrotism was related to epilepsy; ibid., 62.

[128] Holden, *The Sphygmograph*, 86.

on Burdon-Sanderson's writings, that the sphygmograph might be used to predict a "departure from perfect health," prognosis in certain diseases, and the "calculation of endurance in prolonged mental labor." Notions of mental fatigue and intellectual exhaustion were beginning to engage medical scientists in Europe and America and were closely linked to emerging theories of neurasthenia. In his 1888 work, *A Practical Treatise on Nervous Exhaustion (Neurasthenia)*, American neurologist George Miller Beard asserted that "mental labor in cerebrasthenia [is] more exhausting than physical."[129]

Holden reassured his readers that, with patience and training, "sphygmographic hieroglyphs," like those of Egypt (or "even the facial features of a barbarous nation") were decipherable. Emphasizing the desideratum of objectivity, he referred to the "impartial pen of the Sphygmograph." Taking advantage of "the facilities afforded as medical adviser to Newark's Mutual Benefit Life Insurance Company, and [his position] as clinical physician for diseases of the chest at Newark's St. Michael's Hospital, he had recorded and studied thousands of tracings.[130]

Holden began his gallery of sphygmograms with a tracing from a "physician of middle age, in robust health." Among his subjects was Miss G., aged eighteen, who was petite, vigorous, and free of organic disease; her palpitations and "simple functional disorders" were "probably due to inordinate dancing." In this case the sphygmograph confirmed normality. Mr. M., age 32, of sanguino-nervous temperament, usually robust and vigorous, suffered "occasional cardiac disturbances from abuse of tobacco," as well as "nervous hyperaesthesia." In Holden's analysis, the tracing revealed telltale abnormalities.[131]

He proceeded to a more conventional series of tracings in various cardiac disorders including palpitations due to "dissipation," valvular disorders, cardiac hypertrophy, and "threatened apoplexy." Tracings were taken before and after treatment in some of these subjects. In the case of a patient with pericarditis and effusion (inflammation of the membrane around the heart with fluid accumulation), in which one might expect muting of the cardiac impulse, serial sphygmographic tracings had the potential to be of prognostic value.[132]

---

[129] Anson Rabinbach, *The Human Motor: Energy, Fatigue, and the Origins of Modernity* (Berkeley: University of California Press, 1992), 146–53; George M. Beard, *A Practical Treatise on Nervous Exhaustion (Neurasthenia): Its Symptoms, Nature, Sequences, Treatment* (New York, E. B. Treat, 1988), 136.

[130] Holden, *The Sphygmograph*, 9, 87–89.

[131] Ibid., 91–100.

[132] Ibid., 101–12.

In subsequent chapters, Holden reviewed tracings in patients with nervous system disorders and respiratory diseases. In a patient with asthma, then considered a nervous disorder affecting the bronchi and lungs, he noted that "the similarity of the tracings to those taken from my own arteries, while under the influence of certain nervous sedatives, is well marked." He was referring to his experiments (to be described later in the chapter) with a number of pharmaceuticals.[133] Among his "singular cases" was a long-term study of a saloonkeeper with "a quotidian ague [daily fever and chills] running somewhat rapidly into a remittent fever" with apparant recovery. Holden took some forty tracings as he followed the case along.

In another "singular case," a middle-aged woman with chronic "ovaritis" (inflammation of the ovary) was found to have a circulatory disturbance evident on her sphygmographic tracings, which Holden arributed to the diseased ovaries at a time when vague disorders of the female organs were though to influence a host of psychological and physiological abnormalities.[134]

He was also interested in aneurysms (then taken to be any structural abnormality of an artery but now defined more narrowly as a ballooning of the wall of an artery), an area of study popular with all sphygmographers, in part because the tracings were of proven value in localization of the vascular defect.[135]

A chapter entitled "Phthisis" (tuberculosis) presented tracings in tubercular patients in different stages of the illness. Holden, who saw a great deal of tuberculosis in his practice, was familiar with the insurance aspects of the disease. He was perhaps hoping to find some characteristic patterns linking tuberculosis to the pulse tracing. He considered a weak heart and "atonic capillaries" to be typical of all stages of tuberculosis.[136]

THEORIES OF ARTERIAL TENSION

Holden, influenced no doubt by Burdon-Sanderson's work, was also interested in arterial tension. (The pathbreaking work of Frederik Akbar

---

[133] Ibid., 113–20.

[134] Ibid., 121–27.

[135] Ibid., 130–32.

[136] Ibid., 128–30. From the modern perspective, advanced lung disease could be expected to put a strain on the right side of the heart, but this was unlikely to cause pathognomonic changes in the radial pulse (a left heart function) until the disease was extremely far advanced.

Mahomed in England was not published until later in the 1870s; see Chapter 3). In a chapter entitled "Compressibility or Tension" Holden wrote: "All observers have felt the need of some means, not only of readily bringing proper pressure to bear upon the artery, but of instantaneously and accurately recording it."[137] Holden was aware that "the highest degree [of applied pressure by the sphygmograph] which the artery will bear without obliteration is by no means the measure of tension, nor may it give the tracing of greatest amplitude." In an oversimplification, he equated the "amount of tension" in the arteries with the "extent of accumulation of blood in them," and from there "infer[red] the amount in the veins, the conducting power of the capillaries, and the condition of the heart." Citing Dalton, Holden qualified his emphasis on blood volume by recalling the role of the sympathetic nervous system in controlling vascular tone. Limited by the science of his day, Holden did not arrive at a satisfactory concept of hypertension.[138]

Holden included over two hundred tracings taken from patients with the wide-ranging clinical conditions described in his book. Anstie and Burdon-Sanderson would likely have faulted his method of applying pressure on the radial artery by simply pressing down the sphymograph over the wrist. (British investigators stressed the importance of a confined hyperextended wrist, in some cases firmly strapped into a cradle.) The resulting tracings appear confusing and uninterpretable to the casual observer. Holden himself referred to his "sphygmographic hieroglyphics" not once, but twice, in the early pages of his book. The tracings, he said, were "culled with care" and may "thus be of the more assistance to any who desire to pursue the complex yet interesting study of sphymographic hieroglyphics."[139]

Holden viewed the arterial pulse recording as a potential window into the entire vascular system: arteries, veins, and capillaries. His studies with his artificial heart, though not included in his book, confirmed that the radial artery might have much to reveal about the workings of the heart itself. Once the "hierglyphics themselves" were understood, the investigator could begin to parse features of the pulse wave "such as are due to elasticity, contractility or locomotion of the vessel itself, the relative tension of the venous and arterial systems, the condition of the capillary

---

[137] Ibid., 79.

[138] Ibid., 80–85. Theories about the underlying mechanisms of hypertension continue to be revised today.

[139] Ibid., 10.

structures, etc."[140] His emphasis on the clinical features connected with each tracing are evidence that he understood that the sphygmographic tracings could not stand alone: interpretation had to be made in conjuction with the clinical picture.

PHARMACEUTICAL INVESTIGATIONS AND SELF-EXPERIMENTATION

Holden's boldest work with the sphygmographic was described in the last section of his monograph, entitled "Investigations Made with the Sphygmograph into the Action of Certain Medications upon a Healthy Pulse." He studied the effects of four pharmaceutical agents (cannabis, gelseminum, aconite, and quinine) on his own pulse tracing and that of at least one volunteer. Pharmaceutical research had advanced in Europe in the nineteenth century, as drugs such as emetine, strychnine, and morphine were isolated in pure form from plant extracts. Self-experimentation was common—almost required—of the responsible and ethical experimenter. The apothecary assistant who first isolated morphine in 1806 came close to killing himself with the unexpectedly potent derivative of opium.

Particularly in Germany, pharmaceutical research advanced rapidly after mid-century. *Materia medica* (the study of the plants and minerals used to prepare medicines) gave way to research-based pharmacology in textbooks and medical school curricula. Cardioactive drugs, such as atropine, physostigmine, amyl nitrate, and nitroglycerine, joined digitalis, a plant preparation dating to the late eighteenth century, in the practitioner's armamentarium.[141] Medical botany, formerly the backbone of the *materia medica*, became the province of homeopaths and herbalists. Modern American pharmaceutical research began with the founding of professorships of pharmacology at medical schools such as Johns Hopkins, where, in 1893, the European-trained John Jacob Abel was appointed the first professor of pharmacology in the United States.

For many practitioners, the old drugs of the heroic armamentarium served quite well for most purposes; for some incurious doctors, the old drugs served quite well for virtually *all* purposes. But for the up-and-coming generation of physicians, the 1870s were years of great promise in therapeutics. Motivated physicians, often armed with post-graduate

---

[140] Ibid., 37.
[141] Miles Weatherall, "Drug Therapies," in *Companion Encyclopedia of the History of Medicine*, ed. W. F. Bynum and Roy Porter (London: Routledge, 1993), 918–21.

training in Europe and familiar with the medical literature, felt free to experiment on patients (or themselves) with new agents, or, as in Holden's case, apply new methods to the study of old drugs.

In conducting his own pharmaceutical experiments, Holden used a method of observation that seems to have been borrowed from the homeopathic ritual of drug "provings." The homeopathic theories and pharmaceutical rituals of German physician Samuel Hahnemann were introduced into the United States prior to the Civil War by converts to his medical system and German immigrant physicians fleeing revolutions in Europe. As a center of German immigration, Newark had a large number of German-American physicians and homeopaths. In 1866, there were some sixty homeopaths in New Jersey according to the Medical Society of New Jersey and about six hundred "regular" physicians. Holden appears to have been cautiously receptive to homeopathic remedies that seemed to him to be sound.[142]

In a proving, the subject took a specified dose of a drug and recorded every bodily sensation, however trivial, for hours or days. The homeopaths (marginalized and excluded by "regular" physicians from mainstream professional societies) claimed the ability to tease out those symptoms and sensations that were due to the administered drug. They then applied the homeopathic principles of infinitesimals and "like cures like" to prepare and prescribe highly diluted dosages of the same drug. Holden did not subscribe to homeopathy, but he did attempt to note every bodily sensation that followed the dose of a drug he wished to test.

Holden's experiments drew the attention of homeopath Timothy F. Allen, editor of the exhaustive twelve volume reference work, *The Encyclopedia of Pure Materia Medica: A Record of the Positive Effects of Drugs upon the Healthy Human Organism*. Holden's sphygmographic experiments on cannabis indica and gelseminum (see below) were reprinted verbatim as authoritative "provings" along with several of his sphygmographic tracings.[143] It is likely that Holden was unaware that his work was being appropriated by homeopath Allen; had he granted permission for inclusion

---

[142] Holden, *The Sphygmograph*, 151–53; Edgar Holden, "Gelseminum for Hectic," *Medical Record* (New York) 15 (1879): 202–3; For a brief description of "provings," see Rothstein, *American Physicians in the 19th Century*, 154–56.

[143] Note on Holden's experiments with cannabis in Timothy F. Allen, ed. *The Encyclopedia of Pure Materia Medica: A Record of the Positive Effects of Drugs upon the Healthy Human Organism* (New York: Boericke and Tafel, 1875, 1876), 2:489–92; reproduced syphymograms between 2:492–93. Note on Holden's experiments with gelseminum (gelsemium) appear on 4:386; reproduced sphygmograms between 4:396–97.

of his experiments in a homeopathic reference work, he might have faced censure from his colleagues in the Medical Society of New Jersey.

THE PHARMACEUTICAL AUTHORITY AND THE ROLE OF THE SPHYGMOGRAPH

Holden emphasized the potential of the sphygmograph for identifying physiological effects of drugs *before* the patient experienced symptoms and *before* the physician could detect signs of efficacy or toxicity. Sphygmographic changes, in contemporary terms, could serve as "guides to the exhibition of drugs." (Historian Charles E. Rosenberg explains the use of the commonly used expression, "exhibition of drugs" as a "sacramental role in the ritual of healing" that doctor, patient, and family all witnessed.)[144] Holden was also hopeful that the device might prove useful in the study and treatment of poisoning.

The traditional source of therapeutic authority was cumulative and personal experience at the bedside. Medications such as calomel (a toxic mercurial laxative), the "sheet rock of therapy," or tartar emetic (an antimony preparation) *worked*, as Rosenberg noted, "by providing visible and predictable physiological effects."[145] In the new system of scientific medicine, therapies *worked* because they were found to work in the laboratory, or because objective signs such as the pulse or temperature normalized. In Holden's self-experiments with the sphygmograph, changes in his inscribed pulse wave often preceded any detectable symptoms or signs. The sphygmograph, in this case, was the source of authority, even more reliable than the physician-subject himself in detecting subtle departures from normal.

These ideas had great promise and appeal. Joel Seaverns of Boston told the Norfolk (Massachusetts) District Medical Society in 1871 that modern science would be the key to the introduction of new drugs. Older empirical remedies would be confirmed and justified by new physiological and pharmaceutical science. Seaverns was hopeful that the physiology and bacteriology laboratories would help solve "the long vexed question" of the

---

[144] Holden, *The Sphygmograph*, 133; Charles E. Rosenberg, "The Therapeutic Revolution: Medicine, Meaning, and Social Change in Nineteenth-Century America," in *The Therapeutic Revolution: Essays in the Social History of Medicine*, ed. Morris J. Vogel and Charles E. Rosenberg (Philadelphia: University of Pennsylvania Press, 1979), 10.

[145] Rosenberg, "Therapeutic Revolution," 15. Homeopathy fluorished in part because it's useless but harmless dilute drugs were more palatable to patients than the useless but harmful and toxic preparations of mainstream practice.

healing power of pharmaceuticals versus the healing power of nature. He looked forward to the promise of a new effective armamentarium. The physician of the future would be more valued for his therapeutic skills, replacing the iconic master physician "who is great in diagnosis."[146]

CANNABIS

In his first set of self-experiments, Holden took varying doses of an alcoholic extract of *Cannabis indica*, usually in the evening, and recorded his symptoms and his pulse over a few hours. On one occasion, he began a trial of cannabis while "feeling not [as] well as usual owing to overwork," confirming that this was indeed private science by a busy practitioner. His recorded responses to various doses included "lightness," "nervous and excited," "drowsy and calm," "an indefinable sensation of comfort," and "slightly exhilarated." During the fourth and last trial, using a fresh alcoholic extract of cannabis, Holden experienced "terrific excitement, twitchings, dreams . . . painful insomnia, and feeling of desperate recklessness." The following morning, he felt hungover with "head swollen, confusion of ideas." Serial sphygmographic tracings, performed by and on himself, "exhibited great weakness of cardiac power." To the modern eye, such self-experimentation conducted by an obviously impaired experimenter/subject could have little validity. Holden concluded that "the nervous system was broken down by the excitement of reaction, a state lasting for 12 hours."[147]

GELSEMINUM

In a second set of drug trials, Holden experimented with an extract of *gelseminum* [also *gelsemium*] *semipervirens* or yellow jessamine. Although gelseminum was usually relegated to the homeopathic and eclectic armamentaria, Holden had "a somewhat large personal experience" with the drug, having found it useful in "puerperal eclampsia [toxemia of

---

[146] Joel Seaverns, "Recent Advances in Medicine and Their Influence on Therapeutics," *Boston Medical and Surgical Journal*, n.s., 8 (1871): 113–20.

[147] Holden, *The Sphygmograph*, 133–49. A British prescribing guide, republished in the United States in 1855, indicates that Indian hemp (*Cannabis sativa*) or the European variety (*Cannabis indica*) were used for their "narcotic, anodyne, and antispasmodic" properties. They were known to produce "a peculiar kind of delirium and catalepsy." Henry Beasley, *The Book of Prescriptions* (Philadelphia: Lindsay & Blakiston, 1855), 116–17.

pregnancy] and the convulsive disorders of children, the neuralgic and congestive affections of the uterus or ovaries, and particularly in cardiac and pulmonary disease, where sedation and reduction in frequency of the pulse have been desired."[148]

Holden was familiar with the medical literature, and was aware that the eminent Jacob M. DaCosta of Philadelphia had an "unfavorable opinion . . . as to [gelseminum's] action in irritable heart," a functional cardiac disorder seen often in Civil War soldiers, as it was "supposed to have properties as a cardiac sedative" but often had no effect at all.[149] Popular in America for a wide range of symptoms, gelseminum was known to cause paralysis in high doses and fatalities had been reported. Citing a 1873 entry in the *Proceedings of the American Pharmaceutical Association*, authoritative British authors, writing in *The Lancet*, cited progressive neurological and cardiorespiratory deterioration following toxic doses.[150] Holden, always well-informed, would have proceeded with due caution.

Following a self-administered dose, Holden noted "a peculiar sense of weight over forehead," "constriction at the base of the tongue," "peculiar slowness of respiration" (seven per minute), and "giddiness." The sphygmograph, he stressed, showed the "action of the remedy often long prior to the exhibition of any sensible or physiologic effect." The tracings showed fluctuations in arterial tension and "nervous stimulation," in addition to a rather ominous "irregularity of impulse and of rhythm" reflecting the "effect of the poison on the heart." The sphygmographic changes persisted after the drug's detectable symptomatic effects had worn off.[151]

Holden continued to place considerable faith in gelseminum (as used by sensible adherents to "dogmas or favored tenets," a reference to homeopaths). He later reasoned that gelseminum, as a respiratory sedative, would prove particulalry useful in the "hectic" fevers associated with consumption (tuberculosis). His article, "Gelseminum for Hectic," was published in the *Medical Record* (New York) in 1879. Holden was careful

---

[148] Holden, *The Sphygmograph*, 151–53; Holden, "Gelseminum for Hectic," 202–3.

[149] Jacob M. DaCosta, "On Irritable Heart: A Clinical Study of a Form of Functional Cardiac Disorder and Its Consequences," *American Journal of the Medical Sciences* 61 (1871): 45–46.

[150] Sydney Ringer and William Murrell, "On Gelseminum Semipervirens," *Lancet* 2 (1875): 907. In his article published in 1879, Holden acknowledged the serious side effects, but considered toxicity dose-related. Holden, "Gelseminum for Hectic," 202–3.

[151] Holden, *The Sphygmograph*, 150–53.

to qualify his professional brush with homeopathy, citing his discussions with homeopaths of "common sense."[152]

ACONITE

In a third series of drug experiments, Holden administered aconite (monkshood) to both himself and a healthy eighteen-year-old woman. Aconite was a popular and fairly toxic drug classified as an "arterial sedative" and anodyne (analgesic). The author of a mid-century prescription book warned, "A slight increase in the quantity or frequency of the dose may be attended with fatal effects."[153] Physicians routinely used "arterial sedatives," including aconite, to reduce febrile or overstimulated states; such drugs were considered a substitute for phlebotomy (bloodletting), with the goal of relaxing the arteries while preserving the circulating blood volume.[154] The female subject experienced dizziness and changes in her sphygmographic tracings. In himself, Holden recorded slowing of the pulse, "fullness in carotids," faintness, and "cerebral excitement." The serial sphygmograms showed that aconite, unlike gelseminum, "while primarily showing a stage of exctiement, yet reduces the heart's action as to frequency of beat without increasing arterial tension."[155]

QUININE

Holden's fourth and final set of drug experiments involved quinine, a well-established specific remedy in malarial fevers and a drug widely overused as a non-specific tonic. Cinchona, or "bark" had long been known as an effective agent for malaria, often called "intermittent fever" or "ague." Quinine was isolated from the cinchona bark in 1820, and by the middle of the century was being used indiscriminately for a wide variety of fevers and inflammations; it was known to depress cardiac action. By the 1870s, quinine was something of a panacea, not only for fevers, but also as a tonic. Toxicity, referred to as "cinchonism," was frequently seen with the large doses often prescribed; symptoms included gastrointestinal irritation,

---

[152] Holden, "Gelseminum for Hectic," 202–3.
[153] Beasley, *Book of Prescriptions*, 31.
[154] Rothstein, *American Physicians*, 187. Veratrum viride, an extract of false hellebore, was similarly used to relax the arteries and carried significant toxicity.
[155] Holden, *The Sphygmograph*, 154–57.

weakening of the pulse, nervousness, tinnitus (ringing in the ears), and visual disturbances.[156]

Holden self-administered the drug both in a single large dose and as multiple small doses. The sphygmographic changes, which preceded the onset of symptoms, included decreased pulse rate, decreased tension, and the development of a "vibratile character" to the tracings. Symptoms of neck tension and excitement of the nervous system were superimposed on the "fatigue and excitement due to the arduous work of the day just closed." Holden passed a bad night indeed, his sleep disturbed by "nervous jactitation [thrashing] and twitching," urinary frequency and "vesical [bladder] spasm after each attempt," and "severe neuralgic or congestive pain under the left nipple." Upon awakening, he felt "all the sensations common to a man after a night of dissipation and excess." The sphygmographic tracings reflected in their changing wave forms the alarming symptoms.[157] With that unhappy experiment, Holden concluded his venture into self-experimentation with vasoactive drugs.

A CAUTIOUS ASSESSMENT

In summarizing the results of his work with the sphygmograph prior to the publication of his book, Holden frankly admitted the "somewhat diffuse exposition of the subject," but offered three conclusions. Firstly, his modification of the instrument "exhibits a new and wider field as within its scope." Secondly, he felt that he had contributed to showing the "value of a knowledge of the minute peculiarities of the arterial current, in connection with the determination of the condition of both the vascular and nervous system." Thirdly, he believed that he had demonstrated "the power of the sphygmograph to develop this knowledge [i.e., of arterial blood flow] and correctly record it." He anticipated, wrongly as it turned out, that "both the pathological and physiological indications afforded by the instrument are of great importance" and "deeper meaning probably lies in the tracings than has yet been revealed."[158]

It is evident in retrospect that Holden overinterpreted many of the tracings, failing to take into consideration the vagaries of the instrument. In analyzing the recorded pulsewave patterns, Holden considered the patient's history and always sought to correlate stethoscopic findings with

---

[156] For a discussion of quinine, See Rothstein, *American Physicians*, 187–89.

[157] Holden, *The Sphygmograph*, 158–61.

[158] Ibid., 162–63.

sphygmographic tracings. Warning about the dangers of overreliance on the sphygmograph in making a diagnosis, he wrote:

> The reader is desired not to consider the tracings of cases as the universal and invariable exponents of individual diseases. Such could only be obtained after long and patient investigation into every variety and phase of disease, and is equivalent to making a new symptomatology, a task indeed for a generation of observers. They will, however, probably prove in all cases suggestive of the pathological conditions involved.[159]

Holden admitted that the novice might easily become discouraged by the apparently cryptic tracings: "To the professional reader, who looks over a multitude of sphygmographic tracings, the first impression is not infrequently one of disappointment. There is a sameness at first apparent, which would tend to suggest the inefficiency of the instrument as a means of diagnosis, or even of ordinary usefulness."[160] And much work remained to be done, most importantly, in his view, the completion of a "dictionary"—a sort of atlas:

> . . . to which each individual tracing, can be referred for interpretation, and towards this object these [i.e., his own] tracings are a contribution. . . . Careful scrutiny and comparison [of tracings in his book] are invited, since the more minutely they have been studied by myself the more firmly has the conviction grown that our present attempts at translation [from tracing to diagnosis] are defective, and that there yet may be found new keys that will unlock features of new interest.[161]

His work to date, Holden continued, was merely a "tangible starting point for other observers" in a field which was heretofore "pathless and virtually unexplored," something of a misstatement in view of the work of Burdon-Sanderson and others.[162] Holden invited the reader to judge for himself: "Whether the [technical] defects that have so nearly wrecked the science of Sphygmography, ere it had well begun its career, have been fully corrected by the means described or not [i.e., Holden's changes and

---

[159] Ibid., 10.
[160] Ibid., 87.
[161] Ibid., 89.
[162] Ibid., 9–10.

modifications], the reader, who will patiently review the results obtained, will be able to judge." Furthermore, he stressed that his own instrument was less expensive and provided a "more ready applicability."[163] At the time his book appeared (1874), the sphygmograph remained a work in progress. Within a few years, Holden would become increasingly pessimistic about the sphygmograph.

REVIEWS AND SALES OF THE HOLDEN MONOGRAPH

Dalton (writing as J.C.D.), having judged Holden's essay for the Stevens Prize, wrote a lukewarm review of *The Sphygmograph: Its Physiological and Pathological Indications* for the *American Journal of the Medical Sciences*. Without committing himself to any predictions about the sphygmograph, Dalton described Holden's work as "interesting," and lauded the careful selection of tracings to "illustrate all the important points to which the reader's attention is directed."[164]

Holden's monograph was more enthusiastically reviewed in the Montreal-based *Canadian Medical and Surgical Journal*. The lengthy unsigned review described Holden's modifications to the Marey sphygmograph and cited his "entirely original" results:

> This study is well worth the attention of every physician wishing to keep up the knowledge of his times, and we therefore cordially recommend Dr. Holden's essay. . . . We are glad to learn that one of these instruments according to Dr. Holden's pattern has already been ordered from Boston for the Montreal General Hospital, for use by the Attending Staff and Clinical Classes.[165]

The monograph probably sold several hundred copies, judging by its presence in many archival collections. The copy at the College of Physicians of Philadelphia was owned by Edward Hartshorne, a well-educated Philadelphia physician with two years of post-graduate observation in

---

[163] Ibid., 28.

[164] J[ohn] C[all] D[alton], "*The Sphygmograph: Its Physiological and Pathological Indications*, by Edgar Holden" (review), *American Journal of the Medical Sciences* 67 (1874): 478–80.

[165] "*The Sphygmograph: Its Physiological and Pathological Indications*, by Edgar Holden" (review), *Canada Medical and Surgical Journal* 2 (1874): 492–95.

European schools and hospitals. Hartshorne distinguished himself in Philadelphia medical circles as a prison physician, physician to asylums for the insane, and surgeon. He published articles in respected medical journals and lectured on medical jurisprudence. He was attending surgeon at Wills Hospital for the Blind and Lame and at the Pennsylvania Hospital and served as a manager in the latter hospital as well as the Episcopal Hospital of Philadelphia. In short, Hartshorne was a member of the elite medical community of Philadelphia practitioners. His memorialist recalled that Hartshorne "was ever ready to avail himself of new discoveries applicable in practice."[166] Holden's book was not published until Hartshorne was fifty-six years old. Whether or not Hartshorne used his sphygmograph in practice or read Holden's book in any detail is unknown. But he seems to have been the sort of engaged urban practitioner who might have been attracted to the promising new technology of the sphygmograph.

It is not known how many Holden model sphygmographs were constructed; there is no evidence that other physicians in the United States used the Holden instrument despite its appearance in a number of medical/surgical catalogues, usually in the company of better-known instruments. At least one Holden sphygmograph was on order, as noted, by the Montreal General Hospital. No examples of any Holden instruments have been located in museums or private collections, including the collection of five sphygmographs at the College of Physicians of Philadelphia.[167]

APPLICATIONS IN MEDICAL PRACTICE

Holden was called in consultation from time to time by his Essex County colleagues and he used his sphygmograph in a number of cases. In a paper on cardiac pathology read before the New Jersey Academy of Medicine in 1875, Holden recalled the case of a forty-five-year old physician with presumed acute pericarditis (inflammation of the sac around the heart). When first seen by Holden in consultation, there had been "no particle of amelioration" from "antiphlogistic and counter-irritant treatment." Holden

---

[166] Henry Hartshorne, "Memoir of Edward Hartshorne, A.M., M.D., (1818–1885), Read October 6, 1886." *Transactions of the College of Physicians of Philadelphia* 16 (1887): 425–34.

[167] Of the seven sphygmographs in the photographic section of Naqvi and Blaufox's *Blood Pressure Measurement* there is no Holden instrument. N. H. Naqvi and M. D. Blaufox, *Blood Pressure Measurement: An Illustrated History* (New York: Parthenon, 1998), 108–12; information about College of Physicians collection, courtesy late curator Gretchen Worden.

took a thorough history, conducted a detailed cardiovascular examination, and used his sphygmograph to record a pulse tracing. This "verified the belief [i.e. Holden's belief based on clinical examination] that the disease was not in [the patient's] heart." He astutely diagnosed quinine toxicity due to vigorous self-prescribing of tonic quinine by the overworked and exhausted doctor. Holden may have been particularly alert to quinine toxicity after his own unfortunate sphygmographic experiment with self-administration of the drug. The patient recovered with discontinuation of quinine, although Holden attributed improvement to medicinal alcohol and strychnia. The paper was later published in the *American Journal of the Medical Sciences*.[168]

In a case of severe cardiac disease due to a damaged aortic valve, Holden's evaluation included a sphygmographic tracing that showed "impulse exaggerated and some increase of arterial tension." He successfully administered amyl nitrite when the clinical conditions worsened and appeared hopeless. He followed the case for about a month, but did not repeat the sphymographic study.[169] The key point in these case reports is Holden's use of the sphygmograph in his capacity as a consultant and his reliance on a detailed patient history and physical examination, with the sphygmograph providing confirmatory evidence.

HOLDEN'S HONORARY DOCTORATE

Holden's work with the sphygmograph earned him modest renown and an honorary doctorate from Princeton in 1874. His nomination was supported by Princeton trustee Samuel Pennington, a Newark physician and bank president, who stressed in his letter of support addressed to Rev. Dr. McCosh (James McCosh, president of Princeton from 1868 to 1888) that the sphygmograph work had "cost Dr. H. much study, labor and expense." But Holden, continued Pennington, looked for "no pecuniary reward from his instrument or his book, very properly regarding it unprofessional to take out a patent." The petition was successful and Holden was accordingly awarded the advanced degree.[170]

---

[168] Edgar Holden, "Anomalies in Cardiac Pathology," *American Journal of the Medical Sciences* 70 (1875): 97–98; quinine experiments in Holden, *The Sphygmograph*, 158–61.

[169] Edgar Holden, "Successful (Internal) Use of Nitrite of Amyl in Dilated Heart with Aortic Regurgitation," *Medical Record* (New York) 13 (1878): 324–25.

[170] S. H. Pennington, Newark, to Rev. Dr. McCosh, Princeton, March 25, 1874, Alumni Records, Undergraduate, Box 116 (Class of 1859), Folder "Holden, Edgar," Princeton University Archives–Rare Books and Special Collections.

Unlike many honorary degrees, Holden's was well and truly earned; his work with the sphygmograph was equal to any academic work of the day. He justifiably added the degree "Ph.D." after his name on many of his later publications. Perhaps most telling is the title page of the family copy of *The Sphygmograph*; after the author's name, Edgar Holden, A.M., M.D., was added lightly in pencil—either by Holden or his wife—"PhD."[171]

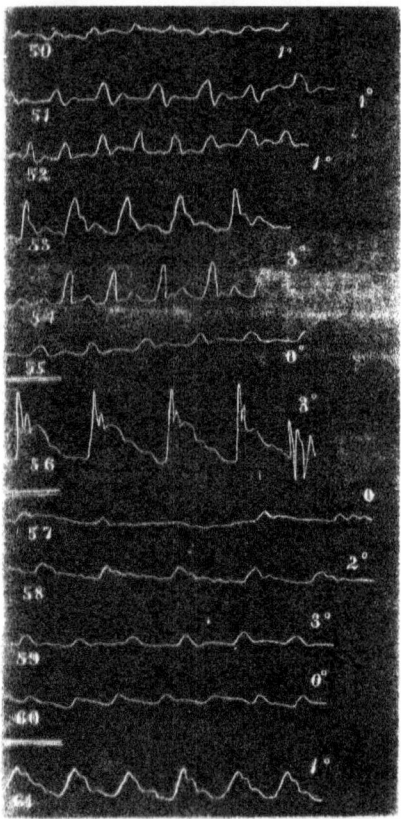

FIGURE 44: Holden's "sphygmographic hieroglyphics," a sample series of tracings in cases of pericarditis with effusion (inflamed sac around the heart with fluid build-up, tracings 50–55); dropsical stage of cardiac hypertrophy with regurgitation (severe heart failure with valve disease, tracing 56); slight cardiac hypertrophy and a heart murmur (tracings 57–60). The subtle distinctions in each tracing are difficult to appreciate. Edgar Holden, *The Sphygmograph: Its Physiological and Pathological Indications -- The Essay to Which was Awarded the*

---

[171] William B. Birdsall, family collection.

"Sphygmographic Hieroglyphics":
The Amateur Science of Edgar Holden

Stevens Triennial Prize, by the College of Physicians and Surgeons, New York, April, 1873 (Philadelphia: Lindsay & Blakiston, 1874), following page 169.

"ERRORS OF THE SPHYGMOGRAPH"

From Holden's earliest articles and his book on the sphygmograph, hints of frustration—tempered with hope for the future—were evident. As early as 1871, he observed with an air of frustration that the essentials of the sphygmograph were simple, but practical application difficult: "Refine the parts to a marvelous degree of delicacy, obtain the movements of the lever over the artery, and move the paper or other receiver with the utmost precision, yet, apply the pen to the paper and the infinitesimal friction stops its movement; a hair, even, will render it motionless."[172]

In 1877, Holden published one final article on the sphygmograph. The title tells the story. "Errors of the Sphygmograph" was a combined valedictory ode to his brief but intense venture into physiological research, a requiem for the sphygmograph, and an avuncular charge to the next generation. "It seemed appropriate," he wrote, "that one who, in a measure a pioneer, had so pressed an unproved science before the profession should abandon the field to other workers." Holden invoked the *accoucheur* (medical attendant at a birth) metaphor so beloved by physicians of the day: "That, as a science, [sphygmography] is yet hardly more than embryonic, is evident; and that through differences among its *accoucheurs* it may never survive delivery, seems its present greatest danger." His earlier hope that pathognomonic tracings would aid in the diagnosis of specific diseases was never realized. The sphygmograph, he declared, "never can become, the sole means of determining disease." Attempts to establish characteristic patterns was apt to lead to errors of "comparison, observation, and of interpretation." The chief fault was not so much the limited technology, but rather that "too much is expected of it."[173]

McBRIDE: AN ENTHUSIASTIC AMERICAN VOICE

Not every American sphygmograph user was as pessimistic as Holden about the future of the instrument. Thomas A. McBride, gifted young New York graduate of the College of Physicians and Surgeons, was intimately familiar with the European literature. McBride summarized the status

---

[172] Holden, "Circulatory Physiology and the Sphygmograph," 48.
[173] Edgar Holden, "Errors of the Sphygmograph," *New York Medical Journal* 26 (1877): 498–99.

of the sphygmograph in the *Archives of Medicine*, an American journal, in 1879. Most physicians, wrote McBride, look on the sphygmograph as a toy or as a complicated piece of machinery. But it was his belief that many of the problems had been solved and the limitations of the instrument understood. Although he listed the Holden sphygmograph among his references, McBride did not comment on it in the text. He favored the classic Marey sphygmograph, a British modification of the Marey sphygmograph, and a novel American instrument developed by Vermont physician Erasmus Pond. (see Chapter 6)

The sphygmograph, McBride said, "should be in every-day use . . . of greatest value and assistance to the general practitioner." Attention must be paid, however, to each element of the pulse tracing. The physician must note the pressure applied to the artery (taking several tracings at various pressures) and the conditions under which the tracing was recorded. McBride closed by predicting that tracings made (and interpreted) with such care "will than fill their proper part in the induction which furnishes the diagnosis, prognosis or indications for therapeusis, and sphygmographic observations, will receive the attention and consideration which they deserve."[174]

Edgar Holden deserves lasting credit for recognizing almost immediately the potential promise of the newly invented Marey sphygmograph and for proceeding with sophisticated experiments with his own modified instrument. The fact that the technology ultimately proved disappointing, both in Europe and America, does not detract from his position as America's first sphygmograph man.

Holden's sphygmograph was created and lived its short life in a uniquely American practice and research environment. The following chapters describe the research of Alonzo T. Keyt of Cincinnati and the commercial efforts of Erasmus A. Pond of Rutland, Vermont, sphygmograph men whose American practice and research environments were distinctly different from those of Holden.

---

[174] Thomas A. McBride, "The Utility of the Sphygmograph in Medicine." *Archives of Medicine* 1 (1879): 184; 196–97.

Chapter 5

Alonzo Thrasher Keyt:
The Elegant Chrono-Cardio-Sphygmograph

While Edgar Holden simply modified the Marey sphygmograph, two American sphygmograph men independently developed novel instruments. Alonzo Thrasher Keyt of Cincinnati, Ohio, created an elegant instrument with which he conducted detailed experiments in cardiovascular physiology. His research, including investigations on healthy volunteers and clinical studies of hospital patients, led to a series of articles in prominent regional and national medical journals. Erasmus Allington Pond of Rutland, Vermont, successfully marketed his portable sphygmograph model, though he had little interest in physiological or clinical investigations. Keyt, through his research, and Pond, through his commercial efforts, gained the attention of European sphygmographers. The events surrounding the inventions and experiments of these unremarked physicians tell us much about American medical research in the late nineteenth century.[1] Pond's work with the sphygmograph is the subject of Chapter 6.

It was not unusual for local practitioners in nineteenth-century America to experiment with new medical therapies and technologies. Not only surgeons, but general practitioners as well, needed "craft knowledge" and had to "learn how to play with new instruments and devices to make them work." Devices that allowed examiners to detect the inner workings

---

[1] Sandra W. Moss, "Profiles in Cardiology: Alonzo Thrasher Keyt," *Clinical Cardiology* 29 (2006): 471–73; Sandra W. Moss, "The Sphygmograph in America: Writing the Pulse," *American Journal of Cardiology* 97 (2006): 580–87.

of the body "symbolized their newfound power" rooted in science and technology. New devices or modifications of older instruments were often discussed at local medical society meetings and were the frequent subject of brief reports in journals and published transactions. Particularly in the United States, the introduction of handmade devices reflected the practical nature of clinical medicine.[2]

PORTRAIT OF ALONZO THRASHER KEYT

Ohio sphygmograph man Alonzo Thrasher Keyt (1827–1885) was a master tinkerer, as were sphygmograph men everywhere. Keyt was a graduate of the Medical College of Ohio. He was selected by competitive examination for an internship at the Cincinnati Hospital, an early sign of promise. Setting up practice in Walnut Hills, a small settlement just outside Cincinnati, he supported his large family as a general practitioner.

Keyt was known locally as a careful diagnostician. "Although as gentle as a woman," Keyt was "bold and resourceful" in an emergency and "excelled as an obstetrician" who was skilled in the use of forceps and the management of difficult labors. He was an active member of the Ohio State Medical Society and the American Medical Association, where he presented some of his research. Keyt was described by his devoted son-in-law, Asa B. Isham, M.D., as "sedate, almost grave, slow and deliberate in action, in accordance with the Dutch blood coursing in his veins."[3] Certainly, he seemed to have been suited for a life in research. However, like the vast majority of contemporary physicians, he relied on general medical practice for his income.

THE KEYT SPHYGMOSCOPE: REINVENTING THE HÉRISSON SPHYGMOMETER

Keyt began his own inventive work by devising a simple sphygmoscope (sphygmometer) in the summer of 1874 "and in the early autumn I showed

---

[2] Joel D. Howell (ed.), "Introduction," in *Technology and American Medical Practice: An Anthology of Sources* (New York: Garland, 1988), xi.

[3] Asa B. Isham, "A Sketch of the Life and Work of Alonzo Thrasher Keyt," *Philadelphia Monthly Medical Journal*, 1 (1899): 726–27; A[sa] B. I[sham], "Keyt, Alonzo Thrasher," in *A Cyclopedia of American Medical Biography*, ed. Howard A. Kelly (Philadelphia: W. B. Saunders, 1912), 2:65–66; [Asa B. Isham], "Alonzo Thrasher Keyt," in *Daniel Drake and His Followers—Historical and Biographical Sketches, 1785-1909*, ed. Otto Juettner, 463–65. Cincinnati: Harvey Publishing, 1909.

to friends the beautiful undulations in the glass tube caused by pulsations of the artery."[4] Keyt's non-recording sphygmoscopes (and his later recording sphygmographs) were constructed on the principle of hydraulic displacement in response to the movements of the artery or the cardiac impulse. In his simple sphygmoscope, conceived in mid-1874, a vertical glass column was marked off in quarter inches and was fitted over a brass bulb filled with water and covered at the bottom by a rubber membrane. The membrane was pressed against an artery (or the chest wall overlying the cardiac apex) and and the water rose and fell in the narrow glass tube with each pulsation: "These undulations are true and exact pulsations of the artery, transferred to the liquid in the tube."[5]

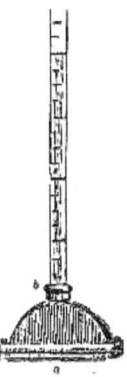

FIGURE 45: Keyt sphygmometer (sphygmoscope) incorporating a sensor of brass covered with a thin rubber membrane and filled with water. When the instrument was pressed down on the radial artery or over the cardiac apex, fluid rose and fell in a glass tube allowing the physician to see the fluctuations of the pulse or the impulse of the heart against the chest wall. Alonzo Thrasher Keyt, "The New Sphygmograph; Or, Instrument Adapted as a Sphygmograph, Sphygmometer, Cardiograph, Cardiometer, and to Other Uses," *New York Medical Journal* 23 (1876): 28.

This appears to have been an independent reinvention, as Keyt was unaware at the time of the Hérisson sphygmoscope or of any other similar device. Hérisson's sphygmoscope, described in his monograph of 1835,

---

[4] Alonzo T. Keyt, "The New Sphygmograph" (correspondence), *New York Medical Journal* 23 (1876): 507

[5] Alonzo T. Keyt, "The New Sphygmograph; Or, Instrument Adapted as a Sphygmograph, Sphgymometer, Cardiograph, Cardiometer, and to Other Use," *New York Medical Journal* 23 (1876): Ibid., 28–31.

was generally not mentioned in articles by Burdon-Sanderson, Anstie, Holden, Pond, or Keyt. Hérisson's original work, in French or in either of the two English translations (British and American), may not have been available to Keyt working in Cincinnati (see Chapter 2). Keyt's son-in-law Isham noted, "In 1874 Dr. A. T. Keyt devised a sphygmometer, at that time unaware that M. le Docteur Hérisson, in 1835, had constructed an instrument similar in principle but different in mechanism." Keyt also commented on the Scott Alison sphygmoscopes of two decades earlier (1856), noting that he (Keyt) was gratified to learn that Scott Alison had invented a similar instrument, something of a retrospective confirmation of the validity of Keyt's independent invention.[6]

Keyt's first improvment on his original sphygmogsope was designed to amplify the pulsatile rise and fall of the water in the glass tubing. He shortened the glass column so that the liquid pulsations peaked just above the upper rim, now expanded into a small cone shape. A thin elastic membrane was fitted over the conic upper margin of the glass column. The pulsations were transmitted via a pin and lever from the elastic membrane and amplified such that the observer could watch the swing of the tip of the lever rather than the rise and fall of the liquid column.[7]

A NEW SPHYGMOGRAPH—IMPROVING ON MAREY, DISMISSING HOLDEN

From sphygmoscope to sphygmograph was a logical step for someone with Keyt's wide knowledge of the literature and a passion for technology and pulse study. In his first major paper in an Eastern medical journal (*New York Medical Journal*, January 1876), he was dutifully respectful of Marey's sphygmograph ("a very fair instrument"). But, based on his own experience with the Marey device, found much to criticize.[8] A posthumous biographical sketch by Isham explains that in 1873, "Dr. Keyt's attention was attracted to the consideration of the graphic method in the portrayal of the movements of the circulation," at which point he began experimenting with the Marey sphygmograph. But he found "M. Mavy's [sic, referring

---

[6] For Hérisson's and Scott Alison's sphygmoscopes or sphygmometers, see Chapter 2. Alonzo T. Keyt, *Sphygmography and Cardiography: Physiological and Clinical*, ed. Asa B. Isham and M. H. Keyt (New York: G. P. Putnam's Sons, 1887), 3; Asa B. Isham, M.D. and M. H. Keyt, M.D. (probably a son) edited Keyt's published articles and combined them into the monograph posthumously; Keyt, "New Sphygmograph," 56.

[7] Keyt, "New Sphygmograph," 29–39.

[8] Ibid., 26–27.

to Marey] spring instrument" insensitive, claiming that the Marey spring mechanism "did not furnish all the undulations of the blood-column to the slide [smoked-glass recording strip]."[9]

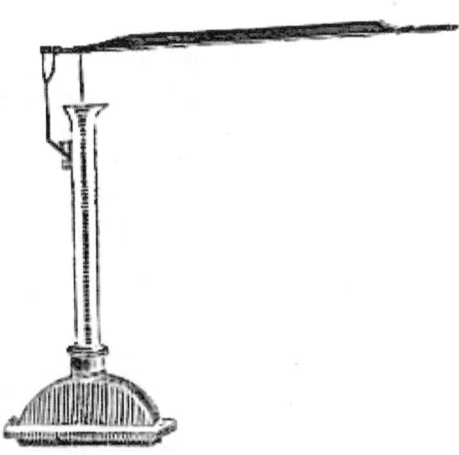

FIGURE 46: The modified Keyt sphygmometer incorporating a wide upright tube filled with water to the brim. A thin elastic membrane covered the top of the tube and moved slightly as the water impinged against it with each pulse beat. The movement of the membrane was multiplied by an attached lever, so that observers could see the wide swing of the free end of the lever. Alonzo Thrasher Keyt, "The New Sphygmograph; Or, Instrument Adapted as a Sphygmograph, Sphygmometer, Cardiograph, Cardiometer, and to Other Uses," *New York Medical Journal* 23 (1876): 29.

Keyt judged the Marey sphygmograph difficult and time-consuming to use, applicable only to the radial artery (the usual site of palpating the pulse in the wrist), and possessing no refinement whatever in its "crude and very defective" provision for estimating the compressibility of the pulse. Furthermore, he proclaimed that the Marey sphygmograph "was not growing in favor with the profession," which was true for general practitioners, but failed to recognize its spotty popularity among research and specialty oriented elite physicians.

Keyt went on to criticize "our countryman" Holden's adaptations. Keyt was familiar with the Holden sphygmograph only through the latter's published monograph. He was unimpressed: "The tracings of this instrument, as published, certainly do not commend it. In a comparative

---

[9] I[sham], "Keyt, Alonzo Thrasher," 66.

estimate, I conceive that Holden's possesses no advantages over Marey's, and in point of fidelity of delineation is far inferior to it." As noted in the previous chapter Holden would effectively abandoned research with his sphygmograph by 1877, having publishing his discouraging valedictory article, "Errors of the Sphygmograph," in that year.

Keyt set out to design a sphygmograph combining convenience, adaptability, facility, and variety of use, with delicacy, precision, and truthfulness of delineation; and withal a simple and correct index of the pressure at which the tracings were taken."[10]

"SPHYGMOGRAPH/SPHYGMOMETER/ CARDIOGRAPH/CARDIOMETER"

In the latter half of 1874, Keyt designed a novel sphygmograph and recorded his first radial pulse tracing in December. By March 1875 his sphygmograph was in "good working order" and he was recording pulse tracings in patients.[11] He demonstrated his sphygmograph at the May 1875 meeting of the American Medical Association. An abstract of his paper (written by a Dr. Bartlett, secretary of the Section on Practical Medicine, Physiology, and Materia Medica; there was no illustration) was published in the *Medical Record* (New York). Keyt took care to emphasize the original design of his device while recognizing earlier sphygmographs designed by Marey:

> It is true, [Keyt] remarked, that the tambour polygraph [of Marey] and mercurial kymograph have points of suggestiveness, yet there is such a difference between these instruments and [my] own—difference in principle, in construction, in operation, and in results—that [I] did not hesitate to speak of the instrument which [I] presented as a new and distinct invention.[12]

In a lengthy 1876 article for the *New York Medical Journal*, evidently designed to introduce his sphygmograph (and himself) to the Eastern

---

[10] Keyt, "New Sphygmograph," 26–27.
[11] Keyt, "The New Sphygmograph" (correspondence), 507.
[12] Alonzo T. Keyt, "A New Sphygmograph—Elastic Membrane and Liquids for Transmitting the Pulsations of the Artery (abstract)," *Medical Record* (New York) 10 (1875): 365.

metropolitan medical establishment, Keyt detailed the evolution of his sphygmoscope into a novel and elegant sphygmograph, characterizing his creation as "an instrument adapted as a sphygmograph, sphygmometer, cardiograph, cardiometer, and to other uses."[13]

One arm of the apparatus consisted of the simple calibrated glass column (the vertical column could be folded to a horizontal position when not in use.) On the second arm was mounted a small reservoir capped by an elastic disc. A pin fixed in the disc moved a lever, the distal end of which inscribed the tracing—thus, a sphygmograph and a sphygmoscope in a single apparatus. The rubber-covered sensor (the portion of the instrument placed directly upon the artery, called by Keyt "the basal membrane") was connected by tubing and stopcocks to the arms of the instrument. The various tubes, chambers, and reservoirs were filled with water.

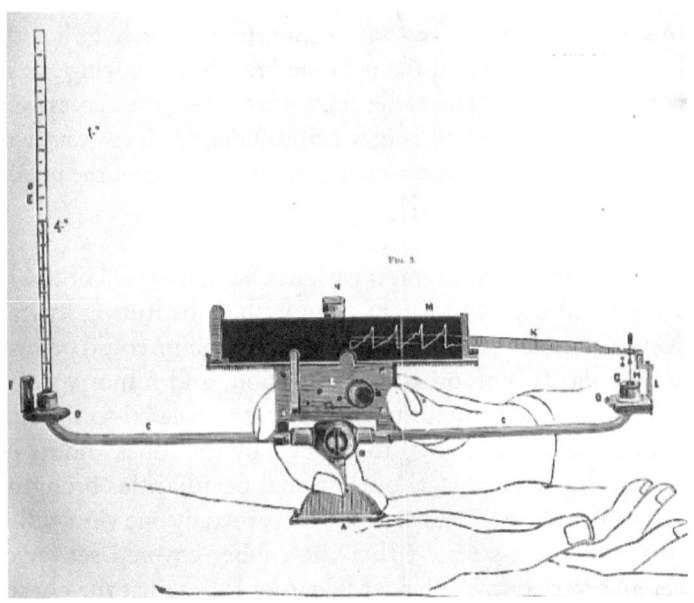

FIGURE 47: The basic Keyt sphygmograph with sphygmometer. By means of a stopcock, the operator could record a sphygmogram (right arm) or observe the pulse rising and falling in the sphygmometer (left arm). Alonzo Thrasher Keyt, "The New Sphygmograph; Or, Instrument Adapted as a Sphygmograph, Sphygmometer, Cardiograph, Cardiometer, and to Other Uses," *New York Medical Journal* 23 (1876): 31.

---

[13] Keyt, "The New Sphygmograph," 26.

Keyt evidently constructed (or more likely had constructed to his specifications by a local craftsman) several such standardized sphygmographs, referring to "uniformity in the instruments."[14] He added detailed (and somewhat daunting) directions for preparing the instrument for use and applying it to the artery. The column of water on one arm of the instrument (essentially a sphygmoscope or sphygmometer) served as a guide to determining the time at which the sphgymograph on the other arm of the instrument should be activated and a sphygmogram recorded:

> We place the base [the sensor pressed down upon the artery] lengthwise over the artery, hold it steady, and bear down gradually, keeping the eye in the mean time on the column in the tube. This will be seen to rise, pulsating as it rises. When the point of pressure is reached which yields the greatest sweep of oscillation, we reverse the stopcock, cutting off and holding this column *in situ* and restoring connection between the liquid in the base and that in the opposite branch, the tracing lever is set in motion. The same force that eased the successive undulations in the tube is now turned upon the lever, causing its movements [and producing a permanet tracing of the pulse waves—a sphygmogram].[15]

This early Keyt sphygmograph was, in effect, a hybrid of the Hérisson sphygmoscope and the Marey sphygmograph, substituting hydraulics for springs. Keyt claimed that with his sphygmograph he could determine the amplitude, regularity, compressibility, tension, and minor waves of each pulseform: "Thus all the qualities of the pulse revealed to the fingers are faithfully and beautifully shown to the eye, by the tubes and its pulsating column; and, more than this, the additional peculiarities brought to light by the sphygmograph may here often be discerned by one who will carefully look for them."[16] Keyt stressed that the rubber-covered sensor could be placed over an artery or over the cardiac impulse against the chest wall (in the recumbent patient), thus a "cardiograph" recording a "cardiogram." A simple elbow tube could be added to allow for "cardiograms" in the upright position.[17]

---

[14] Ibid., 34.
[15] Ibid., 35.
[16] Ibid., 30–38; quotation 38.
[17] Ibid., 39–40.

Tracings of Keyt's own pulse and that of a cardiac patient using both the Marey and Keyt sphygmographs were included in the article (Keyt was experienced in the use of the Marey sphygmograph). He was pleased to note that the tracings with the Keyt instrument were as good as those with the Marey sphygmograph: "Happily both instruments, differing as the principle of mechanism, give substantially the same result, which we may accept as confirmatory that both are good instruments. One proves the other." And, he added modestly, perhaps his own sphygmograph gave slightly better definition of the pulse waves.[18]

If placed over the chest wall, the instrument could record respiratory excursions, thus functioning as a pneumograph. Using two sphygmographs simultaneously, he could record paired arterial pulsations or paired cardiac and arterial pulsations. Like other sphygmographers, Keyt recorded serial pulses in various types of fevers. His article of some thirty pages was a *tour de force* of original thinking; what his instruments lacked in practicality, they made up for in beauty of design, clarity of recordings, and potential value to research in cardiovascular disease and clinical application.[19]

After his death, his son-in-law and biographer rhapsodized—with justification—over the quality of Keyt's sphygmograms: "This gave beautiful tracings, delineating perfectly in the sphygmogram all the pulse-waves, as well as also cardiogram, or tracings of the movements of the heart. For the first time became available for study and complete description the perfect human cardiogram and sphygmogram."[20]

KEYT'S MASTERPIECE: THE CHRONO-CARDIO-SPHYGMOGRAPH

Keyt soon came to believe that the standard sphygmographic tracings made by his predecessors had little clinical value. In the introduction to a compendium of Keyt's collected works the editors (a physician son and son-in-law) dismissed earlier instruments ("single sphygmographs" that recorded only a single pulse or a cardiac impulse), which had "contributed comparatively little of real value."[21]

---

[18] Ibid., 41–45.
[19] Ibid., 45–56.
[20] Isham, "Sketch of the Life and Work of Alonzo Thrasher Keyt," 727.
[21] Keyt, *Sphygmography and Cardiography*, 16. This was a somewhat myopic assessment, as the Keyts seemed to disregard the vital work of Mahomed, for example, who worked with a modified simple spygmograph to document essential hypertension; see

What was required, in Keyt's view, was a double (dual function) sphygmograph, with one component recording the apical pulsation of the heart (thus a cardiograph) and the other *simultaneously* recording an arterial pulsation (this might be the carotid artery or any other artery such as the brachial or radial in the upper extremity). The evolution, construction, and application of this new instrument was the subject of Keyt's detailed paper in the July 1877 *New York Medical Journal*.

On a single portable frame, Keyt mounted two sphymometers, two sphygmographs to record pulsations on a moving smoked glass plate, a pair of sensors for the heart and an artery, and an inscribing clockwork chronometer. The "output" of this intricate construction consisted of three simultaneously recorded tracks: a cardiac tracing, an arterial tracing (or two arterial tracings if an arterial abnormality was suspected), and a time line marked off in fifths of a second. The instrument itself was an elegant piece of mechanical and hydraulic engineering. Aesthetically, it was an *objet d'art*, with its tall glass columns and the visual impression of equipoise at the base.[22]

WATER OR AIR?

Keyt's complex cardiosphygmograph was, like his earlier devices, a hydraulic instrument, with water filling the tubes and columns. Keyt would later experiment with both water and air as mediums of transmission, comparing tracings made on himself and volunteers. Simultaneous pulse tracings of his right and left radial arteries—one with an air-filled column and the other with a water-filled column showed that both water and air could transmit the pulsations of the artery to the recording system. However, the hydraulic system produced a much higher amplitude pulse wave. He concluded: "Water transmits movements with much greater power than air, which gives it a wider range of appplication, embracing feeble movements that air is incapable of inscribing."[23]

Chapter 3).

[22] Alonzo T. Keyt, "Cardiographic and Sphygmographic Studies," *New York Medical Journal* 26 (1877): 24–26.

[23] Alonzo T. Keyt, "Experiments to Determine the Relative Merits of Water and Air as Media of Transmission for Sphygmographs," *Medical Record* (New York) 18 (1880): 479–82, quotation 482.

Alonzo Thrasher Keyt:
The Elegant Chrono-Cardio-Sphygmograph

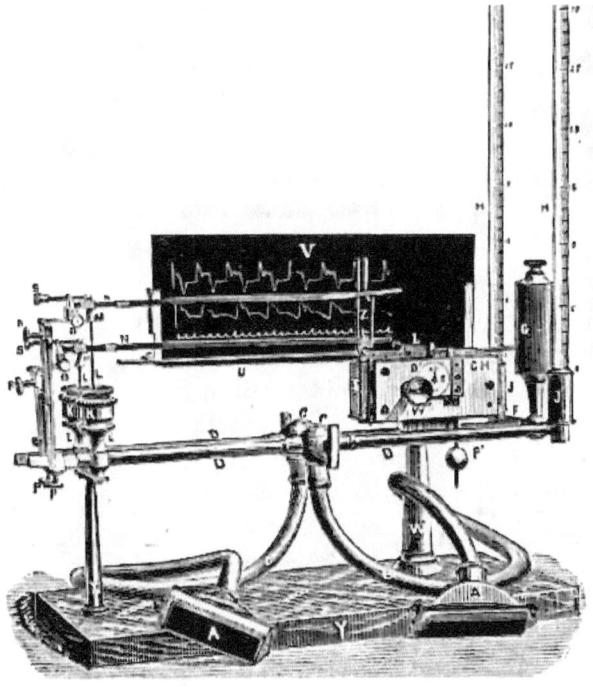

FIGURE 48: The Keyt chrono-cardio-sphygmograph, featuring two glass columns, two sphygmographs (or one cardiograph and one sphygmograph), an inscribing chronometer marking off time in fifths of a second, and two sensors. Tubes and columns were filled with water. The instrument simultaneously recorded a cardiac and a pulse tracing (or two pulse tracings) as well as time intervals. Alonzo T. Keyt, "Cardiographic and Sphygmographic Studies (I)," *New York Medical Journal* 26 (1877): 24.

EXPERIMENTING WITH THE SPHYGMOGRAPH

By 1877, Keyt was beginning to position himself as an expert and authority:

> My qualification for accurate work in this line of inquiry arises mainly from my experience in the use of certain instrumental devices and combinations, invented by myself, and peculiarly adapted to the purpose intended. In addition, I claim for myself a keen interest in the work and the excercise of scrupulous care at every step of its execution.[24]

---

[24] Alonzo T. Keyt, "Cardiographic and Sphygmographic Studies," 20.

Keyt began his experimental work with a vivisection experiment (the mark of a true experimental physiologist in the European tradition) on a living turtle with a portion of its lower shell removed. No doubt the turtle was chosen because of its slow heart rate. Keyt was able to correlate the cardiographic waves with the filling (diastole) and pumping (systole) cycles of the heart. He also recorded (through the chest wall) the pulsations of the heart of a toad and a kitten, noting the effects of respiration on the cardiac waves in the latter animal.[25]

Sphygmographic tracings together with auscultation of the heart sounds in a healthy human volunteer confirmed the evidence of his animal studies—proving to his satisfaction that the upstroke of the curve correlated with systole (contraction of the left ventricle as it pumps blood into the arterial circulation) and the downstroke with diastole (relaxation and filling of the left ventricle). Keyt considered it essential to demonstrate conclusively the correlation of the cardiac cycle with the basic upward and downward portions of the sphygmographic curve: "Until the relationship of the graphic lines to these two chief conditions of the heart's action is established, there can be no trustworthy interpretation of the cardiac and arterial pulse curves." Only then could detailed interpretation of the pulse curve be attempted.[26]

CARDIOVASCULAR INTERVALS IN SPHYGMOGRAPHIC TRIALS

Keyt's goal was to use his device to analyze with mathematical precision the sequence of cardiovascular (heart to artery) events in a range of suspected cardiac pathologies, both for research purposes and for clinical diagnosis. The movement of the carriage, upon which was mounted the smoked glass plate (inscriptions of pulsations were made by styluses scratching into the smoked glass), could be speeded up or slowed down. The smoked glass plate moving at an average velocity past the recording stylus could hold about seven or eight cardiac or pulse beats. With a faster carriage speed, fewer pulsations were recorded but, since the waveforms were spread out, more detailed study was possible. With a slower carriage speed, more pulsations could be recorded on a fixed length of smoked glass allowing for more information about cardiac rhythm. Keyt's device allowed him to discover sequences of events far beyond the ability of the most

---

[25] Ibid., 22–23.
[26] Ibid., 23–25.

careful physical examination by the standard methods of pulse palpation with the finger and auscultation of the heart with the stethoscope.

Unlike earlier sphygmographers who focused on interpreting the shapes—the peaks and valleys within each recorded arterial pulsation—Keyt was more interested in the timing of the cardiac impulse as it moved from the heart into the arterial circulation. It was such intervals, detectable with his double cardiosphygmograph, that Keyt believed would reveal the pathophysiology of such conditions as heart failure and valvular diseases of the heart. Armed with this information, he could apply his sphygmocardiograph to the diagnosis of puzzling cases at the bedside.

"MEDICAL FRIEND" AND "LITTLE SUBJECTS"

Keyt's first subject was a healthy young "medical friend," possibly Isham, his physician son-in-law. As a physician, the subject was able to assist in holding the cardiac sensing device in position. Keyt made dual tracings of the cardiac impulse and arteries both close to the heart (carotid) and more distal arteries in the arms and legs. Upon removing the smoked glass from the carriage, Keyt used a compass to mark key events and determine the delay in fractions of a second between cardiac and arterial tracings. The calculation of various intervals and ratios was exacting and tedious work. Keyt's lengthy and detailed explanation of his procedures for evaluating simultaneous tracings was, in fact, discouragingly complex.[27]

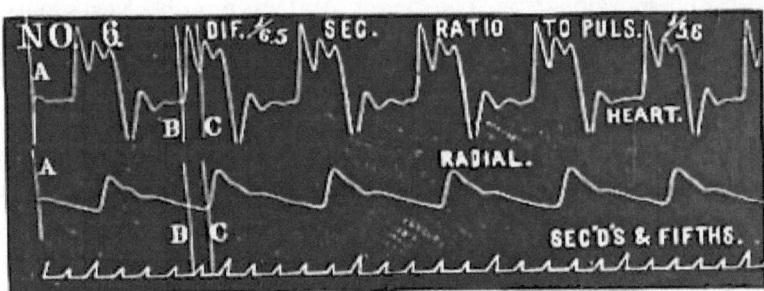

FIGURE 49: Sample tracing made with the Keyt chrono-cardio-sphygmograph. The cardiac impulse is on the top line with the arterial pulse recording below it (in this case the radial artery). At the bottom is the time recorder in seconds (large ticks) and fifths of a second (small ticks). The lines marked BC defined

---

[27] Ibid., 24–36.

the time intervals between cardiac contraction and arterial impulse. Alonzo T. Keyt, "Cardiographic and Sphygmographic Studies (I)," *New York Medical Journal* 26 (1877): 27.

In 1878, Keyt briefly extended his study of normal subjects to children (or perhaps only one child). The child named Asa, probably a grandchild, was the the four-year-old "little subject." Keyt recorded the temporal arterial and ventricular waves. He chose the temporal artery (in front of the ear) because holding the pressure sensor over the carotid artery (in the neck) would cause "annoyance to the child." Not wishing to "enforce upon the little subject undesirable restraint," Keyt took only one set of tracings. Comparing the child's tracing to those of an adult male, he concluded that the mean velocity of the pulse wave increases with age.[28]

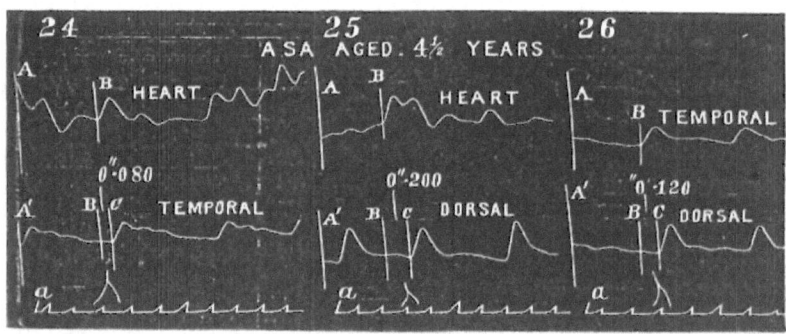

FIGURE 50: Trace of a child's pulse and cardiac impulse made with the Keyt chrono-cardio-sphygmograph. The subject (Asa) was probably Keyt's four-year-old grandson. Alonzo T. Keyt, "Cardiographic and Sphygmographic Studies (III),: *New York Medical Journal*, 28 (1878): 34.

An imaginative man, Keyt studied a normal (sleeping) infant, trying to correlate pulsations of the fontanel (the soft area between the unclosed fissures of the infant skull) with the pulsations of the heart and great vessels. His studies seemed to show that the rise and fall of the fontanel was not due solely to direct transmission of the cardiac output through the cerebral arteries. Either the entire brain rose with each heartbeat or the cranial arteries fill in "anticipationof the waves from the heart." Today, we would call this autoregulation, a term not in use in Keyt's time. He drew attention to a sphygmographic study of brain pulsations conducted on an older child with a traumatic skull injury with permanent loss of an area of

---

[28] Keyt, *Sphygmography and Cardiography*, 50–54.

bone. The research was conducted by New York physician Mary Putnam Jacobi, whose work with the sphygmograph is discussed in Chapter 7.[29]

SPHYGMOGRAPHIC STUDIES OF DISTANCE WALKERS

Keyt also explored the effects of exercise on the pulse tracing by studying professional distance walkers, reporting his results in 1878. Perhaps he took his cue from an article by Frederick Akbar Mahomed in England (cited by Keyt), who recorded tracings of a British distance walker, as reported in the American edition of *Lancet* in 1876. Keyt recorded the pulse waves of Bertha Von Hillern of Cincinnati, a woman who walked one hundred miles in twenty-eight hours, and of Daniel O'Leary, "the champion pedestrian of the world," during a two hundred mile walk completed over fifty-eight hours in Cincinnati. Hillern's radial pulse was studied at miles seventy-three and ninety-eight. The pulse wave was interpreted as being of low volume, decreased arterial tone, decreased blood pressure, and "reduced action of the heart." In his studies on O'Leary, Keyt was able to record both cardiac and arterial pulsation. He found O'Leary's circulation to be typical of what we would now call the athletic heart: "His circulation under exercise suffers no strain, no disturbance, but keeps on in the even tenor of its flow and movements." His low arterial tension was seen as an advantage as his heart pumped against relatively low resistance, always "equal to its work" and never "goaded to undue exertion."[30]

CARDIAC TO ARTERIAL INTERVALS: A WINDOW INTO CARDIOVASCULAR PHYSIOLOGY AND PATHOLOGY

Keyt's primary interest was the measurement of the interval in fractions of a second between cardiac contraction and the generation of the various components of the arterial (sphygmographic) wave. In his 1877 article in the *New York Medical Journal*, he stressed the value of his twinned

---

[29] Ibid., 142–48.
[30] Ibid., 130–41. Keyt included "Observations on Bertha Von Hillern's Pulse," *Cincinnati Clinic* [sic] (1878), and "O'Leary's Pulsations," *Cincinnati Lancet and Clinic* (1878) in a list of his publications to date: Alonzo T. Keyt, "The Claims of the Graphic Method," *Cincinnati Lancet and Clinic* n.s. 8 (1882): 484.

sphygmograph–cardiograph in representing "the form, relation, duration, and succession of the movements pertaining to the same pulsations, as they emanate from the heart and display themselves in different arteries."[31] Such studies had obvious application to clinical conditions such as cardiac valvular stenosis (narrowing).

Few men in Europe and none in America were applying the sphygmograph to such quantitative studies. In the early 1870s, A. H. Garrod at Cambridge had published several such studies, and Keyt was familiar with Garrod's work (see Chapter 3).[32] One of Keyt's earliest research interests with respect to human cardiophysiology was the determination of the interval between the beginning of ventricular contraction of the ventricle and the opening of the aortic valve (detected as the pulse wave in the carotid artery adjusted for the brief time it takes the blood to reach the carotid artery). He called this interval (which Garrod termed "syspasis") the "presphygmic interval." Although others, including Garrod, had attempted to measure such "heart–carotid interval[s]," their instruments lacked the precision of Keyt's chrono-cardio-sphygmograph.[33]

Keyt maintained that his meticulous methods "admit[ted] of no material fallacy." He found that the presphygmic interval varied with the time of day and between individuals. Other sphygmographers had found such variations in normal subjects a source of frustration, but Keyt was not so easily discouraged. He found that abnormalities in the presphygmic interval were more pronounced in patients with structural heart disease. He continued to seek methods of determining the presence of such organic defects (such as abnormalities of the aortic valve) by the detection of abnormal intervals.[34] As noted earlier, precise measurement of these intervals, etched onto the smoked glass plate, required a painstaking and tedious system of marking the sequential events using a calibrated compass.[35]

---

[31] Keyt, "Cardiographic and Sphygmographic Studies," 29.
[32] Keyt, *Sphygmography and Cardiography*, 76, 79.
[33] A. H. Garrod, "On Some Points Connected to the Circulation of the Blood, Arrived at from a Study of the Sphygmographic Trace," *Proceedings of the Royal Society of London* 23 (1874–75): 140–51; Alonzo T. Keyt, "The Presphygmic Interval, or Time Required to Start the Arterial Pulse after the Beginning of the Systole of the Ventricle," *Boston Medical and Surgical Journal* 102 (1880): 409–13; Keyt, *Sphygmography and Cardiography*, 76.
[34] Keyt, "Presphygmic Interval," 411.
[35] Keyt, "Cardiographic and Sphygmographic Studies," 28–29.

CLINICAL APPLICATIONS

In the late nineteenth century, hospitalized patients were often expected to consent to participation in medical studies, some of which were painful and dangerous. Keyt's sphygmographic studies were without risk for patients; at worst, the instrument was a trifle frightening and the required extension of the wrist (if the radial artery was examined) or pressure on the carotid artery transiently uncomfortable. In the clinical research environment of the times, his studies were benign, non-invasive, and possibly of value in contributing to a diagnosis for his own patients and patients referred by his fellow physicians.[36] From a practical standpoint, Keyt was able to provide advice and consultation to local physicians faced with difficult diagnostic dilemmas in cardiovascular cases. For example, in 1880, he was asked to evaluate a hospitalized Cincinnati patient with "enormous delay of the pulse."[37]

In 1879, he applied his sphygmograph to the study of aneurysms, calling into the question the conventional wisdom that a deformed pulse wave in a distal artery was attributable to aneurysmal deformity in the more proximal vessel. Isham (his physician son-in-law) invited him to study a critically injured and paralyzed patient to help resolve the issue. Keyt arrived at the interesting conclusion that pulse deformities and delays in distal vessels could be due to neurovascular abnormalities in conditions such as paralysis and concluded that pulse delays are not specific indicators of aneurysm.[38] There were surely many other consultations that were not reported in the medical literature.

From the mid-1870s until his death in 1885, Keyt applied his system to the clinical study of diseased hearts and blood vessels. Mechanical disorders of the mitral and aortic valves had always attracted sphygmographers, and Keyt was no exception. Rheumatic heart disease was common at the time and frequently affected the heart valves, causing considerable morbidity and mortality. Congenital valve diseases as well as valvular complications of syphilitic aortitis were common and untreatable causes of valvular abnormalities. Keyt used his cardiosphygmograph to evaluate valvular heart diseases such as aortic stenosis, which might be expected to cause delays in transmission of the pulse.[39]

---

[36] Susan E. Lederer, *Subjected to Science: Human Experimentation in America before the Second World War* (Baltimore, Johns Hopkins University Press, 1995), 9.

[37] Alonzo T. Keyt, "Enormous Delay of the Pulse," *Medical Record* (New York) 17 (1880): 169–70.

[38] Alonzo T. Keyt, "The Sphygmographic Indications in Aneurism" *Medical Record* (New York) 16 (1879): 507–11.

[39] Alonzo T. Keyt, "Cardio-Sphygmographic History of Aortic Obstructive Lesion," *Medical Record* (New York) 19 (1881): 621–24.

Isham remarked, "To him is due the discovery that an abnormal delay of the pulse-wave followed upon mitral regurgitation [a leaky mitral valve]. The value of this revelation to the practical physician is obvious."[40]

THE CHALLENGE OF COMPLEX CASES

Keyt welcomed complex cases that, in his view, were impossible to decipher without the aid of his cardiosphygmograph. His fellow clinicians had no diagnostic tools beyond their stethoscopes and Marey-type sphygmographs to complement their skills in physical examination.

In May 1880, he published a short article in the *Boston Medical and Surgical Journal* (forerunner of the *New England Journal of Medicine*) introducing his compound sphygmograph to the Boston medical community.[41] Several months later, in the same journal, he showed how he applied his device to the diagnosis of complex cardiovascular disorders. He presented the case of a middle-aged man with marked cardiac symptoms and an abnormal examination marked by systolic and diastolic murmurs. In 1878 and again in 1879, Keyt had recorded cardiac and arterial pulsations in this patient. The text was accompanied by clear tracings marked with his calibrated compass and measurements of cardiac contraction to arterial pulse intervals. He explained that the images included in the article, which were very clear in black ink on a white background, were transferred from his original white on black tracings; he trusted to "photographic transfer and skilful engraving" to make the highly accurate images for publication.

At the post-mortem examination in 1880, Keyt confirmed his suspected diagnoses of aortic valve insufficiency (regurgitation) and aortic artery aneurysm. With precise measurements of cardiac to artery intervals and some rather complex reasoning, he concluded:

> So in our case the ordinary signs and symptoms, at the first examination, were sufficient to determine the presence of large aortic insufficiency. Accepting this, the want of abnormal precipitation of the carotid and subclavian pulses enabled me to arrive at the diagnosis of coexisting aortic aneurism before there were any other indications of this condition.[42]

---

[40] Isham, "Keyt, Alonzo Thrasher," 66.
[41] Alonzo T. Keyt, "The Compound Sphygmograph," *Boston Medical and Surgical Journal* 102 (1880): 484–85.
[42] Alonzo T. Keyt, "The Influence of Aortic Aneurism and Aortic Insufficiency, Singly

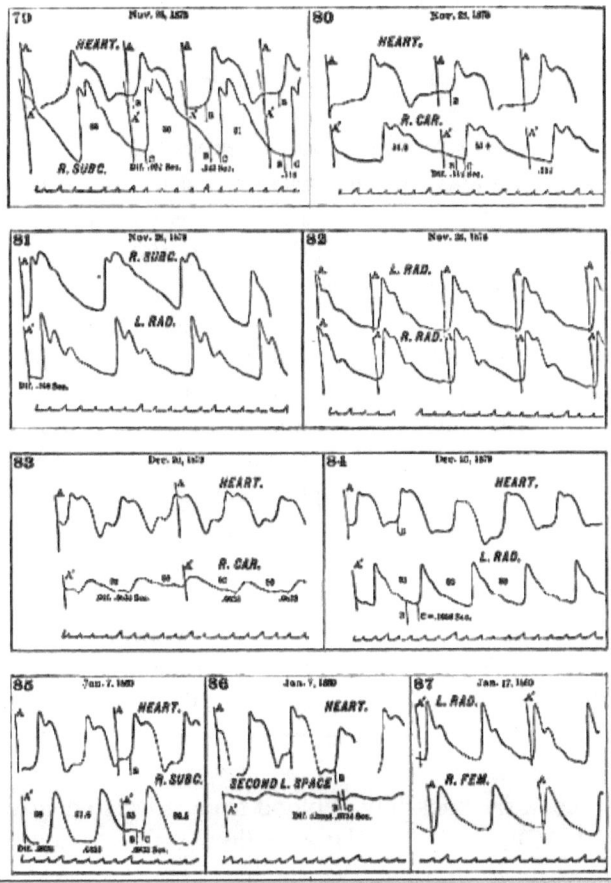

FIGURE 51: Serial "cardio-sphygmograms" in a patient with valvular heart disease and an aortic aneurysm. Keyt's markings (vertical lines labeled A), made with a calibrated compass, allowed him to calculate intervals (in fractions of a second) between cardiac and arterial events. These intervals were a window into disorders of the heart (such as valvular abnormalities) and the arteries (such as aneurysms). Alonzo T. Keyt, "The Influence of Aortic Aneurism and Aortic Insufficiency, Singly and Combined, on the Retardation of the Pulse," *Boston Medical and Surgical Journal* 103 (1880): 317.

---

and Combined, on the Retardation of the Pulse," *Boston Medical and Surgical Journal* 103 (1880): 315–18; quotation, 318.

LATER CARDIOSPHYGMOGRAPHIC STUDIES

In the 1881 *Boston Medical and Surgical Journal*, Keyt reviewed the cardiac physiology as visualized by his cardio-sphygmograph. Few general practitioners would have understood—or had the skill to apply to the problems of daily practice—his detailed exposition invoking sequential cardiac events spanning mere fractions of a second. Advising the reader to "study at his leisure" the tracings (in a previous issue of the *Journal*), which showed in detail the "components of the cardiac and pulse waves related to the cardiac cycle," Keyt concluded:

> Thus by this method a group of interesting and important facts come easily within our reach—facts physiological and clinical which a few years ago were entirely hidden from view for the want of the proper devices to disclose them; but now that the multiple simultaneous graphic method has been developed and made practical, results are already manifest and richest revelations await to reward its freer application.[43]

Keyt felt justified in challenging the mechanism of a heart murmur described in 1862 by Austin Flint, professor of the principles and practice of medicine at Belleview Hospital and the Medical College (New York). Flint was America's premier expert in the area of clinical cardiac diagnosis. Flint attributed the murmur (still referred to today as the Austin Flint murmur) to a disturbance in the backflow of blood from a diseased aortic valve to a healthy mitral valve, causing the latter to flutter. Taking care to document his great respect for Flint, Keyt was convinced that the murmur emanated from the aortic valve itself.[44] Although still controversial, current thinking, supported by modern cardiac imaging technology, is in agreement with Flint: the murmur is due to abnormal flow from the diseased aortic valve impinging on a normal mitral valve.[45]

---

[43] Alonzo T. Keyt, "The Mechanism of the Cardiac and Arterial Traces, and Some of the Teachings of Cardio-Sphygmography," *Boston Medical and Surgical Journal* 105 (1881): 297.

[44] Alonzo T. Keyt. "A New Interpretation of Flint's Mitral Direct or Presystolic Murmur without Mitral Lesions," *Boston Medical and Surgical Journal* 109 (1883): 30–31.

[45] Robin A. P. Weir and Henry J. Dargie, "Images in Clinical Medicine: Austin Flint Murmur," *New England Journal of Medicine* 359 (2008): e11; http://www.nejm.org/doi/full/10.1056/NEJMicm072437#t=article (accessed 27 January 2017).

A MODEST NATIONAL STAGE

Keyt was aware that northeastern medical journals carried more prestige and would likely win him a larger audience than local publication in Cincinnati journals. Many of his twenty-two original articles up to 1882 were published jointly in the *Cincinnati Lancet* (or *Lancet and Clinic*) and a New York or Boston journal. A list of his publications to date, which he appended to an 1882 article in the *Cincinnati Lancet and Clinic*, included the following: *Cincinnati Lancet and Clinic* (13), *New York Medical Journal* (5), *Medical Record* (New York) (4), *Boston Medical and Surgical Journal* (4), and *New York Archives of Medicine* (1). A one-page description and illustration of his compound sphygmograph was published by the prestigious *Lancet* (London) in 1880.[46] In 1882, the first volume of the *Journal of the America Medical Association* published a series of three articles by Keyt. The *Journal* likely had little international cachet in its early years, but was destined to become an authoritative American medical journal.[47]

CARDIOGRAPHY

Departing from his interest in simultaeous cardiosphygmography—a pulse tracing and a cardiac impulse tracing—Keyt focused on the cardiac impulse itself in an article for the *Journal of the American Medical Association* in 1885, the year of his death. The paper had been presented at the annual meeting of the Association, further evidence of Keyt's pursuit of national attention to his work. He observed that cardiography—the recording of the left ventricular impulse against the chest wall—was less well studied than sphygmography. Once again, to be clear, the resulting "cardiogram" is not to be confused with the electrocardiogram (EKG or ECG), which would not be introduced into clinical medicine until the twentieth century. Keyt's explanation of the events of the cardiac cycle was precise and

---

[46] Keyt, "Claims of the Graphic Method,", 484–86; Alonzo T. Keyt, "The Compound Sphygmograph," *Lancet* 2 (1880): 50.

[47] Alonzo T. Keyt, "An Experimental Inquiry into the Causes of the Variations of Pulse-Wave Velocity and Duration of the Cardio-Aortic or Presphygmic Interval Observed in Man (I)," *Journal of the American Medical Association* 1 (1883): 437–46; Alonzo T. Keyt, "Facts and New Experiments in Illustration of the Variations of Pulse-Wave Velocity in Man, and Bearing Upon the Elucidation of the Causes Which Produce Them (II)," *Journal of the American Medical Association* 1: 605–12; "The Causes of the Variations of the Cardio-Aortic or 'Pre-Sphygmic' Interval (III)," *Journal of the American Medical Association* 1: 661–68.

(typically) complex. For the physician interested in cardiac physiology, Keyt's cardiograph could elucidate the "form and chronometry of the heart's pulsations. . . . supplying a void in our knowledge of the finer physiology of the heart's movements."[48]

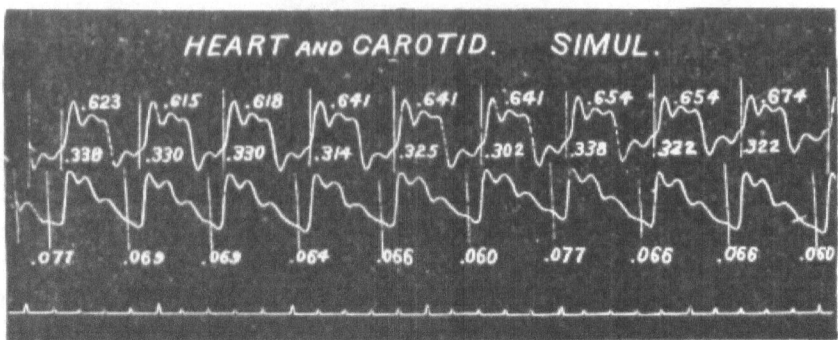

FIGURE 52: Detailed study of the cardio-carotid interval. Keyt demonstrated that the time from cardiac contraction to arrival of the pulse in the carotid artery (less than a tenth of a second), varies slightly even as the heart rate remains constant. This illustrates the delicacy of Keyt's elegant cardiosphygmograph, his interest in elucidating cardiovascular physiology, and his compulsive attention to detail. Alonzo T. Keyt, *Sphygmography and Cardiography, Physiological and Clinical*, edited by Asa B. Isham and M. H. Keyt (New York: G. P. Putnam's Sons, 1887), 128.

Keyt's interest in cardiography was shared by a number of European investigators, including Marey himself. With more sensitive technology, the apexcardiograph, which converted the mechanical force of the phases of cardiac contraction and relaxation into an electrical readout, enjoyed moderate popularity among cardiologists in the mid-twentieth century. Apexcardiograms looked remarkably similar to the recordings of the cardiac impulse against the chest wall recorded by Keyt's cardiograph. In recent decades, echocardiography, using ultrasound rather than pressure transducers has replaced apexcardiography.[49]

---

[48] Alonzo T. Keyt, "Cardiography," *Journal of the American Medical Association* 5 (1885): 141–45; quotation, 145.

[49] For example, see Keyt, *Sphygmography and Cardiography*, 60 and the sample apexcardiogram at https://commons.wikimedia.org/wiki/File:Apex-cardiogram.jpg.

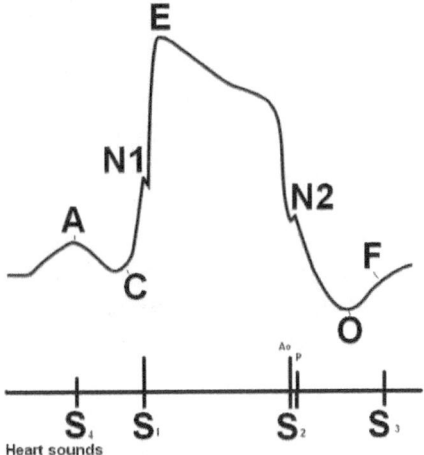

FIGURE 53: Schematic of an apexcardiogram similar to recordings used clinically in the 1960s. Apexcardiograms were often correlated with simultaneous heart sounds (indicated here by S1 to S4) and murmurs (phonocardiogram), and EKG tracings. Compare to "heart" recording by Keyt, figure 52. https://commons.wikimedia.org/wiki/File:Apex-cardiogram.JPG (accessed 29 January 2017).

KEYT'S EUROPEAN CONNECTIONS

Rather than ally himself intellectually with British sphygmographers, Keyt considered himself a colleague of Marey and his French disciples. In the *Cincinnati Lancet and Clinic* for 1882, Keyt stressed his allegiance to the European concept of the graphic method and his links to Marey in an article entitled "Claims of the Graphic Method."[50] He proudly reviewed his correspondence with the great man, quoting from Marey's 1881 book, *La circulation du sang à l'état physiologique et dans les maladies*: "One sees there that the traces of the American instrument [referring to Keyt] have undulations a little stronger [than mine]." Keyt continued:

> As before stated, Marey adopts my chronographs [timed tracings] and I in turn have profited by adopting his device for starting and stopping the movement [of the recording paper under the pen] by displacement of air in a rubber tube held in the mouth. . . . it leaves the hands free . . . enabling one

---

[50] Marey published *La méthode graphique dans les sciences expérimentales et principalement en physiologie et en médicine* in 1878.

to successfully experiment on himself or others without an assistant.[51]

Keyt's biographer wrote that Marey himself "employed Doctor Keyt's instrument in preference to his own," adding that François Franck, a pupil of Marey, who apparently carried out studies similar to those of Keyt, had "borne testimony to Dr. Keyt's sphygmograph surpassing all others for fidelity and utility." Marey, it seems, praised Keyt's instrument directly to distinguished American physician and director of the Library of the Surgeon General's Office, John Shaw Billings.[52] Keyt seems to have seen himself as something of a colleague of Marey, a unique source of pride for an American working in the rarified world of sphygmography. The quality of his recordings were undeniably excellent. In an 1882 article for the *Cincinnati Lancet and Clinic*, he recalled:

> Some years ago when my sphygmograph was less perfect then now, I made some comparative experiments—tracing the radial pulses of the same subjects with the two instruments [Marey and Keyt sphygmographs]; Of these experiments Marey says: "The author publishes an interesting series of comparative traces obtained on the same subjects with his instrument and mine . . ." Other and stronger testimony of this distinguished authority I could add as to the correctness and excellence of my traces; but these also speak for themselves.[53]

IN PURSUIT OF A LEGACY

Following Keyt's death, his devoted son-in-law described the qualities that he brought to his sphygmographic investigations: "All the attributes of an investigator in this line of research he possessed, such as marvelous patience, untiring perseverance, strict conscientiousness, delicacy of manipulation, and the inventive skill or genius to overcome the diverse unfavorable elements in the way of the inquiry."

---

[51] Keyt's quotation from Marey's *Circulation du sang* are from Keyt, "Claims of the Graphic Method," 478, 480–82.

[52] Isham, "Sketch of the Life and Work of Alonzo Thrasher Keyt," 727. Franck's comment that Keyt's sphygmograph "surpass[ed] all others for fidelity and utility," was made to a Cincinnati physician, presumably visiting with Franck in France.

[53] Keyt, "Claims of the Graphic Method," 478. Marey cited Keyt's article, "The New Sphygmograph"; the quotation was translated from Marey, *La circulation du sang*, 701.

Despite his dedication and his extenisve body of work, some in major medical journals in Boston and New York, as well as the *Journal of the American Medical Association*, Keyt "remained singularly unnoticed by [his] countrymen"—in the eyes of his son-in-law he was a prophet without honor in his own country. He received just six orders for his compound sphygmograph—one from Marey, one from England, and four from the United States. Of his collected works gathered into book form after his death, a respectable four hundred copies were sold; the remaining six hundred were destroyed in a warehouse fire. He received no invitation to appear before a "learned body" outside of Cincinnati, no honorary degrees, no other honors.

Among Americans, only Nathan S. Davis of Chicago, a pioneer in medical education and the first editor of the *Journal of the American Medical Association*, publicly praised Keyt's research as an "ingeniously conceived, patiently executed, and logically considered series of experimental investigations," as important as any "that have appeared in this or any other country in the past decade." Of European accolades, the loyal Isham recalled in a memorial for his father-in-law, "tidings of encouragement from men of high distinction in medicine" reached Keyt from Paris, Vienna, London, Berlin, Munich, Edinburgh, and other European cities. European physiologists cited Keyt as an authority on pulse wave velocities and the timing of the cardiac cycle.[54]

Keyt would have been deeply gratified—had he known—that Alfred H. Garrod of Cambridge, who had done early work on the "presphygmic interval," greatly admired his work (see Chapter 3). A biographer wrote of Garrod, who died in 1879: "Nothing gave [Garrod] greater pleasure during his last illness than the fact that conclusions the same as some of his own most cherished ideas and discoveries, connected with the circulation of the blood, had been arrived at independently by an American physiologist [Keyt] with no knowledge of his previous work on the same subject."[55]

---

[54] Isham, "Sketch of the Life and Work of Alonzo Thrasher Keyt," 727–29; quotation 727. The editorial commentary, almost certainly by editor Nathan S. Davis in this first volume of the *Journal of the American Medical Association*, was from "Original Investigations," *Journal of the American Medical Association* 1 (1883): 708–9. Isham attributed the unsigned commentary to Davis; this is probably correct, since Davis would likely have personally overseen every aspect of the first volume of the *Journal*.

[55] W. A. Forbes, "Biographical Notice," in *The Collected Scientific Papers of the late Henry Garrod, M.A., F.R.S.*, (London: R. H. Porter, 1881): xii–xiii.

THE KEYT SPHYGMOGRAPH IN INSURANCE RISK ASSESSMENT

Prior to his father-in-law's death, Isham himself published an article in the respected *American Journal of the Medical Sciences* promoting the use of the sphygmograph in life insurance evaluations. Isham, in addition to his medical practice, was professor of physiology at the Cincinnati College of Medicine and Surgery. It appears that Isham relied on tracings taken by his late father-in-law in cases they had observed together. Isham stressed the value of the sphygmograph in diagnosing occult valvular disease in applicants for life insurance. He anticipated that in the hands of a consultant, sphygmography could clear up questions about heart murmurs discovered during routine insurance examinations. This would allow the company medical director to consider accepting an applicant with what is now called an "innocent murmur" without increased risk to the company. In Isham's words, it was the duty of medical examiners towards the company "to recommend only clean risks." However, by denying insurance to a man (applicants were mainly men) with a benign murmur, "the applicant and his assigns are injured in that they are deprived of the benefits [of] life insurance . . . to which they should be entitled [as men in excellent health].[56]

In fact, sphygmography never figured in insurance underwriting. Emphasis by insurance company medical directors such as Edgar Holden, himself a leading American sphygmograph man (Chapter 4), was on careful physical examination of the heart and lungs and a detailed history by the often poorly-trained physicians who contracted with national companies to perform examinations on local applicants.

Sphygmography did not turn out to be the key to determining "soundness" that Burdon-Sanderson, Holden, Keyt, and Isham had envisioned. That distinction would go to the sphygmomanometer—the familiar blood pressure cuff—early in the twentieth century.[57] Although Keyt himself had little regard for Holden's sphygmograph, it is interesting that George Van Wagenen, Holden's successor as head of the medical department at Newark's Mutual Benefit Life Insurance Company, observed in 1915 that the sphygmomanometers of the day, however imperfect,

---

[56] Asa B. Isham, "Value of Cardio-sphygmography for the Determination of Cardiac Valvular Conditions and of Aneurism, Particularly for Examiners in Life Insurance," *American Journal of the Medical Sciences* 84 (1882): 119. Isham's professorship noted in [Isham], "Alonzo Thrasher Keyt," in *Daniel Drake and His Followers*, 465.

[57] Sandra W. Moss, *Edgar Holden, M.D., of Newark, New Jersey: Provincial Physician on a National Stage* (XLibris, 2014), 357–61.

had been of "inestimable value to use, particularly in that class of case which have defied our usual methods of insurance examination."[58] Van Wagenen was of the generation that fulfilled the hopes of men like Isham for an instrument that would guide life insurance companies in approving applicants.

"A STUPENDOUS TASK"

Keyt's dedication to his sphygmographic studies required an almost super-human effort—a "stupendous task"—as his son-in-law described in a memorial biography. The family home was in the suburbs (of Cinncinati), and Keyt would have had to travel some miles into the center of town to find hospitalized subjects suitable for his studies. He supported his family (a wife and seven children) by general medical practice. The fact that he had considerable obstetric skills, excelling in attendance upon "difficult labors," suggests that he was often called out at night and that his time was rarely his own. Isham's analysis of Keyt's selfless devotion to his sphygmographic research, while laden with expressions of intense devotion, seems fair:

> Tracings were taken of every one who would submit to the application of the instrument... Cases of valvular and orificial [refering to the space or opening between the leaflets of the heart valves] heart-disease were sought for, the hospitals were hunted over for aneurysmal dilatations and growths obstructing the circulation, almost all forms of disease were put under contribution. Numerous tracings were taken of all, and, in many cases, again and again. The mortality lists were watched, autopsies interceded for and the findings eagerly noted. Distance, time or expense were not considered if a postmortem could but be obtained.[59]

In his last published article, which appeared in the *Journal of the American Medical Association* in 1885, Keyt continued to hold out great hope for simultaneous cardiosphygmography. Unlike so many American and

---

[58] George A. Van Wagenen, "Report of the Committee on the Blood Pressure Test," *Abstract of the Proceedings of the Annual Meeting of the Association of Life Insurance Medical Directors of America* (1912–1914): 243.

[59] Isham, "Sketch of the Life and Work of Alonzo Thrasher Keyt," 727–28.

British sphygmographers, he never became discouraged by the intricacies and uncertainties of sphygmography.[60] Keyt died suddenly in 1885 of "cardiac paralysis" occasioned, according to the autopsy (performed by Isham), by overwork. His obituary in the *Journal of the American Medical Association*, almost certainly written by the ever-faithful Isham, noted tersely that he was "better known in Europe than in his own country."[61] Keyt's beautiful chrono-cardio-sphygmograph died with its inventor.

GLIMPSING THE FUTURE: THE PASSION FOR NUMERIC OBJECTIVITY

In his studies of the precise chronometry of sequential cardiac and arterial events, Keyt anticipated the passion for numeric objectivity that characterizes modern diagnostic cardiology. For example, modern electrocardiographic reports routinely include a number of timed events such as the PR and QT intervals, QRS width, a vector analysis of the electrical axis, and often a numeric analysis of wave heights in support of a diagnosis of cardiac hypertrophy. As with the Keyt cardiosphygmograph, the subjective impressions of the cardiologist regarding wave shape is also critical to correct diagnosis. Echocardiography relies on precise measurement, in this case the dimensions of cardiac structures such as valves and thickness of the heart muscle. Exercise stress tests, too, generate numerical data in addition to subjective evaluation of the shape of electrocardiographic waves. Though hampered by the relatively primitive technology of his time, Keyt nevertheless glimpsed the future.

---

[60] Keyt, "Cardiography," 145. For this article, Keyt added a recording of respiratory excursions to his polygraphic tracings.

[61] "Alonzo T. Keyt" (obituary), *Journal of the American Medical Association* 5 (1885): 615–16.

Chapter 6

Erasmus Allington Pond: The Practical Portable Sphygmograph

Erasmus Allington Pond, a native of Massachusetts, pursued a peripatetic medical education, studying with preceptors in Massachusetts and South Carolina, as well as Baltimore. He attended lectures at Maryland University and Tremont Medical School (Boston), and received his M.D. degree from the medical department of Harvard in 1853. Pond settled in Rutland, Vermont, opening a general practice and joining a number of state and national pharmaceutical and medical organizations, including the American Association for the Advancement of Science. He treated patients with diseases of the heart and arteries at the Rutland Dispensary, a facility devoted to providing medical advice for the poor and post-graduate training for physicians. In 1885, he served as president of the Rutland County Medical and Surgical Society.[1] His 1889 obituary in the *Boston Medial and Surgical Journal* listed Pond as a former president of the Vermont State Medical Society.[2] However, a search through the *Transactions of the Vermont State Medical Society* confirmed his membership and appointment to several committees, but there is no evidence that he ever served as president.[3]

---

[1] H. P. Smith and W. S. Rann, *History of Rutland County, Vermont* (Syracuse NY: D. Mason, 1886), 240, 385.

[2] "Erasmus A. Pond" (obituary), *Boston Medical and Surgical Journal* 120 (1889): 572; "Recent Deaths," *New York Medical Journal* 49 (1889): 635.

[3] Confirmed by telephone communication with the Vermont Medical Society, 31 August

A lengthy scientific article written by Pond for the Vermont State Medical Society was published in the *Transactions of the Vermont Medical Society* in 1864. The published paper, previously read before the society, described Pond's harrowing and heart-wrenching experiences during several diphtheria epidemics. Of interest is his mention of a report delivered to the Society in 1863 in which he reviewed his treatment of a child dying of diphtheria. In desperation, Pond performed a tracheotomy on the child, who subsequently recovered.[4]

THE CONSTRUCTION OF THE POND SPHYGMOSCOPES

Pond's studies of the pulse began in the mid 1870s. According to a report published in December 1875 (submitted to the *Boston Medical and Surgical Journal* by James R. Chadwick, secretary of the Suffolk District Medical Society), Pond demonstrated his "new sphygmoscope" before the Suffolk District Medical Society (Boston area) in November 1875. The compact size and potentially low cost promised to obviate the obstacles presented to the practitioner by the bulky sphygmoscopes of earlier workers.

Pond's simple Hérisson style sphygmoscope model consisted of a calibrated glass tube, three to six inches long, with a flared base. The open lower end was covered with a thin rubber membrane, which was pressed down upon the artery by the operator. Alternatively, the entire device could be strapped to the arm. Physicians could follow the pulsations in the artery by observing the rise and fall of a colored liquid in the glass tube. Pond's son, Dr. Wallace R. Pond of Stockton, California, was credited with perfecting the instrument by fitting the thin calibrated tube into a larger tube that acted as a reservoir for the liquid. The smaller tube acted as a piston, "regulating the heights of the vibrating column and showing the motions of the pulse." Atop the calibrated tube, an "annular tube," the exact nature of which is unclear from the illustrations, "will indicate sumultaneously the pressure and the vibrations."[5]

---

31 2016.

[4] Erasmus A. Pond, "Diphtheria," *Transactions of the Vermont Medical Society* (1864): 53–64.

[5] James R. Chadwick, "Proceedings of the Suffolk County District Medical Society: A New Sphygmoscope," *Boston Medical and Surgical Journal* 93 (1875): 740–42.

Erasmus Allington Pond:
The Practical Portable Sphygmograph

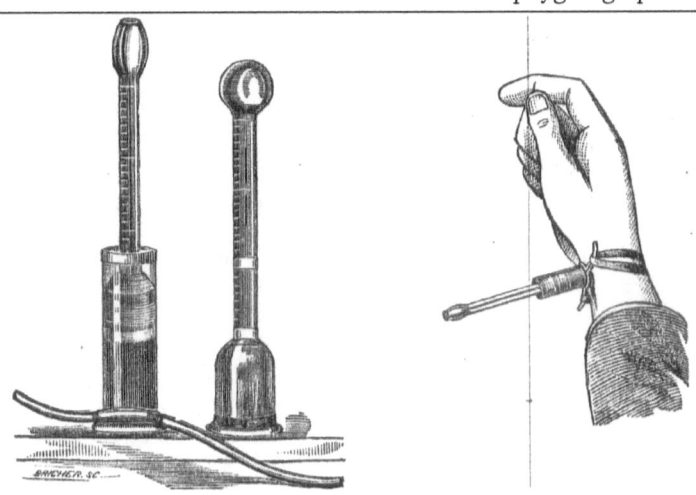

FIGURE 54: Pond sphygmoscope demonstrated before the Suffolk District Medical Society, November 1875. James R. Chadwick, "Proceedings of the Suffolk District Medical Society: A New Sphygmoscope," *Boston Medical and Surgical Journal* 93 (1875): 741.

Pond had an affinity for patenting his medical devices. Detailed drawings of several Pond sphygmoscopes appear in the United States Patent Office records (United States Patent No. 161,821, 6 April 1875). Wallace R. Pond also patented a sphygmoscope design (United States Patent No. 167,785, 14 September 1875).[6]

APPLYING THE POND SPHYGMOSCOPE

The senior Pond had cleverly used his sphygmoscope to follow a case of senile gangrene. Just as modern ultrasound devices are used to detect pulses along the course of a blocked artery or vein, Pond applied his sphygmoscope to the femoral artery above the gangrenous foot, tracing the pulsations as far distally toward the foot as possible and thus determining the point at which the vessel was occluded. He evidently was among the first to see the practical value of using a sphygmoscope to determine the level at which an amputation, if necessary, might best be performed.

---

[6] Erasmus A. Pond, "Sphygmoscopes, U.S. Patent No. 161821, 6 April 1875," United States Patent and Trade Office, www.google.com/patents/US161821 (accessed 2 February 2017); Wallace R. Pond, "Sphygmoscope, U.S. Patent No. 167785, 14 September 1875," United States Patent and Trade Office, www.google.com/patents/US167785 (accessed 1 February 2017).

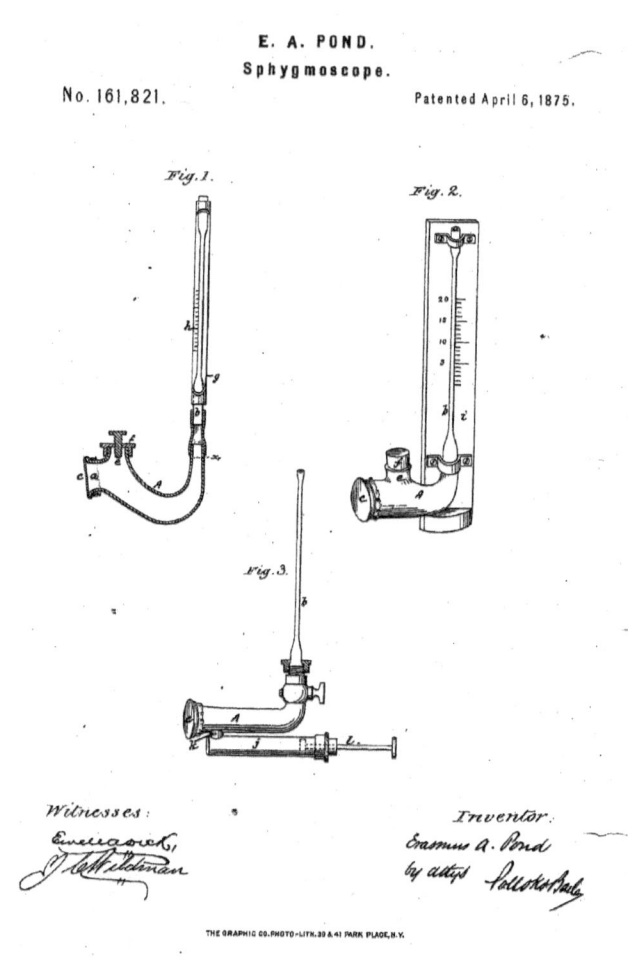

FIGURE 55: Early Pond sphygmoscopes. U.S. Patent No. 161,821, 6 April 1875; www.google.com/patents/US161,821.

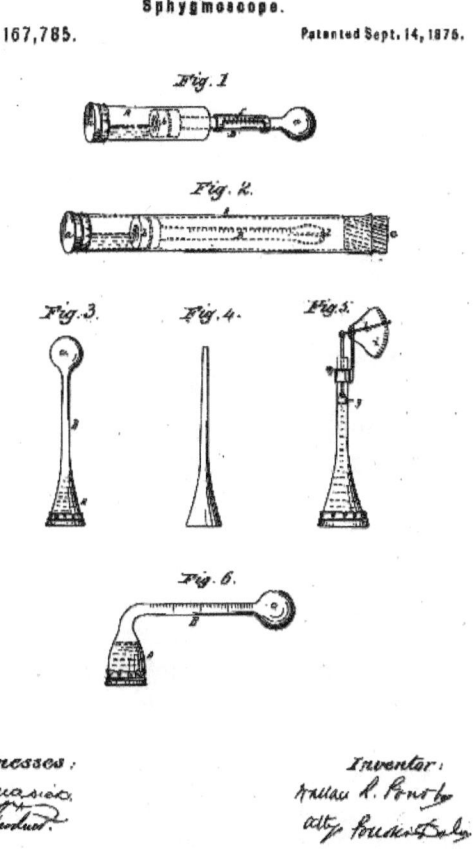

FIGURE 56: Pond sphygmoscopes. U.S. Patent No. 167,785, 14 September 1875; www.google.com/patents/US167785.

Eager to demonstrate other practical applications of the new device, Pond went beyond pulse study for its own sake and tried out his instrument in laboring women. He found that the sphygmoscope "heralds every pain and indicates the general strength of the woman." He also monitored the pulse during anesthesia, perhaps using the sphygmoscope as a guide in dosing of anesthetic gas. He studied the "brain" pulse, perhaps a reference to the alterations in the peripheral pulse secondary to brain damage or a recording of the pulse in the infant fontanelle. In typhoid fever and diphtheria he observed a "jiggling pulse," which he attributed to "paralysis of the heart."[7] Such scattered applications betray a lack of depth; yet Pond's enthusiasm and creativity is undeniable. His sphygmoscope, like that of Alonzo T. Keyt, appears to have been an independent re-invention of the Hérisson sphygmoscope.

THE J. B. UPHAM PRIORITY CONTROVERSY

A physician in the audience at Pond's presentation to the Suffolk District Medical Society rose to protest that Pond's sphygmoscope was identical with that "invented by [Somerville] Scott Allison [sic, the correct spelling is Alison], which had been made familiar to the profession in Boston by the brilliant experiments made with it in this city several years ago by Dr. J. B. Upham." Scott Alison had, in fact, introduced his sphygmoscope in 1856 in a paper to the Royal Society; a detailed report on the paper was later published in the *Proceedings* (see Chapter 2, Figure 10). The protester, a man with a long memory, was correct—J. B. Upham of Boston did indeed present the Alison sphygmoscope to an earlier Boston audience at some date prior to 1861. In his book published in London in 1861, Scott Alison cited a reference by Upham in the *Boston Medical and Surgical Journal* to "the delicate and beautiful instrument of Dr. [Somerville] Scott Allison [sic], of London, called the sphygmoscope."[8]

Scott Alison credited Upham with an ingenious adaptation that no doubt delighted his Boston audience. Upham applied "an electro-magnetic machine with a bell attached to it. As the liquid in the sphygmoscope rises, it breaks contact in the electro-magnetic machine, and a hammer falling upon

---

[7] Chadwick, "Proceedings of the Suffolk County District Medical Society," 741–42.

[8] Ibid., 742 (see Chapter 4 for an account of Upham's presentation); Somerville Scott Alison, "A Description of a New Sphygmoscope, an Instrument for Indicating the Movements of the Heart and Blood-Vessels; With an Account of Observations Obtained by the Aid of that Instrument," *Proceedings of the Royal Society of London* 8 (1856–57): 18–26; the paper was reported upon by G. O. Rees for the *Proceedings*.

a bell, a sound is instantly obtained." Further, Upham had transmitted the signals over telegraph wires some three miles from Boston to Cambridge.[9]

Pond, who was touchy about priority, responded that he and his son had constructed over twenty different instruments over the previous few years, and that he was unfamiliar with either Upham or Alison. Thus, Pond had in fact reinvented the Scott Alison sphygmoscope, which itself was an independent reinvention of the Hérisson sphygmoscope.

FROM POND SPHYGMOSCOPE TO POND SPHYGMOGRAPH

Pond, of course, realized that his sphygmoscope, though its fluctuations could be observed by several physicians, was not a sphygmograph—that is, it had no recording component and thus created no permanent record. But even as he demonstrated his improved sphygmoscope to his Boston audience, Pond was at work on a sphygmograph of his own. He had, as he mentioned to his Boston audience, "affixed to his pattern [i.e., the sphygmoscope], a recording apparatus, so that it was now both a sphygmoscope and a sphygmograph." The claim took up exactly one sentence at the end of his sphygmoscope presentation and was not accompanied by an exhibit or demonstration; nor were there any tracings published with the report. However, he was clearly on his way to designing what would prove to be his practical, popular, compact, handy (and marketable) sphygmograph of novel design.[10] Perhaps he feared that his active patent applications might be hijacked if he revealed too many details of the work in progress.

Like Keyt's instrument, Pond's sphygmograph used hydraulics rather than springs to transmit pulse waves. The device was described by an admiring Staten Island physician and president of the Richmond County Medical Society in 1877:

> By far the most sensitive and satisfactory instrument which I have seen is one constructed by Dr. E. A. Pond, of Rutland, Vermont, in which the arterial waves are transmitted through a film of India-rubber to a column of water bearing a float, the rise and fall of which move a lightly-balanced lever terminating

---

[9] Somerville Scott Alison, *The Physical Examination of the Chest in Pulmonary Consumption* (London: John Churchill, 1861), 346–47.
[10] Chadwick, "Proceedings of the Suffolk County District Medical Society," 742.

in a flail-jointed needle, whose point, resting on a smoked slip of mica, records the pulse-tracing.[11]

Graphics from two patent applications illustrate the evolution of the Pond sphygmograph from 1876 to 1878 (U.S. Patent No.183205, 10 October 1876; U.S. Patent No. 205412, 25 June 1878).[12]

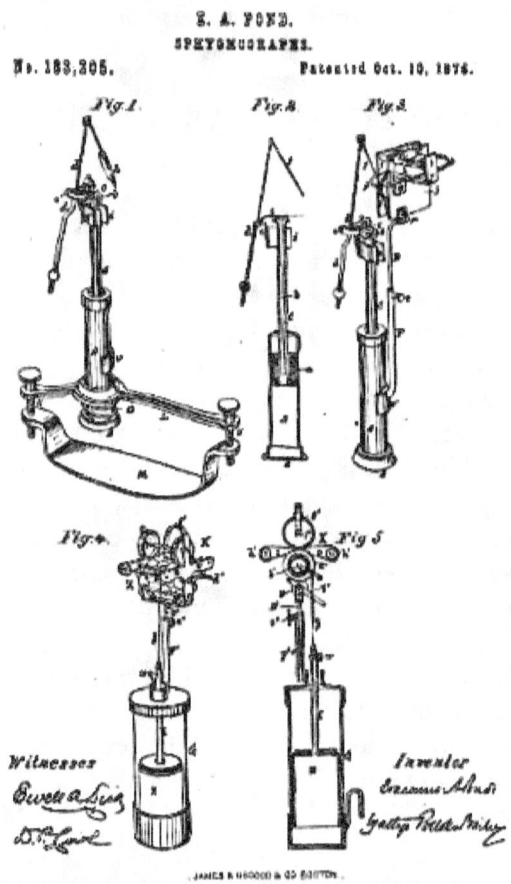

FIGURE 57: Pond sphygmograph, U.S. Patent No. 183,205, 10 October 1876; www.google.com/patents/US183205.

---

[11] Alfred L. Carroll, "The Clinical Use of the Sphygmograph," *New York Medical Journal* 26 (1877): 255–56.

[12] Erasmus A. Pond, "Sphygmographs, U.S. Patent No. 183205, 10 October 1876," United States Patent and Trade Office, www.google.com/patents/US183205; "Sphygmograph, U.S. Patent No. 205412, 25 June 1878," United States Patent and Trade Office, www.google.com/patents/US205412 (both accessed 1 February 2017).

Erasmus Allington Pond:
The Practical Portable Sphygmograph

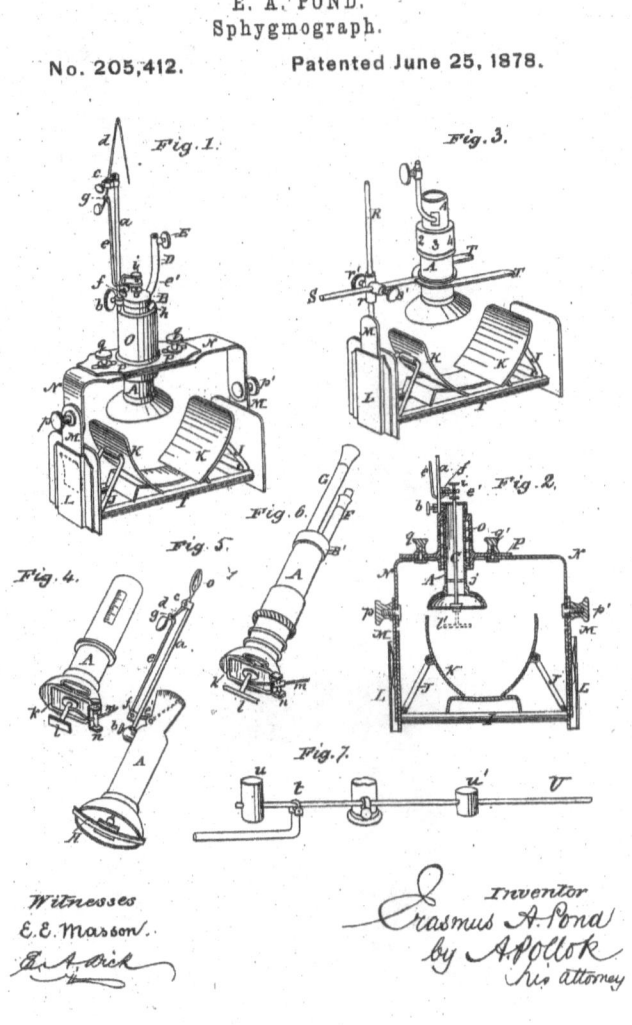

FIGURE 58: Pond sphygmograph. U.S. Patent No. 205,412, 25 June 1878; www.google.com/patents/US205412.

A contemporary medical supply catalogue, the prestigious George Tiemann & Co.'s *American Armamentarium Chirurgicum*, included a detailed description of the Pond instrument. The sensor (the component placed directly over the artery or the cardiac impulse) was a rubber diaphragm stretched over the bottom of a fluid-filled concentric pair of vertical tubes, the inner tube acting as a piston. (Later, the option of a metal button sensor was added as an alternative to the rubber diaphragm.) Inside the tubing was a free glass float which responded to any movement of the fluid in the tube or vibration of the rubber sensor at the base of the tube. A delicate needle and counterpoise mechanism transmitted the movements of the glass float to a recording strip. As with all sphygmographs, the recording strip was propelled by a clockwork mechanism. Like the Keyt model, it was a hydraulic system. A cradle was provided for the patient's wrist.[13]

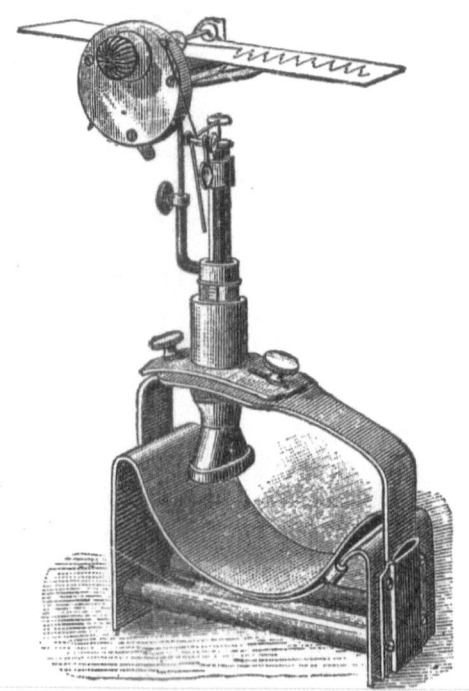

FIGURE 59: Commercial Pond sphygmograph. George Tiemann. *The American Armamentarium Chirurgicum*. New York: George Tiemann (ca. 1879): I:87.

---

[13] George Tiemann & Co., *The American Armamentarium Chirurgicum: George Tiemann & Co.* (New York: George Tiemann & Co., ca. 1879), I:87.

KEYT AND POND BATTLE OVER PRIORITY

The similarity of Pond's instrument to the first Keyt sphygmograph is striking, although there is sufficient evidence to justify the conclusion that each man, Pond in Vermont and Keyt in Cincinnati, worked independently to create similar, but not identical, sphygmoscopes and sphygmographs of a type distinctly different from the spring operated instruments of Marey and Holden.

A battle over priority, fought out through letters to the editor in the *New York Medical Journal*, ensued in 1876. Keyt had ended his lengthy article entitled "The New Sphygmograph" (published in the January 1876 issue of the *New York Medical Journal* and graced with multiple tracings) with the claim that he could find no precedent for his instrument: "After a pretty thorough enquiry as to instruments employed in the study of the circulation, I find nothing to imply that the combination is not new.... Whenever it becomes apparent that my combination has been put in practice prior to 1875, I will cheerfully renounce priority, but must still assert originality of invention."[14]

In response, Wallace R. Pond fired off a letter to the same journal (dated January 1876 and published in the March 1876 issue) referring to Keyt's "able article." Once past the niceties, he went on to cite patent applications and the November 1875 mention of the sphygmograph before the Suffolk District Medical Society. The senior Pond, wrote his son, had been demonstrating his sphygmoscope and sphygmograph since late 1874, "as many of his friends can testify, who, in company with himself, made numerous experiments with them, fascinated by the beauty and delicacy of their working and the simplicity of their construction." Pond's son had likewise been demonstrating the instruments in California. He finished with none-too-subtle innuendo: "I would not for a moment doubt the honesty of Dr. Keyt in his assertion of originality, though the latter portion of his article would lead one to suppose that he was not entirely ignorant of Dr. Pond's claim."[15] It should be noted that Pond's first sphygmograph patent was granted in October 1876 (based on a search of online federal patent records); at the time of the dispute he did not hold the patent, though he probably applied for it early in 1876.[16]

---

[14] Alonzo Thrasher Keyt, "The New Sphygmograph; Or, Instrument Adapted as a Sphygmograph, Sphygmometer, Cardiograph, Cardiometer, and to Other Uses," *New York Medical Journal* 23 (1876): 56.

[15] Wallace R. Pond, "Correspondence," *New York Medical Journal* 23 (1876): 288–90.

[16] Unfortunately, United States patent records available on line prior to 1976

Keyt was well-read in the pertinent American, British, and Continental medical literature. He apparently read the *Boston Medical and Surgical Journal*, but would have focused on major articles and not the appended proceedings of the Suffolk County Medical Society (under the heading of "A New Sphygmoscope") at the back of the issue. Keyt in turned fired back in a letter to the editor of the *New York Medical Journal* (dated March 1876 and published in the May 1876 issue), claiming priority—and the high professional ground. He got right to the point:

> I'm sure I never heard of Dr. E. A. Pond, of Rutland, Vermont, or of Dr. Wallace R. Pond, of San Francisco, California, until their names appeared in the last issue of the *New York Medical Journal*. I do not consider there is any question of priority between Dr. Pond and myself. The distinctive features of my invetion have, I trust, been sufficiently set forth in my descriptive article. Whenever a mechanism is produced which, upon trial, proves superior to my sphygmograph, I shall be ready to hail it; for excellence of invention concerns us as physicians more than priority in the use of a principle.[17]

Pond, as Keyt correctly pointed out, had merely mentioned his sphygmograph in his presentation to the Suffolk District Medical Society (as reported in the December 1875 issue of the *Boston Medical and Surgical Journal*) but provided no details of construction, no images, and no tracings. The assertion that the Pond sphygmograph was demonstrated before his professional friends does not constitute priority.

Why the epistolary parrying initiated by the Ponds? The answer probably lies in their plans to patent and market the sphygmograph, for which they would need to establish some priority. In fact, the Keyt and Pond designs, while based on similar hydraulic principles, were sufficiently distinct to make both easily patentable. Setting aside the patents pursued by the Ponds, true priority—through the time-honored route of a detailed publication in a respected medical journal—clearly belongs to Keyt. The mere mention by the Ponds of a sphygmograph in an advanced stage of

---

contain images without accompanying text; the date of original application is not given on the images related to the Pond sphygmograph; https://www.uspto.gov/patents-application-process/search-patents.

[17] Alonzo T. Keyt, "The New Sphygmograph" (Correspondence), *New York Medical Journal* 23 (1876): 506.

development, patented or not, does not establish priority in the eyes of the medical community, and certainly not in the eyes of the American Medical Association, which frowned upon patents.

SPHYGMOGRAPH PATENTS AND THE ETHICS OF THE AMERICAN MEDICAL ASSOCIATION

Keyt's letter in response to the Ponds' assertion of priority, written hastily and with considerable pique, opened with a telling comment: "In a communication published in the March 1876 number of your Journal [*New York Medical Journal*], I find that a claimant armed with a *patent* has arisen for my new sphygmograph."[18] The work "patent" was italicized in the *Journal* and probably underlined by Keyt in his letter. He stressed that his presentation at the May 1875 meeting of the American Medical Association was on record in the form of an abstract in the *Medical Record* (New York). Having reviewed the extant literature on sphygmographs, Keyt felt justified in referring to his instrument as "a new one, and believed that designation to be appropriate and just."[19] He concluded in response to the Ponds' claim of priority rather testily: "I worked independently at the problem and produced an efficient mechanism. It would be humiliating if the principles of this mechanism should now, on the threshold of their usefulness, be fettered by a *patent*."[20]

In fact, Pond may have been withholding information about his sphygmographs from his medical peers pending patent grants and potential marketing. As noted earlier, in his talk before the Suffolk County Medical Society, at a meeting held in November 1875 and reported in December 1875 in the *Boston Medical and Surgical Journal*, Pond focused solely on his sphygmoscope (by that date, patents on his sphygmoscopes—but not his sphygmograph—had been granted). Only when challenged by an audience member about the priority of his sphygmoscope, did he utter the word "sphygmograph."[21]

According to historian of medical technology Audrey B. Davis, physicians did not adopt the usual procedures associated with inventors.

---

[18] Ibid., 506 (italics in original).
[19] Alonzo T. Keyt, "A New Sphygmograph—Elastic Membrane and Liquids for Transmitting the Pulsations of the Artery" (Abstract of a paper read before the American Medical Association, May 1875), *Medical Record* (New York) 10 (1875): 365.
[20] Keyt, "New Sphygmograph," 507; italics in original.
[21] Chadwick, "Proceedings of the Suffolk County District Medical Society," 742.

For example, taking out a patent was viewed with opprobrium, at least in theory. The inventor's name on the instrument was considered a sufficient and ethically proper reward. Certainly, Keyt was openly contemptuous of Pond's reference to patent protection. Manufacturers could "appease inventors" and perhaps cash in on professional recognition by naming a new device or modification for the inventor. Physician inventors would garner some modest glory, while the manufacturer garnered the royalties and income.[22]

Taking out patents was clearly proscribed by the American Medical Association's Code of Ethics, although how closely this was adhered to is uncertain. The Code of Ethics of the American Medical Association was adopted at the founding meeting of the organization (the National Medical Convention) in Philadelphia, May 1847. In the section entitled, "Of the Duties of Physicians to Each Other, and to the Profession at Large," subheading "Duties for the Support of Professional Character," is found the following injunction: "Equally derogatory [a reference to advertising medical services] to professional character is it for a physician to hold a patent for any surgical instrument or medicine."[23]

Some respectable American physicians, no doubt many American Medical Association members among them, were critical of the restriction. A correspondent to the *Medical Record* (New York) in 1876 commented on the display by medical instrument manufacturers at the Centennial Exhibition. The correspondent thought that the medical profession deserved much of the credit for inventing and modifying these instruments so proudly displayed by the manufacturers. The instrument makers charged a fee to the inventor for fashioning the device or instrument. Once the product was sold, the manufacturer kept all the profits. The correspondent suggested that the manufacturer might be made to share some of the profits with the inventors, perhaps as a royalty. This plan, he concluded, "would save the dignity of the profession, and though not so remunerative as the holding of a patent, it would nevertheless give a physician some pecuniary

---

[22] Audrey B. Davis, *Medicine and Its Technology: An Introduction to the History of Medical Instrumentation* (Westport CT: Greenwood Press, 1981), 240–41.

[23] American Medical Association, *Code of Ethics of the American Medical Association, Adopted May, 1847* (Philadelphia: P. K. and T. G. Collins, 1848, 16. This booklet was printed privately for the Philadelphia Delegation to the National Convention held in Philadelphia in May, 1847, The relevant secion on patents is Chaper 2, Article 1, Paragraph 4. https://archive.org/stream/63310410R.nlm.nih.gov/63310410R#page/n7/mode/2up (accessed 9 September 2016).

recompense for the outlay of his time and means, and for the labor of his brain."[24]

Pond was not a member of the American Medical Association according to directories published in 1874 and 1878.[25] He was a member of the state medical society of Vermont (state medical societies were constituent members of the American Medical Association), but that organization was small and probably wielded little authority. He was certainly not constrained by the Code of Ethics, rushing as he had to patent his instruments.[26]

KEYT'S PATENT: "HE COUNTED NOT HIS WORK FOR GAIN"

Keyt, wrote his son-in-law, "guided his conduct by the Hippocratic Oath and the code of ethics of the American Medical Association."[27] In his tart 1876 response to Pond's claim of priority ("a claimant armed with a *patent*"), Keyt seemed to hold a low opinion of patents by physicians. However, he did take out a patent on his "chrono-cardio-sphygmograph" in 1878, possibly to protect his good name and claim of priority in the wake of his fight with Pond. The patent document was headed "sphygmometer," but the drawings clearly indicate the Keyt sphygmograph recording a sphygmogram, as well as the cardiac sensors for simultaneous arterial and cardiac tracings, and the timer marking off seconds and fifths of a second. The patent was registered on 14 May 1878.[28]

---

[24] "Medical Patents" (editorial), *Medical Record* (New York) 11 (1876): 816.

[25] Samuel W. Butler (comp.) *Medical Register and Directory of the United States* (Philadelphia: Office of the Medical and Surgical Reporter, 1874, 1878).

[26] Pond also received patents for a pill-making machine and improvements in the pill-making machine in 1852 and 1855; Erasmus A. Pond, "Pill Machine, U.S. Patent No. 9455, 7 December 1852," United States Patent and Trade Office, www.google.com/patents/US9455; "Pill Machine, U.S. Patent No. 12960, 29 May 1855," United States Patent and Trade Office, www.google.com/patents/US12960 (both accessed 2 February 2017).

[27] Asa B. Isham, "A Sketch of the Life and Work of Alonzo Thrasher Keyt," *Philadelphia Monthly Medical Journal*, 1 (1899): 726.

[28] Alonzo T. Keyt, "Sphygmometer, U.S. patent No. 203548, 14 May 1878." United States Patent and Trade Office, www.google.com/patents/US203548 (accessed 3 February 2017).

Writing the Pulse

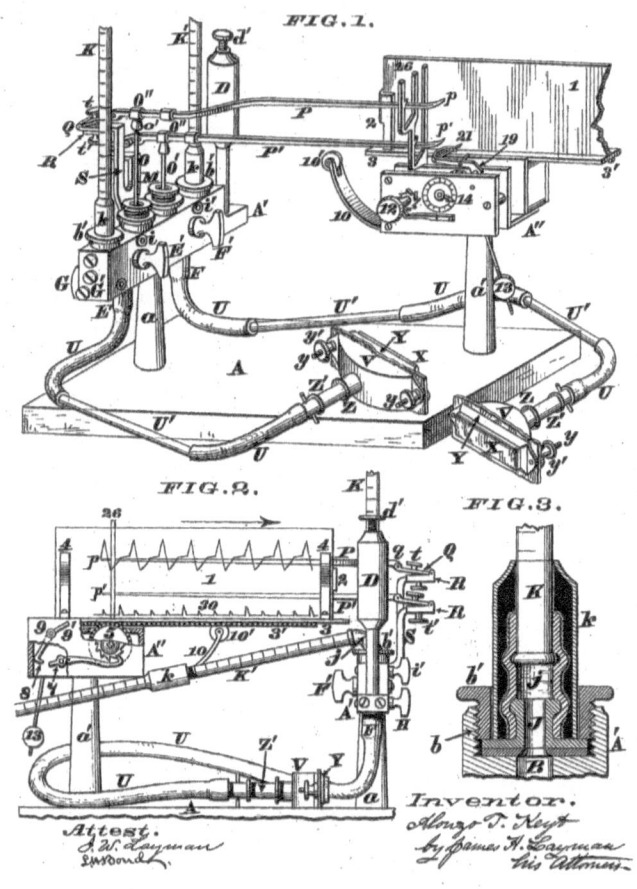

FIGURE 60: Alonzo T. Keyt's patent document (first of three pages) for his chrono-cardio-sphygmograph, with the incorrect title of "Sphygmometer." U.S. Patent No. 203,548, 14 May 1878. www.google.com/patents/US203548.

The major instrument catalogues in the collection of the New York Academy of Medicine show no record of the Keyt sphygmograph, although it is possible that Keyt attempted to market his sphygmograph in Europe. He sold but a handful of sphygmographs; acceptance of his concept and design rather than money would have been the prime reward in Keyt's eyes. His son-in-law and biographer, wrote in 1899:

> In the furtherance of his researches Dr. Keyt spent thousands of dollars, he suffered much pecuniary loss by forgetfulness of calls, and he shortened his life by his assiduous labor. . . . But he counted not his work for gain. He wrought from a pure love for science, and was happy when he brought to light a new fact for the information of the profession and the world.[29]

HOLDEN: "NO PECUNIARY REWARD"

Edgar Holden took the high road with regard to patents, though his sphygmograph appeared in many instrument catalogs of the day. If indeed any Holden sphygmographs were sold, the profits likely went to the instrument companies. Holden received a well-earned honorary doctorate from Princeton University in 1874 for his work with the sphygmograph. In the letter of recommendation written by a distinguished alumnus and trustee (also a physician), it was stressed that Holden looked for "no pecuniary reward from his instrument or his book, very properly regarding it unprofessional to take out a patent."[30] The honorary degree would be its own reward.

POPULAR APPEAL OF THE POND SPHYGMOGRAPH

Alone of the three American sphygmograph men, Pond achieved commercial success, both in Europe and America. He improved and perfected his sphygmograph, but seemed to have had little interest in pursuing cardiovascular studies as Keyt had done—and would continue to do—for the rest of his life. Pond did read a paper on the sphygmograph

---

[29] Isham, "Sketch of the Life and Work of Alonzo Thrasher Keyt," 729.
[30] S. H. Pennington, Newark, to Rev. Dr. McCosh, Princeton, 25 March 1874. Alumni Records, Class of 1859, Box 116. Seeley G. Mudd Manuscript Library, Princeton University, Princeton, NJ.

before a meeting of the Vermont State Medical Society in 1883, long after the instrument was patented, but the paper does not appear to have been published in the transactions of the society.[31]

The Pond Sphygmograph Company was a small firm located in Rutland Village. Abbott S. Pond, Erasmus Pond's eldest son (probably not a physician), was associated with the company, perhaps on the business and manufacturing side.[32] Since the Pond sphygmograph was marketed through a number of catalogues, it seems likely that the Rutland firm wholesaled directly to instrument houses. It is not known if the company sold directly to physicians.

If an advertisement by the Pond company is to be believed, the Pond sphygmograph proved popular among influential sphgmograph users and innovators both in the United States and Britain. The short-lived *Country Practitioner*, published in rural New Jersey, included a full-page advertisement for the Pond sphygmograph in September 1881. Among the leading sphygmographers cited in testimonials were Frederick Akbar Mahomed of Guy's Hospital (see Chapter 3) ("I have abandoned my own instrument for all ordinary purposes [presumably not for research applications], as all the information I require can be obtained with much greater facility by means of your most ingenious little instrument"); Thomas A. McBride of the College of Physicians and Surgeons in New York ("I think that no physician can be without it"); Mary Putnam Jacobi of New York (see Chapter 7) ("I am in the constant habit of using it or ordinary diagnosis in office practice"); and none other than Edgar Holden of Newark (see Chapter 4) ("I concede to it the preference, not only over my own, but Marey's, Keyt's and every other I have seen").[33]

Pond died in 1889 at age sixty seven after a brief illness. He was recalled in the local popular press as a "beloved physician," although the Vermont Medical Society of which he had been a member did not publish an obituary.[34] His obituary in the *Boston Medical and Surgical Journal* noted that he was "best known to the general medical profession as the inventor of the sphygmograph."[35]

---

[31] *Transactions of the Vermont State Medical Society* (1884): 4.

[32] *Gazetteer and Business Directory of Rutland Vermont for 1881–82*, (Syracuse, NY: Journal Office, 1881), 464.

[33] "Pond's Improved Sphygmograph" (advertisement), *The Country Practitioner* 3 (1881): np.

[34] "Dr. E. A. Pond Dead," *Burlington Free Press*, May 31, 1889. Clipping courtesy Sylvia Bugbee, University of Vermont Libraries.

[35] "Erasmus A. Pond" (obituary), 572.

Today, the Pond sphygmograph is found in limited numbers in instrument collections. One example is extant at the Mütter Museum of the College of Physicians of Philadelphia.[36] It was less successful than the compact Dudgeon sphygmograph introduced in England in 1881 and marketed in American catalogues (see Chapter 7). British homeopath and inventor Robert Dudgeon, who reviewed the key features of many instruments in an 1882 monograph, found the Pond sphygmograph limited by its insensitive and uncalibrated rubber sensor, as well as its top-heavy construction (the recording strip and clockwork mechanism hovered over the rest of the instrument).[37]

PHILADELPHIA TRIALS OF THE POND SPHYGMOGRAPH

An early review of Pond's commercially available instrument by Philadelphia physician Frank Woodbury was presented before the Philadelphia County Medical Society and published in that city's *Medical and Surgical Reporter* in 1878. (Pond had exhibited the instrument in 1876 at the International Medical Congress held in Philadelphia.) At the request of prominent Philadelphia physician Jacob Mendes DaCosta of Jefferson Medical College, Woodbury "made some trials" of the instrument on the wards of the Pennsylvania Hospital. Woodbury stressed the ease of applying the instrument to an artery (or over the heart) and obtaining a reading, although practice was required due to the "delicacy of construction."

Woodbury also learned that Pond had since added a "governor" to the watch movement controlling the speed at which the paper or glass (limited to about six inches) moved under the recording stylus, so that the tracing could be taken at any speed. This would be a convenient feature in cases where the examiner wished to "spread out" the pulse wave for closer examination. In cases with a very slow heartbeat or if there was a question of an irregular heartbeat, decreasing the velocity of the carriage allowed the recording of more beats. Woodbury found the instrument far superior to Marey's sphygmograph. He displayed several tracings taken in various disease states (the single tracing printed in the article was of Dr. Pond's normal pulse). DaCosta was "much pleased" with the tracings and declared them the "finest he had ever seen." Woodbury's conclusion echoed the opinions of Burdon-Sanderson and Holden: although the

---

[36] Courtesy, Gretchen Worden, late curator, Mütter Museum, Philadelphia.
[37] Robert E. Dudgeon, *The Sphygmograph: Its History and Use as an Aid to Diagnosis in Ordinary Practice* (London: Baillière, Tindall, & Cox, 1882), 23–24.

sphygmograph could not itself make a definitive diagnosis of any disease, "it offers corroborative testimony which is capable of strongly confirming impressions arising from the usual methods of physical examination."[38]

PRAISE FROM NEW YORK

Writing in 1879, McBride of New York, visiting physician to the Presbyterian Hospital and editor of the *American Journal of Neurology and Psychiatry*, described the recently improved Pond sphygmograph. He noted the resemblance of the Pond instrument to one invented by Maurice Longuet of France, as originally described in the *Bulletin de l'Academie de Médicine* (Paris) in 1868. The Longuet instrument involved a taut string leading from a sensor and passing over a wheel and thence to a recording pencil; the structure was vertical and thus had somewhat the appearance of the Pond sphygmograph. McBride praised the compactness ("can be carried in one's pocket conveniently"), affordability, and ease of use of the Pond sphygmograph. A tracing could be made in three to five minutes (a decided improvement over other instruments) "without disturbing the patient in the slightest."[39]

THE VISIONS OF THREE AMERICAN SPHYGMOGRAPH MEN

Pond seemed not to have pursued experiments or clinical studies beyond the sphygmoscope trials mentioned in his address to the Suffolk County Medical Society in 1875. If he had pursued such studies, if only to calibrate the instrument, he did not publish the results. A survey of the *Transactions of the Vermont Medical Society* located only one very brief

---

[38] Frank Woodbury, "Pond's American Sphygmograph," *Medical and Surgical Reporter* 38 (1878); 493–94.

[39] Thomas A. McBride, "The Utility of the Sphygmograph in Medicine," *Archives of Medicine* 1 (1879): 186–87; Dudgeon. *The Sphygmograph*, 17–18. The Longuet sphygmograph was originally described in detail by [Louis-Jules] Béhier, "A New Perfected Sphygmograph," *Bulletin de l'Académie Impériale de Médicine* 33 (1868): 962–64. It is very unlikely that Pond was aware of Longuet's work. The Languet sphygmograph was not found in any of the American catalogues at the New York Academy of Medicine. An illustration of the Longuet device appears at https://commons.wikimedia.org/wiki/File:Sphygmographe_de_Longuet.jpg (accessed 2 February 2017).

note about Pond's sphygmoscope. At the annual meeting of the Vermont Medical Society in 1876, Pond "showed his new sphygmoscope."[40]

The *Index Catalogue of the Library of the Surgeon General* lists no publications for Pond except for two instruction manuals related to his sphygmograph. The first manual listed in the *Index Catalogue* was *Pond's Improved Sphygmograph*, ten pages in length and published in Rutland in 1877, probably by the Pond Sphygmograph Company. A second manual, *Pond's Perfected Sphygmograph*, emphasizing "simple, portable, practical," was thirty-one pages long and published by Parke, Davis & Co. at an unknown date, but likely later than 1877.[41]

Of the three leading American sphygograph men—Holden, Pond, and Keyt—it was Keyt who had the clearest vision. Holden, who merely modified the Marey sphygmograph, was ultimately frustrated by waveform analysis and voiced his discouragement in his 1877 article, "Errors of the Sphygmograph," in the *New York Medical Journal*.[42] Pond, though his portable sphygmograph seemed to enjoy considerable commercial success, had no apparent interest in medical research. As noted in the previous chapter, only Keyt, although hampered by the technology of his day and the formidable complexity of his compound sphygmograph, glimpsed, however vaguely, the future place of technology and mathematical precision in cardiovascular diagnosis.

"YANKEE INGENUITY"

The sphygmograph entered American consciousness through European journals and monographs. The instrument itself first entered the country in the hands of returning American medical graduates, traveling physicians, and quite likely through orders submitted to European instrument makers. Of the American sphygmographs, only the Pond instrument gained any degree of popularity in the American market. Although the work of Marey,

---

[40] "Proceedings of the Sixty-fourth Annual Meeting [of the Vermont Medical Society] at Montpelier, October 11th and 12th, 1876," *Transactions of the Vermont Medical Society* (1864–1876): 421.

[41] *Pond's Improved Sphygmograph*, 10 pp, Rutland: Tuttle & Co., 1877; *Pond's Perfected Sphygmograph*, 31 pp. Detroit MI: Parke Davis & Co., n.d.; cited in *Index Catalog, Library of the Surgeon-General's Office*, Series 1, 11:493, Series 1, 13:387. It is unknown whether Pond's relationship to Parke, Davis & Co. extended beyond the manual. Parke, Davis & Co. seemed to limit their production to pharmaceuticals during this period.

[42] Edgar Holden, "Errors of the Sphygmograph," *New York Medical Journal* 26 (1877): 498–504.

Burdon-Sanderson, and Mahomed and other European sphygmograph men was well-regarded in American publications, neither American research nor American physicians quite counted in Europe. This may have led both Holden and Keyt to pepper their articles with European names and, somewhat self-consciously, to address a European audience. That little of lasting scientific or practical value would emerge from their experiments was not foreseeable at the time. Twentieth-century investigators with more advanced technology would provide better answers to the questions posed by the nineteenth-century sphygmograph men.

Although Holden and Keyt might be labeled provincials by some, both men boldly engaged a far more organized and powerful British and European research system, even as they labored in the vineyards of general medical practice. For his part, Pond (the most provincial of the three Americans) correctly predicted that his sphygmographs could compete commercially with the American and European models on the market.

"Yankee ingenuity" characterized these and other American tinkerers in medical technology. American medical research was coming of age, led to a large extent by amateur researchers. The American sphygmograph men were neither disciples nor students—they saw themselves as their own masters, as pragmatic inventors and improvers. In the course of the next few decades, as research became professionalized within the medical schools and universities, American medical science would come to dominate western medicine.

The expression "Yankee ingenuity" suggests that Americans were somehow more inventive than Europeans. Of course, the American sphygmograph men were no more ingenious or inventive than the Europeans who inspired their work and there is nothing identifiably "Yankee" about the sphygmograph. But the fact that they worked alone and always outside institutional boundaries sets them apart from the Europeans. None of the three American sphygmograph men were involved in major medical metropolitan organizations such as the College of Physicians of Philadelphia or the New York Academy of Medicine, and none could be counted among the American elite. All belonged to local, state, and/or national medical societies, but the American Medical Association was hardly a prestigious international scientific organization in the 1870s. Aside from collaborations between Keyt with his son-in-law and Pond with his son, all three men worked alone, without the benefits of research academies or collegial discussion. None of the Americans published articles in European journals except for a brief article by Keyt in the *Lancet* (London) initially published in the *Boston Medical and Surgical Journal*.[43]

---

[43] Alonzo T. Keyt, "The Compound Sphygmograph," *Lancet* 2 (1880): 50; Alonzo

Holden appears to have been content with the attention his work received among associates and colleagues; his publications (and the honorary doctorate at Princeton) were apparently their own reward. Keyt, however, felt the snub by his own countrymen quite acutely, even bitterly. As noted in an earlier chapter, his devoted son-in-law and memorialist considered Keyt a prophet unheeded in his own land. For Pond, a dedicated and eclectic tinkerer given to taking out patents, the cachet of a patent and modest commercial success appears to have been sufficient reward.

Compared to the emerging American research establishment typified by John Call Dalton in New York, Harvard physiology professor Henry Pickering Bowditch in Boston, George Hammond in Philadelphia (see Chapter 7), and Silas Weir Mitchell also in Philadelphia, the American sphygmograph men were even further removed physically and culturally from the Continental and British research culture. Their quintessential "Yankee" quality was their self-confident assumption that ordinary, non-elite, and decidedly uninvited American practitioners from Newark, Cincinnati, and Rutland should participate in a research project that elite Europeans claimed for their own.

A "TECHNOLOGY DIALOGUE"

While necessarily based in European antecedents, the work of Holden, Keyt, and Pond was sophisticated, original, and often quite ingenious. The "technology dialogue" between Europe and America on the subject of the sphygmograph was complicated.[44] Holden drew heavily on the work of Marey in France and Burdon-Sanderson in England. However, his modified Marey sphygmograph and his experimental work had little impact in Europe (or America for that matter). He abandoned the sphygmograph within a few years and turned his multiple talents to other medical fields. Keyt appears to have conducted a limited correspondence with Charles François-Franck, a student and colleague of Marey. Keyt's biographer noted that Marey praised the Keyt apparatus and "François-Franck, a pupil of Marey, has also borne testimony to Dr. Keyt's sphygmograph

---

T. Keyt, "The Compound Sphygmograph," *Boston Medical and Surgical Journal* 102 (1880): 484–85. The identical articles were limited to a description and image of the Keyt compound sphygmograph; no experimental work or sample tracings were included.

[44] For a discussion of the concept of technological dialogue (or dialectic), see Arnold Pacey, *Technology in World Civilization* (Cambridge MA: Massachusetts Institute of Technology Press, 1998), vii–viii.

surpassing all others for fidelity and utility." Keyt cited his indebtedness to the research of François-Franck in an article on the effect of cardiac valvular disease on sphygmographic tracings.[45]

Pond, after a few initial experiments, lost interest in the sphygmograph as a research or clinical tool. Although he demonstrated the device before local medical audiences, he published no original articles (the few published reports of his work were written by third parties) and does not appear to have had any correspondence with European investigators.[46] Aside from two pamphlets published under the auspices of his sphygmograph factory, there was no entry in the *Index Catalogue* for any publication in a medical journal describing Pond's clinical or research work with his sphygmograph.

Nevertheless, Pond's practical sphygmograph, manufactured in his own small company in Rutland, Vermont, penetrated the European—or at least the British—market. For example, Dudgeon (British inventor of another popular portable sphygmograph) was familiar with the Pond sphygmograph, which may have influenced his own portable design.[47] London physician and sanitarian Benjamin Ward Richardson found the Pond spygmograph "wanting" and introduced his modified Dudgeon sphygmograph.[48] As noted earlier, if an advertisement by Pond in a minor New Jersey medical journal (*The Country Practitioner*) is to be believed, Frederick Akbar Mahomed of Guy's Hospital, who made great advances in the study of hypertension using his modified Marey sphygmograph, adopted the Pond sphygmograph for ordinary clinical use.[49] In 1890, William Broadbent, a distinguished British sphygmographer, observed in a monograph on the subject that the American Pond sphygmograph, like the British Dudgeon, was "handy and convenient, but a gratuitous provision for exaggeration and for extraneous jerks and vibrations exists in [the lever mechanism]."[50] Ironically, though he had only a passing and minor intellectual engagement with the sphygmograph, Pond had the greatest impact on Europeans, who knew nothing of him except his name on the patented Pond sphygmograph.

---

[45] Isham, "Sketch of the Life and Work of Alonzo Thrasher Keyt," 727. Alonzo T. Keyt, "The Influence of Aortic Aneurism and Aortic Insufficiency, Singly and Combined, on the Retardation of the Pulse," *Boston Medical and Surgical Journal* 103 (1880): 315–16.

[46] Chadwick, "Proceedings of the Suffolk County District Medical Society," 740–42.

[47] Dudgeon, *The Sphygmograph*, 23–24.

[48] B[enjamin] W[ard] Richardson, "A Standard Sphygmograph," in A. S. Aloe Co., *Aloe's Illustrated and Priced Catalogue of Superior Surgical Instruments, Physician's Supplies and Hospital Furnishings*, 6th ed., 354–55. St. Louis: A. S. Aloe Co., ca. 1893;

[49] "Pond's Improved Sphygmograph," *Country Practitioner*, n.p.

[50] William H. Broadbent, *The Pulse* (London: Cassell, 1890), 33.

CHAPTER 7

The Sphygmograph in America: Research, Marketing, and Application

This chapter surveys the career of the sphygmograph and derivative instruments in American practice and research in the closing decades of the nineteenth century and the early decades of the twentieth century. The experiences of a variety of "end-users" of one or another of the commercially available instruments help define the limited applicability and acceptance of the sphygmograph in American medical research and practice.

AMERICAN ASSESSMENTS OF EUROPEAN AND AMERICAN SPHYGMOGRAPHS

In 1879, New York consultant Thomas A. McBride capably reviewed the current uses of the sphygmograph. In his opinion, only the sphygmographs of Marey, Mahomed, and Pond "claimed the attention of the profession at present."[1] McBride maintained that the sphygmograph was not a mere toy for specialists. Its limited use was due to "the great cost of the instrument," time expended in taking recordings, "apparently widely different traces obtained in the same pathological conditions by various observers," and

---

[1] Thomas A. McBride, "The Utility of the Sphygmograph in Medicine," *Archives of Medicine* 1 (1879): 198; "Dr. Thomas Alexander McBride" (obituary), *New York Times*, 7 September 1886.

the disparities in interpretation of the tracings. These problems, ventured McBride, seemed to have been solved:

> Now that the significance of the elements of the pulse-trace is determined, and that the importance of measuring the amount of pressure employed to develop the pulse-trace is appreciated, and that it is realized that the pulse-trace is seldom pathognomonic or diagnostic of diseased conditions, and that the inferences of the observer must be based upon the significance of each factor of the pulse-trace, the amount of pressure employed, and the conditions under which the observation is taken, the sphygmograph is proving to be of the greatest practical use in medicine.[2]

McBride's cheerful optimism aside, such a highly qualified encomium can hardly have been encouraging to busy American general practitioners. Most experts in sphygmography stressed the unsuitability of the instrument for the average practitioner. For those general practitioners who kept up with the medical literature, sphygmographic tracings in medical articles might have appeared instructive and interesting, but hardly relevant to daily practice.

At about the same time, Alfred Carroll, president of the Richmond County (Staten Island, New York) Medical Society, spoke to the members on "The Clinical Use of the Sphygmograph." Carroll was perhaps typical of up-to-date urban practitioners who read the literature and were enthusiastic about introducing new technology into their practices. The sphygmograph, like the thermometer, extended the human senses. Just as the thermometer detected low grade fevers unappreciable by touching the skin, so the sphygmograph "comes to our assistance, giving its visible delineation of the phenomena which we partly know [by physical examination], and showing us others which we could not discover in its absence." Among the sphygmographs Carroll cited as "well known" were those of Marey, Burdon-Sanderson, Anstie, Mahomed, and Holden. He was familiar with (or had at least seen) several of these models, but the most "sensitive and satisfactory" instrument in his experience was that of Pond (aee Chapter 6). Carroll evidently had personal experience with the sphygmograph, citing his examination of patients with rheumatic endocarditis, thoracic aneurysm, and arrhythmias. He illustrated his article with several of his own tracings.[3]

---

[2] McBride, "Utility of the Sphygmograph," 184–85.
[3] Alfred L. Carroll, "The Clinical Use of the Sphygmograph," *New York Medical Journal*

Despite occasional enthusiasts like McBride and Carroll, there were few American voices raised in favor of sphygmography in general practice. In 1882, the *Lancet* (London) published an editorial plea for more general use of the sphygmograph by private practitioners. The editorial was reprinted in the *Medical and Surgical Reporter* (Philadelphia). The writer claimed for the sphygmograph "high practical value even to the busy practitioner." Further, "the discredit into which it has fallen has resulted from the not unnatural enthusiasm of its introducers, who made too much of it, and exaggerated the importance." When "rightly" used, the instrument had much to offer. The *Lancet* editorialist saw the sphygmograph as an instrument which might potentially enhance the status of the profession, stating, "it is of interest to the progress of our art that it should be generally employed."[4] General practitioners among American readers, if they read the Philadelphia journal at all, probably paid little heed.

Some major hospitals may have seen the sphygmograph as an emblem of institutional expertise and sophistication. The Massachusetts General Hospital, seeking to introduce the most up-to-date medical practices, added sphygmographic tracings to some hospital charts in the early 1870s.[5]

As a device that straddled both the physiology lab and a few elite medical practices, the sphygmograph was not a unifying instrument among practitioners. Debates about interpretation and the quality of tracings produced by various models tended to be divisive. At times, sphygmography seemed to be more about the individual instruments and their inventors or champions than about medical science and practice. There was no move to unify around the sphygmograph in the nineteenth century as there was around the laryngoscope and ophthalmoscope. Motivated physicians, particularly in urban centers, could make a living from otolaryngology or ophthalmology by the end of the nineteenth century, but there was no living in sphygmography.

THE SPHYGMOGRAPH: TRICKLING DOWN TO THE PUBLIC

Information about the sphygmograph trickled down sparingly to the educated public during the nineteenth century. As early as 1869, John

---

26 (1877): 254–56, 261–65. The thermometer was introduced into American practice largely through the work of "Éduoard Séguin in the early 1870s.

[4] "The Sphygmograph" (editorial), *Medical and Surgical Reporter* 46 (1882): 378–79.

[5] John Harley Warner, *The Therapeutic Perspective: Medical Practice, Knowledge, and Identity in America, 1820–1885* (Princeton: Princeton University Press, 1997), 156.

Call Dalton of the College of Physicians and Surgeons in New York published an article in *The Galaxy*, a popular general interest magazine, explaining the circulation of the blood in humans and describing the Marey sphygmograph in language easily accessible to the educated adult: "An instrument has been contrived within a few years with which some of the peculiarities of the pulse may be indicated with rather more delicacy than it is possible to perceive them by the finger, and by which they may, at the same time, be registered for future examination." A pulse recording was included, introducing the concept of graphic inscription to the lay reader.[6]

A writer for the literary magazine, *North American Review* (July 1873), summarized a series of talks on the sphygmograph delivered before the British Medical Association in Oxford a year earlier by Frederick Akbar Mahomed of Guy's Hospital. The lectures were illustrated with images (possibly lantern slides). But the article gave no illustrations of either the sphygmograph or a sphygmographic tracing, making it almost impossible for the lay reader to imagine the instrument or its tracings. Furthermore, the author seems to have misjudged the ability of the telegraph to transmit a pulse tracing:

> And if the reader will now attempt to form a mental picture as he goes along with us, we will endeavor to clear up the mystery of the sphygmograph as intelligibly as it can be done without diagrams, at least to give some conception of the simple process by which the heart is made to write out a description of its own ailments at the end of a telegraphic wire a thousand miles away.

Machines capable of transmitting images—primitive facsimile machines—were invented in the 1840s and 1850s, but application was extremely limited. At no point in his multi-part presentation did Mahomed mention transmission by telegraphy and no example of a tracing transmitted by telegraph has been found in the literature consulted for this book. (J. B. Upham in Boston transmitted pulse signals, probably amounting to a simple beep for each pulse wave, by telemetry as early as 1869, but almost certainly did not transmit an actual sphygmogram; see Chapter 4). Despite the engaging prose, the heart could not "write out a description of its own ailments at the end of a telegraphic wire a thousand miles away." Overstating the capabilities of the sphygmograph, the reporter asserted that the "pulse of every individual is as characteristic of him as his intonations or carriage." He concluded with a far more cautious

---

[6] John Call Dalton, "How the Blood Circulates," *The Galaxy* 8 (1869): 673–74.

assertion, reminiscent of the early British and American experience, that the sphygmograph's action "is circumscribed and its value limited. It is the index of the vital and dynamical condition of the circulation alone."[7] The article in the *North American Review* could have done little to enlighten American readers.

In 1884, Joseph C. Hutchinson of New York published *A Treatise of Physiology and Hygiene for Educational Institutions and General Readers*, a compact textbook designed for secondary schools and colleges. In his chapter on the circulation, Hutchison discussed the importance of pulse palpation to the examining physician and continued: "A very ingenious instrument, known as the sphygmograph, or pulse-writer, has recently been invented, by the aid of which the pulse is made to write upon paper its own signature, or rather to sketch its own profile. This instrument shows with great accuracy the difference between the pulse of health and those of disease."

Although he overstated the value of the instrument in diagnosis, Hutchinson captured the essence of the graphic method through his use of such metaphors as "the pulse is made to write upon the paper its own signature" or to "sketch its own profile." A sphygmographic tracing of a normal pulse was provided, with the information that "that part of the trace which is nearly perpendicular coincides with the contraction of the ventricles, while the wavy portion marks their dilatation."[8] The lay reader at once comprehended the novelty and promise of the graphic method—and technology—as applied to clinical medicine.

In general, however, the sphygmograph seems to have enjoyed little cachet among medical consumers. There is no evidence that patients sought out physicians who used the instrument; certainly, it never achieved the status of a fad. If the sphygmographer gained a certain professional status in America, it was most likely in the hands of the proto-specialist—physiologically sophisticated diagnosticians like Edgar Holden or Alonzo Thrasher Keyt—and later the first generation of twentieth-century

---

[7] This is a review and summary of a series of articles by F[rederick] A[kbar] Mahomed in the *London Medical Times and Gazette*, 1872. Frederick Akbar Mahomed, "On the Sphygmograph," *London Medical Times and Gazette* 1 and 2 (1872): 1:62–64, 128–130, 220–22, 250–51, 340–42, 427–29, 569–71; 2:143–45, following page 154 (sample tracings), 324–26. W. O. Johnson, "The Sphygmograph," *North American Review* 117 (1873): 1, 13–17.

[8] Joseph C. Hutchison, *A Treatise of Physiology and Hygiene for Educational Institutions and General Readers* (New York: Clark & Maynard, 1872), 116. It is not clear what "their dilatation" refers to, but it is likely the filling of the ventricles during diastole. In fact, the sphygmogram reflects on the left ventricle, and the plural "ventricles" is misleading.

specialists in cardiology—who were called upon by local general practitioners to offer an opinion in a difficult case.

In a 1921 book designed for the educated public, New York cardiology specialist Louis Faugères Bishop—without actually naming the sphygmograph—admonished potential patients:

> While a superficial examination of the pulse is apt to mislead uninformed people and people who are thoughtless, still with instruments of precision much can be learned by the expert in studying the pulse. A person with heart trouble who can find a physician who will take the time and trouble to make careful tracings of the pulse and study its meaning is foolish indeed if he does not appreciate what is being done for him; he should submit with patience to what may seem tedious repetitions of observation.[9]

WILLIAM HAMMOND'S SPHYGMOGRAPH SPAT

Most American researchers and interested clinicians who took up sphygmography simply used machines developed by others. William Hammond may have been one of the first American adopters of the Marey sphygmograph. During his varied career, Hammond had been a military surgeon conducting experiments at frontier outposts, an early and enthusiastic member of Philadelphia societies for biological experimentation, an unjustly maligned and court-martialed surgeon general during the Civil War, an early practitioner of the fledgling specialty of neurology, and, in his later years, a leading proponent of the vastly misjudged enthusiasm for animal hormonal extracts.[10]

In 1893, Hammond became involved in a vitriolic feud, conducted in the pages of the *New York Medical Journal*, with J. S. Leonhardt, a feisty practitioner from Lincoln, Nebraska. This feud not only exemplifies the occasional public contestations surrounding the sphygmograph, but also highlights one of the greatest problems of the instrument itself: namely, the lack of standardization. Like Keyt of Cincinnati, Leonhardt was a midwestern physician who was not at all intimidated by the Eastern

---

[9] Louis Faugères Bishop, *Heart Troubles: Their Prevention and Relief* (New York: Funk & Wagnalls, 1920), 49–50.

[10] Bonnie E. Blustein, *Preserve Your Love for Science: Life of William A. Hammond, American Neurosurgeon* (Cambridge: Cambridge University Press, 1991), passim.

establishment. Hammond, for his part, claimed almost twenty-eight years of experience with his Marey sphygmograph, purchased in Paris in 1865. In addition, he also used the Pond sphygmograph for twenty years. Leonhardt favored a British Dudgeon sphygmograph.

At the root of the exchange of insults was a dispute over the interpretation of sphygmographs taken in connection with Hammond's research on "Cardine," an extract of animal heart tissue which allegedly acted as a cardiac tonic. Leonhardt questioned Hammond's reading of the sphygmograph tracings published in the original "Cardine" article. Hammond responded by questioning Leonhardt's ability to interpret a normal tracing. The splenetic exchange between Leonhardt and Hammond included charges of pomposity, smugness, intellectual opacity, and incompetence on both sides, concluding in a "challenge for a sphygmographic tournament."[11]

A typical piece of invective by Hammond, who was perhaps miffed by a challenge from a provincial such as Leonhardt, was as follows: "Dr. Leonhardt never having seen any similar sphygmographic tracings, I can well believe his assertion; but if he will kindly take the trouble to consult Marey's *Physiologie médicale de la circulation du sang*, Paris, 1863, he will find not 'several thousand' perhaps, but enough, I think, to convince him that there is even yet something for him to learn on the subject."[12] Leonhardt was not impressed by Hammond's metropolitan authority and was equally acidulous regarding Hammond's article on Cardine: ". . . they are not normal sphygmograms, and that they are unworthy of the least confidence as indicating anything favorable in the circulation—and I challenge their defender to prove the healthy tracings by any rule of sphygmography or process of reasoning whatever. For him to say 'I say they do' is no answer."[13]

Hammond believed that "nothing is more absurd" than comparing the tracings from different machines.[14] This is a key point. One of the

---

[11] William A. Hammond, "Cardine; The Extract of the Heart: Its Preparation and Physiological and Therapeutic Effects," *New York Medical Journal* 57 (1893): 429–31; J. S. Leonhardt, "Organic Juices in Therapeutics," *New York Medical Journal* 57 (1893): 642; William A. Hammond, "A Further Contribution to the Subject of 'Animal Extracts,'" *New York Medical Journal* 58 (1893): 14–15; J. S. Leonhardt, "The Sphygmograph as an Instrument of Precision," *New York Medical Journal* 58 (1893): 225–26; William A. Hammond, "The Sphygmograph as an Instrument of Precision (With Apologies to Dr. Leonhardt)," *New York Medical Journal* 58 (1893), 588–89.

[12] Hammond, "A Further Contribution," 15.

[13] Leonhardt, "The Sphygmograph as an Instrument of Precision," 226.

[14] Hammond, "'The Sphygmograph as an Instrument of Precision' (With Apologies to Dr. Leonhardt)," 589.

insurmountable difficulties that beset the sphygmograph enthusiasts was the inability to standardize different models. Even models by the same manufacturer were idiosyncratic in the hands of individual users. Marey is said to have remarked upon what he called "instruments of chaos."[15] Although the sphygmograph cannot be so glibly dismissed, it was certainly, at least for Hammond and Leonhardt, an instrument of contention.

After almost three decades of experience with the sphygmograph, Hammond appeared to dismiss not only Leonhardt, but the sphygmograph itself: "Now, in regard to the value of the sphygmograph, I have never put much confidence in it. The conditions of its employment are so variable that it is difficult, except in very pronounced cases of disease of functional derangement, to get indications approaching accuracy and that do not vary with each application of the instrument.[16]

MARY PUTNAM JACOBI AND THE BOYLSTON PRIZE

Throughout her professional life, Dr. Mary Putnam Jacobi, the ambitious daughter of a New York publisher, was a champion of high quality medical education for women. The depth and breadth of her medical education far exceeded that of most scientifically inclined male physicians of her day. After earning a pharmacy degree at the New York College of Pharmacy in 1861 and an M.D. degree at the Female Medical College of Pennsylvania in 1864, Putnam completed an internship at the New England Hospital for Women. Acutely aware that her medical education in the United States had not prepared her for a career as a scientific physician, she matriculated at the *École de Médecine* of the University of Paris. She was the first woman to be admitted (despite considerable opposition from many faculty members) and the second to graduate from the institution (1871), having reaseached and written her thesis on the nature of fatty acids.

In 1873, Putnam married Abraham Jacobi, a prominent and powerful New York physician credited with founding pediatrics in America. He helped her gain access to the prestigious medical circles of New York and she was the first woman to be admitted as a member of the elite New

---

[15] Carita Constable Huang, "Instruments of Chaos: The Necessity and Impossibility of Standardizing the Sphygmograph in Late-Nineteenth Century American Medicine," abstract. shot.press.jhu.edu/meeting/huang/htm. Huang's paper was presented at a meeting of the Society for the History of Technology (ca. 2002). This website can no longer be accessed (2016) and the original attribution to Marey was not confirmed.

[16] Hammond, "'The Sphygmograph as an Instrument of Precision,'" 589.

York Academy of Medicine. Her distinguished medical career combined medical practice, a professorship at the Woman's Medical College of the New York Infirmary, medical research and publication in prestigious journals, and advocacy for women's progress in the male-dominated medical profession.[17]

THE BOYLSTON PRIZE: THE SPHYGMOGRAPH AND MENSTRUATION

Harvard University's Boylston Prize Committee announced the topic for the 1876 prize: "Do women require mental and bodily rest during menstruation, and to what extent?" Putnam Jacobi, then in her early thirties and a professor of *materia medica* at the Woman's Medical College of the New York Infirmary, recognized a golden opportunity to refute Harvard professor Edward Clarke's 1873 book *Sex in Education; or, A Fair Chance for the Girls*. Clarke and many of his male colleagues maintained that mental activity, particularly as encountered in higher education, drained nervous force from developing ovaries and uteri, and set the scene for permanent and disabling gynecologic, obstetric, and social dysfunction. The monthly menstrual period was considered a particularly dangerous time, posing an alarming threat to womanhood when proper hygienic principles were flaunted.[18]

Historian Carroll Smith-Rosenberg points out that this was not an academic exercise on Clarke's part. Clarke and other like-thinking physicians (including S. Weir Mitchell in Philadelphia) influenced state legislators and educators. For example, the regents of the University of Wisconsin, drawing on the medical literature (with a dash of nineteenth-century hereditarian dogma) opined in 1877: "[I]t is better that the future matrons of the state should be without a University training than that it should be produced at the fearful expense of ruined health, better that the future mothers of the state should be robust, hearty, healthy, women than that, by over study [sic], they entail upon their descendents the germs of disease."[19]

---

[17] Carla Bittel, *Mary Putnam Jacobi and the Politics of Medicine in Nineteenth-Century America* (Chapel Hill: University of North Carolina Press, 2009), passim; Helen Lefkowitz Horowitz, "The Body in the Library," in *The 'Woman Question' and Higher Education*, ed. Ann Mari May (Cheltenham, England: Edward Elgar Publishing, 2008): 22–26.

[18] Edward Clarke, *Sex in Education; or, A Fair Chance for the Girls* (Boston" James R. Osgood and Co., 1873); Mary Putnam Jacobi, *The Question of Rest for Women during Menstruation* (New York: G.P. Putnam, 1877); Bittel, *Mary Putnam Jacobi*, 122–23.

[19] Board of Regents, University of Wisconsin, *Annual Report for the Year Ending September*

Clarke's demeaning view of fragile womanhood had aroused the ire of Boston woman's rights activist C. Alice Baker, who advised Putnam Jacobi to submit an essay to the prize commitee (all essays were submitted anonymously so that the name and gender of the essayist were not made known to the judges). Putnam Jacobi had previously taken on Clarke in an 1874 essay entitle "Mental Action and Physical Health." It appears that the distinguished physicians on the Boylston Prize Committee had chosen the topic knowing full well that the submitted essays would be a referendum on Clarke's book. In fact, some members of the prize committee were privately critical of Clarke's analysis.[20]

Putnam Jacobi marshalled the best scientific medical tools of her time to present her case. Her handwritten essay effectively used the power of graphic representation to strengthen the medical argument for the resiliance of women. Sphygmographic studies of women were a major component of her refutation of Clarke's theories. Although her scientific approach reflected her rigorous European training, Putnam Jacobi used the sphygmograph as an authoritative technology in a distinctly American setting. Her work suggests that the sphygmograph occupied a position of authority among the top tier of research-oriented American physicians, particularly those who were strongly influenced by European medical science.

THE EVIDENCE PROVIDED BY STATISTICS

(Note: It is not clear to what extent the hand-written prize-winning essay submitted to the Boyston Prize Committee in 1876 differs from the published book (1877), *The Question of Rest for Women during Menstruation*. The analysis that follows is based on the book.)

In laying out her research for her essay on the question of rest for women during menstruation, Jacobi reasoned that if women were indeed ruled by their menstural cycles, then purported rhythmic changes in female physiology (expressed by the contemporary concepts of "nutritive force" or "vital force") should correspond to the menstrual cycle. Based on her research, Jacobi demonstrated—by the scientific standards of her

---

30, 1877 (Madison, 1877), 45; quoted in Caroll Smith-Rosenberg, *Disorderly Conduct: Visions of Gender in America* (New York: Oxford University Press, 1985), 259–60.

[20] Bittel, *Mary Putnam Jacoby*, 123, 126–27.

day—that menstruating women were not disabled or ill and, unless pain or a condition such as a nervous disorder coexisted, rest was not required. To support her thesis, she marshaled three newly authoritative evidentiary methods: statistics, the laboratory, and "instruments of precision."

Using the statistical methods available to her, Putnam Jacobi analyzed the answers to sixteen multi-part (and somewhat subjective) questions, provided by 268 respondents (of one thousand surveyed). Among those surveyed were professional women (teachers and physicians), working class women, and housewives. She distilled her results (with some dozen variables) into tables analyzing family history, exercise, general health, menstrual history, work history, and other factors. Confident in the power of statistics, Putnam Jacobi drew several conclusions from the questionnaires. In summary: "Immunity from menstrual suffering was to be expected in proportion" to childhood health and vigor, family history and vigor, exercise, thoroughness of "mental education," "steadiness of occupation," and marriage "at a suitable time." "As to rest," she continued, "we have seen that the above data do not suffice to inform us of its influence. We can only assert negatively that in a large proportion of cases it has been quite superfluous."[21] While the primitive statistical methods would not pass muster today, they were more than adequate to the standards and methods of surveys in the 1870s.

EVIDENCE SUPPORTED BY THE LABORATORY

Putnam Jacobi turned from statistical analysis of questionnaire responses to the increasingly hegemonic authority of the laboratory and the graphic method. She was as qualified as any clinician of her day to use scientific methods of investigation to argue the cause of equality between the sexes. During her five years in Paris (two as a non-matriculated student), she worked for a time in the microbiology laboratory of Louis-Antoine Ranvier, an assistant to pioneering physiologist Claude Bernard, where she gained skill in microscopy and histology. She also conducted sophisticated chemical experiments on the fatty degeneration of liver tissue and its relation to the body's nutrition. The graduation thesis she would later submit to the medical college in Paris (where she was finally admitted in 1868) was based on this work. At the completion of her formal studies in Paris (1871), she graduated with honors and was awarded a bronze medal

---

[21] Putnam Jacobi, *Question of Rest*, 26–63; summary of results, 62–63.

for her thesis.²² Her scientific education in France prepared her well for her independent laboratory investigations into the question of rest for women during menstruation.

Oxygen consumption, body temperature, carbon dioxide excretion, urea excretion, vital capacity of the lungs, arterial tension, and the dynamic force of muscles were demonstrable and scientific markers for physiological function.²³ Putnam Jacobi selected some of these measurements for her study. Daily urea excretion, considered a measure of nutritional status as reflected in urinary excretion of the end products of protein metabolism, was measured in a few women over a period of months. The results suggested that urea excretion increased premenstrually and decreased at the onset of menses. Putnam Jacobi attributed this to "increased nervous action" and an increased rate of assimilation of nutrients.²⁴

EVIDENCE OF TECHNOLOGY: DYNAMOMETER AND SPHYGMOGRAPH

Clearly aware of the latest technologies in physical diagnosis, Putnam Jacobi used two dynamometer (pressure gauge) models to assess the strength of the muscles in the hand, back, and "loins" in various phases of the menstrual cycle. She supplemented dynamometer studies with weight lifting studies in a small sample of women subjects. The results were inconclusive.²⁵

Finally, she turned to the sphygmograph to demonstrate (or refute) the physiological effects of "rhythmic waves of nutrition or vital force." Putnam Jacobi used a Mahomed sphygmograph (a modified Marey instrument "in which exists a mechanism for varying and accurately estimating the degree of pressure exerted on the artery by the lever of the instrument") to demonstrate arterial tone and volume at various points during the menstrual cycle in a small group of subjects. She used as her guide to arterial physiology a set of "laws" laid out by German physiologist Leonard Landois.²⁶

The American sphygmograph inventors—Edgar Holden, Alonzo T. Keyt, and Erasmus A. Pond—had little influence on their own

---

[22] Bittel, *Mary Putnam Jacobi*, 60–61.
[23] Putnam Jacobi, *Question of Rest*, 115.
[24] Ibid., 142–43, 162.
[25] Ibid., 145–48.
[26] Ibid., 148–49.

countrymen, except perhaps for the occasional purchase of a Pond sphygmograph by interested practitioners. When Putnam Jacobi decided to use a sphygmograph to determine arterial tension, it was the British Mahomed modification of the Marey prototype that she purchased, possibly bringing it back with her from Europe. Holden's monograph was, no doubt, available to her and his modified sphygmograph was offered in catalogues, but neither she nor any other American seems to have been impressed by his minor modifications of the Marey sphygmograph. Putnam Jacobi's work on the problem of the menstural cycle was completed before Holden published his pessimistic 1877 article entitled "Errors of the Sphygmograph" in the *New York Medical Journal*.[27] In all likelihood, her reading of the sphygmographic literature focused primarily on European and British articles and monographs, with little or no attention to the scanty American literature.

Putnam Jacobi's detailed and necessarily subjective analysis of the tracings taken pre-, intra- and post-menstrually in eight women of varying backgrounds and health status, shows an impressive grasp of what Holden liked to call "sphygmographic hieroglyphics." For example, commenting on the pulse curves under various degrees of pressure applied to the radial artery, she wrote: "On December 24, one day before menstruation, the curve is a little more elevated, the summit more rounded, while the line of ascent is more oblique than on either December 22 or January 11, but not too high (compare lines 5 and lines 6 on the three days)."[28] A woman who habitually took to her sofa for four or five days during her menstrual period demonstrated a sinking curve and a short ascension line; a few days later the ascension line was more vertical and "a trifle more fulness [sic] in the artery seems indicated by a little more roundness of the summit."[29] In all, forty-five sphygmographic tracings were reproduced in Putnam Jacobi's monograph.

Such subjectivity and reliance on inexact descriptive terms frustrated many users of the sphygmograph, although Putnam Jacobi seemed to enjoy analyzing the curves and felt confident that the sphygmograph was yielding important and presumably reproducible information. To the modern eye, her readings of sphygmograms were, to be charitable, overinterpreted. She, like the sphygmograph men in Europe and America, expected too much of the technology.

---

[27] Edgar Holden, "Errors of the Sphygmograph," *New York Medical Journal* 26 (1877): 498–504.

[28] Putnam Jacobi, *Question of Rest*, 150.

[29] Ibid., 152.

JUDGING THE EVIDENCE

Whether the Boylston Prize judges followed and understood Putnam Jacobi's analyses of the pulse curves (in all likelihood, none were experienced sphygmographers), they cannot have failed to have been impressed by the pages and pages of carefully labeled tracings taken at four different applied pressures in the eight subjects at various times in their menstrual cycles. Putnam Jacobi summarized her many tracings and concluded that pressure in the arteries increased premenstrually, but decreased sharply a few hours after menstrual flow began, reaching a nadir at the cessation of flow: "in women [there] exists a rhythmic wave of plenitude and tension of the arterial system." Her theoretical analysis of this phenomenon reflected a good grasp of the cardiovascular physiology of the day, focusing on the strength of arterial contraction, blood volume, and the resistance of the arteries (or at least the radial artery). In effect, each menstrual period was a "pregnancy in miniature." The underlying mechanism was postulated to be "an increase in the mass of the circulating fluid."

Putnam Jacobi's knowledge of recent advances in medicine was impressive. What was needed, she commented, was some "measurement of the blood corpuscles" as reported in the recent French literature. "Circumstances beyond our control," she continued, "have hitherto prevented us from pursuing this research, which we propose to do later." Putnam Jacobi demonstrated with considerable force that women's bodies prepared steadily for menstrual hemorrhage by increasing "nutritive strength." Subsequent decreases in various parameters during the menstrual period did not represent depletion or loss of strength, but were rather a return to baseline.[30]

CONCLUSIONS: MENSTRUATING WOMEN ARE GOOD TO GO

Combining her accumulated data questionnaires concerning personal health and menstrual histories, theoretical considerations based on current understandings of physiology, the evidence of the laboratory, and her serial sphygmographic studies, Putnam Jacobi concluded that we can "find no reason to suppose that menstrual rest is desirable or necessary" beyond the adequate rest and short breaks from work that were advisable at all times for women in the interests of general health and improved work efficiency.[31]

---

[30] Ibid., 159–61, 164.
[31] Ibid., 231–32.

Putnam Jacobi's use of diagnostic technology and the laboratory, together with a sophisticated use of contemporary statistical methods, clearly impressed the distinguished male judges of the Boylston competition and struck a blow for advancement of women in society. She chose the subject of fitness during menstruation because she suspected that the research laboratory and new technologies, in which she had invested much of her professional identity, would reveal what she knew to be the truth—that women were equal to men and did not require "management." In assessing the monograph, it might be said that the distaff side of Yankee ingenuity was transplanted from Europe in the service of American women.[32]

Medical technology was not always recruited in support of women's fitness for full partnership in American society. For example, in the late nineteenth century, the hemacytometer, an instrument for measuring the number of red cells in blood, helped define the vague symptom complex of pallor, lethargy, nervous complaints, gastrointestinal irregularities, menstrual disturbances, and apparent maladjustment to the pace of modern society—all subsumed under the diagnostic label of "chlorosis," a malady of young women. A finding of "poor" blood, confirmed by the hemacytometer, justified treatment paradigms that involved removal to a rest home or hospital and an array of dietary and personal hygiene regimens.[33]

THE SPHYGMOGRAPH AND THE WRATH OF THE ANTIVIVISECTIONISTS

Putnam Jacobi was a fearless and self-confident investigator who did not shy away from the accepted laboratory practice of vivisection (dissections and experiments on living and often unanesthetized animals in pursuit of physiological knowledge), a practice vigorously defended by elite physicians against the relentless attacks of the powerful anti-vivisection movement. Her recent biographer writes that she "most forcefully resisted the gendering of experimentatism vis-à-vis the controversial act of live-subject experimentation." She was particularly interested in using animal

---

[32] Despite Putnam Jacobi's powerful essay, women were not admitted to Harvard Medical School until 1945.

[33] Keith Wailoo, "'Chlorosis' Remembered: Disease and the Moral Management of American Woman," in *Drawing Blood: Technology and Disease Identity in Twentieth-Century America* (Baltimore: Johns Hopkins University Press, 1997), 17–45. In time, the hemacytometer and other hematological diagnostic technologies led to the demise of chlorosis as a disease entity by reframing a low blood count as one of several types of anemia.

and human subjects to investigate the physiological effects of medications.³⁴ In 1899, at the request of William W. Keen, president of the American Medical Assocation, she was asked to appear before a Senate committee to defend vivisection and its contributions to medical science, joining elite male physicians from Johns Hopkins, Harvard Medical School, and the United States government. Keen hoped that her appearance as a member of the "humane sex" would be helpful in defense of vivisection.³⁵

Experiments and teaching demonstrations on living subjects ("human vivisection"), blurring the line between the physician's responsibility to patients and the interests of scientific research, were another target of the antivivisectionists. Sydney R. Taber, an attorney and leader of the antivivisection movement, singled out Putnam Jacobi ("one of the most distinguished women in the medical profession") for demonstrating the effects of atropine (a valuable drug, still in use today, with multiple applications and considerable dose-related toxicities) in three healthy women subjects before a class of students at the Woman's College of the New York Infirmary.

He reserved particularly vehement criticism for Putnam Jacobi's experiments on Josie Nolan, a ten-year-old "very healthy Irish boy."³⁶ The sphygmograph figured prominently in these experiments. Young Nolan had suffered a head injury some eighteen months prior to Putnam Jacobi's experiments, leaving him with an open area of the skull bones (2 ½ by 1½ inches) covered by a thick membrane, probably the dura mater (the outer meningeal membrane surrounding the brain) with overlying skin. Pulsations of the membrane were synchronous with the arterial pulse at the wrist and reflected the pulsations of the cranial blood vessels; bulging due to vigorous inhalation was plainly visible over the membrane. Otherwise, the boy was fully recovered. In part, this was a "found" experiment, Putnam Jacobi having done nothing to create the defect (surgeons had previously removed loose fragments of skull immediatedly after the accident). However, by taking advantage of the boy's cranial defect to study the effects of various drugs, she undertook active experimentation. While there was little risk of serious injury, each of the drugs had the potential for unpleasant side effects.

"The case," wrote Putnam Jacobi in her 1878 article in the *American Journal of the Medical Sciences*, "offered a unique opportunity for the study

---

³⁴ Bittel, *Mary Putnam Jacobi*, 110–11.

³⁵ Susan E. Lederer, *Subjected to Science: Human Experimentation in America before the Second World War* (Baltimore: Johns Hopkins University Press, 1995), 57–58.

³⁶ Sydney R. Taber, *Illustrations of Human Vivisection* (Chicago: Vivisetion Reform Society, 1906), 12. Considering the suffering of some animals (and possibly humans) subjected to vivisection, the critics were not without some justification.

of conditions affecting intra-cranial pressure." She adjusted the Mahomed sphygmograph to the boy's head with the sensing lever resting on the membrane and skin overlying the brain. She proceeded to record the pulsations (due to arterial flow from the aorta into the major blood vessels of the brain) in the recumbent boy. She recorded a baseline sphygmogram with no interventions, and then studied the effect of commonly used therapeutic agents including quinine, belladonna (botanical based preparation with atropine-like effects) dosed at intervals for four days prior to study, atropine by injection, coffee, tartar emetic, brandy, potassium bromide, and exercise after ingestion of a full meal. Although she reached no definite conclusions, Putnam Jacobi analyzed each of the rather featureless tracings with respect to intracranial pressure and cerebral blood flow.

There was no notation concerning any ill effects of the drugs upon the boy. A slightly rapid pulse (recorded at 104 per minute) following belladonna was an expected side effect and may have been uncomfortable for the child. Associated symptoms might have included blurry vision, and dry mouth. Tartar emetic, though it did not induce vomiting, might have caused nausea. Quinine has a multitude of side effects particularly with prolonged or high dose administarion.[37] What motivated the mother to agree to the experiments on her son is unclear, but it is possible she received some much-needed remuneration. The child was almost certainly not consulted; clearly he experienced days and perhaps weeks of non-therapeutic dosing of a series of generally safe but potentially harmful pharmaceuticals.

LOUIS FAUGÈRES BISHOP: CLINICAL CARDIOLOGIST

One of America's first full-time clinical cardiologists was Louis Faugères Bishop, Sr., a native of New Brunswick, New Jersey. Obliged to leave the state to attend medical school (New Jersey had no medical schools until the mid-twentieth century), he graduated from the College of Physicians and Surgeons in New York in 1889. Like other promising Jersey-born physicians, Bishop did not return to his native state. He remained in New York, building a reputation as an elite private practitioner specializing in disease of the heart and circulation. He held a professorship of heart and circulatory diseases at Fordham University School of Medicine,

---

[37] Mary Putnam Jacobi, "Sphygmographic Experiments Upon a Human Brain, Exposed by an Opening in the Cranium," *American Journal of the Medical Sciences* 76 (1878): 103–12.

consultancy on diseases of the heart at Lincoln Hospital, and membership in the prestigious New York Academy of Medicine.[38]

By 1908, Bishop was devoting his private practice entirely to cardiology. He was convinced that James Mackenzie's work with the polygraph was the foundation of modern cardiology (see Chapter 3). He visited Mackenzie (unannounced) in his office in Britain, where Mackenzie at once recognized a kindred spirit. Bishop returned to New York with what is believed to have been the first Mackenzie polygraph introduced in the United States. Bishop quickly applied the instrument to his own practice, correlating polygraph readings with tracings from the elecrocardiograph, the latter then in its clinical infancy.[39]

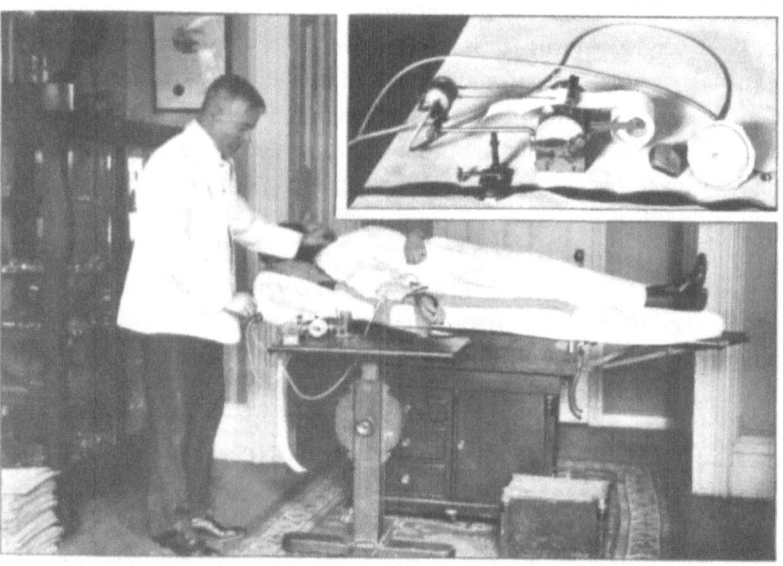

FIGURE 61: Cardiologist Louis Faugères Bishop using a Mackenzie polygraph in his New York office practice ca. 1920 (inset, Mackenzie polygraph). Louis Faugères Bishop, *Heart Troubles: Their Prevention and Relief* (New York: Funk & Wagnalls, 1921), facing page 312.

---

[38] "Louis Faugeres Bishop Sr." (obituary), *Journal of the American Medical Association* 117 (1941): 1458; W. Bruce Fye, *American Cardiology: The History of a Specialty and Its College* (Baltimore: Johns Hopkins University Press, 1996), 24–27.

[39] Louis Faugères Bishop, *Heart Troubles: Their Prevention and Relief* (New York: Funk & Wagnalls, 1920), 302, facing p. 312; Paul Reichert and Louis Faugères Bishop Jr., "Sir James Mackenzie and His Polygraph: The Contribution of Louis Faugères Bishop, Sr.," *American Journal of Cardiology* 24 (1969): 401–3.

In 1918, Bishop's complete heart examination included a Wassermann test for advanced syphilis (a common cause of cardiovascular disease at that time); blood count (to detect increased red cells) and detection of a dark color to the blood (a sign of low oxygen due to inefficient cardiac function); urinalysis (to detect kidney disease, a common factor in heart disease and high blood pressure); "orthodiagram" (a heart radiograph to show the anatomy of the chambers); electrocardiogram (an "autograph of the activities of the heart"), and "polygram" (arterial and venous tracings recorded with the Mackenzie polygraph). He stressed the value of "instruments of precision" and suggested that even the time-honored value of the stethoscope in detecting murmurs might be obviated by application of the advanced technology of his day.[40] Bishop was writing as a full-time cardiology specialist; general practitioners could not be expected to meet such standards. As noted earlier in this chapter, Bishop encouraged cardiac patients to submit to a "tedious" sphygmographic examination to aid in correct diagnosis.[41]

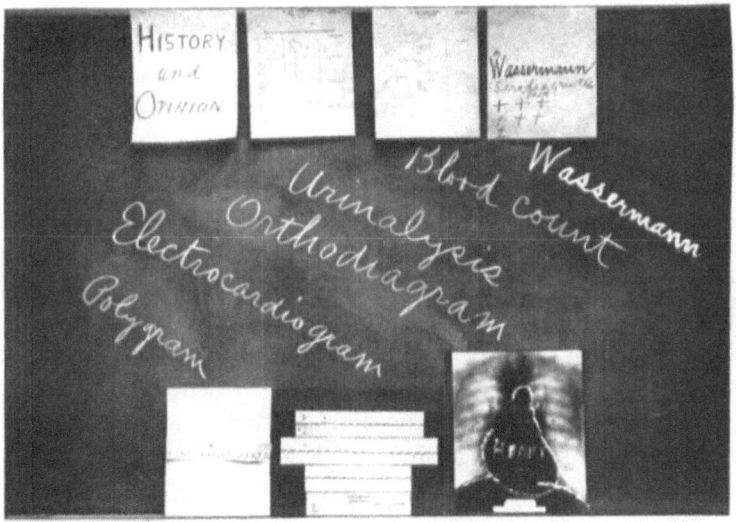

The usual findings in a complete heart examination

FIGURE 62: Elements of a complete cardiac evaluation ca. 1920 according to early clinical cardiologist Louis Faugères Bishop. Tests included a Wasserman test (for syphilis), blood count, urinalysis (to detect kidney disease), orthodiagram (chest X-ray to show heart size and configuration), electrocardiogram, and

---

[40] Bishop, *Heart Troubles*, facing page 188.
[41] Ibid., 49–50.

polygram recorded with Mackenzie's multi-channel polygraph. Louis Faugères Bishop, *Heart Troubles: Their Prevention and Relief* (New York: Funk & Wagnalls, 1921), facing page 188.

PAUL DUDLEY WHITE: A CAUTIOUS APPRAISAL

Harvard's Paul Dudley White, the pre-eminent early-twentieth-century American cardiologist, surveyed the history of the sphygmograph from the vantage point of the early 1930s. He hit upon a key point: the deceptive simplicity of the sphygmograph. Even with more modern sphygmographs, "much training and experience are needed for the satisfactory recording and interpreting of arteriograms, although the technique at first glance may appear simple." Overstating the case somewhat, White wrote that "the new records [of the pulse] added little knowledge beyond that which had already been gained by mere palpation or inspection of the arterial pulse. As a result, sphygmography was abandoned for nearly half a century, except for special studies." Early investigators had expected too much of the sphygmograph, said White, "and the failure of extravagant interpretations to be justified caused its early decline." It is important to note that White and Bishop were writing from the vantage point of three decades of American experience with the electrocardiograph, a perspective that nineteenth-century American sphygmograph men and researchers like Putnam Jacobi did not share and could not imagine.

In his own work, White had found the "improved" instruments, particularly the Mackenzie polygraph, introduced after the turn of the century, to have some value if used carefully. "We realize now," wrote White in 1931, "that the shape and amplitude of the arteriogram [sphygmogram] are complicated not only in themselves but frequently by the addition of artifacts due to the graphic method itself." In fact, nineteenth-century sphygmographers had realized these problems almost immediately, and, like Holden, had grown discouraged. White's 1931 textbook suggests that sphygmograms might yet be of value in studying cardiac arrhythmias if they "cannot be analyzed by ordinary physical examination or where the electrocardiograph is not available." White's classic 1931 cardiology textbook included many pulse tracings and a lengthy discussion of sphygmography presented in the tone of a teaching exercise rather than a guide to current practice. He reluctantly admitted that the sphygmograph had once again fallen into disuse by the early 1930s: "sphygmographs (and polygraphs) are rarely used and have once more, after their revival, returned to accumulate dust upon the shelves."[42]

---

[42] Paul Dudley White, *Heart Disease* (New York: Macmillan Company, 1931), 192–95.

THE DUDGEON SPHYGMOGRAPH IN AMERICA

One late-entry British sphygmograph (ca. 1880) enjoyed popularity in America as well as Britain. A number of American catalogues listed the practical and compact instrument invented by homeopathic physician Robert Ellis Dudgeon, with the pocket model priced at a relatively modest $18.50. Advertisements promoted its ease of use, portability (4 ounces, with dimensions less than 2.5 inches), speed of obtaining a reading ("almost as quickly as the pulse can be felt with the finger"), simplicity of repair, and flexibility of operation. Dudgeon's convenient 1882 pamphlet, *The Sphygmograph: Its History and Use as an Aid to Diagnosis in Ordinary Practice*, featuring a clear brief set of instructions, may have helped popularize the model. The title stressed the applicability to "ordinary practice" rather than research or specialty practice.[43]

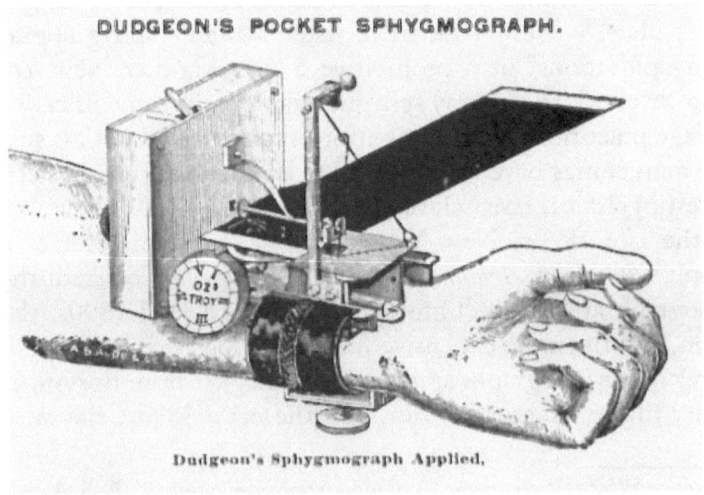

FIGURE 63: British homeopathic physician Robert E. Dudgeon's popular portable sphygmograph. A. S. Aloe Co. *Aloe's Illustrated and Priced Catalogue of Superior Surgical Instruments, Physician's Supplies and Hospital Furnishings*, 6th ed. (St. Louis: A. S. Aloe Co., 1893, 352.

Benjamin Ward Richardson of Britain, whose modified Dudgeon sphygmograph was offered for sale in a St. Louis catalogue (ca. 1893),

---

[43] Robert E. Dudgeon, *The Sphygmograph: Its History and Use as an Aid to Diagnosis in Ordinary Practice* (London: Baillière, Tindall, & Cox, 1882), 67–72.

remarked in the promotional literature that for "all writing purposes, and for perfect convenience, Dr. Dudgeon's Sphygmograph may be taken as well nigh perfect." However, Richardson found that both the Dudgeon and Pond sphygmographs lacked "the means of applying, accurately and easily, the pressure upon the pulse, and of registering the reading so as to be able to obtain a natural standard," with any variations representing "unnatural or morbid variations." Richardson also adjusted the recording surface in his sphygmograph such that calibrated horizontal lines were printed along with the pulse tracings.[44]

SPHYGMOGRAPHS IN AMERICAN INSTRUMENT CATALOGS

American instrument catalogues began to offer sphygmographs in the 1870s. Competition for a limited market seemed to be fairly intense. John Reynders, a New York firm, listed Marey's sphygmograph "for observing pulsations" at a prohibitive $75.[45] Another New York firm offered a "Mercy" (i.e. Marey) sphygmograph at the same price.[46] Clearly, the average practitioner could not afford such a capital outlay, suggesting that the market may have been limited to a few American physicians with an interest in clinical research or specialization.

In the late 1870s, New York's George Tiemann & Co. catalog, the iconic *American Armamentarium Chirurgicum*, offered the Pond sphygmograph at $35.00. Throughout the 1880s and 1890s, the Pond, Dudgeon, and the more expensive Marey (variously designated "Mairey" or "Marez") sphygmographs appeared in catalogues from Boston, Chicago, and other major American cities.[47] In the early 1890s, the A. S. Aloe

---

[44] B[enjamin] W[ard] Richardson, "A Standard Sphygmograph," in A. S. Aloe Co., *Aloe's Illustrated and Priced Catalogue of Superior Surgical Instruments, Physician's Supplies and Hospital Furnishings*, 6th ed. (St. Louis: A.S. Aloe Co., ca. 1893), 352–54. The date was in pencil on the catalogue in the collection of the New York Academy of Medicine.

[45] John Reynders & Co., *Illustrated Catalogue and Price-List of Surgical Instruments* (New York: John Reynders & Co., ca. 1870), 107.

[46] Caswell, Hazard & Co., *Illustrated Catalogue of Surgical Instruments and Appliances* (New York: Caswell, Hazard & Co., 1874), 24.

[47] George Tiemann & Co., *The American Armamentarium Chirurgicum* (New York: George Tiemann & Co., ca. 1879), I:87 (illustration and description), 7 (price list); The Codman & Shurtleff company of Boston also offered a "Mairey" sphygmograph in 1875 for a prohibitive $60, and continued listing it until at least 1890; Codman & Shurtleff, *Catalogue of Surgical Instruments* (Boston, Codman & Shurtleff, 1875), 71; Codman & Shurtleff, *Illustrated Catalogue: Surgical Instruments and Appliances* (Boston:

Co. of St. Louis was offering the Pond instrument for the same price, in addition to the Dudgeon Pocket ($18.50), Holden ($30.00), and Marey ($60.00) sphygmographs.[48] Catalogs that offered the Dudgeon model often appended his relatively straightforward instructions. To put sphygmograph prices in perspective, a physician could purchase an up-to-date binaural stethoscope for $4.50 to $8.00.[49]

No Holden sphygmograph seems to have survived in medical instrument collections. The Holden sphygmograph had originally been manufactured by the George Tiemann Company in New York. The large company, with offices New York (Manhattan) and Brooklyn, included the Holden sphygmograph, together with Marey and Pond models, in its 1879 catalogue, although no price was listed for the Holden model.[50] It is possible that Holden had the company manufacture a single prototype for his own use and others might have been available by special order Although the Holden sphygmograph was advertised in several catalogs, it is doubtful if more than a handful (if any) instruments besides the prototype were ever produced. The similarity to the Marey device (with a few new and modified features), and the appearance of more portable sphygmographs such as the Pond and Dudgeon designs seem to have limited any potential market for Holden's sphygmograph. In 1878, the New York firm of Shepard & Dudley listed the Holden sphygmograph, accompanied by an illustration, for $40. No other sphygmograph was offered by this company, but two other Holden instruments, both respiratory, were offered in the same catalogue.[51] Surprisingly, the Aloe company of St. Louis continued to offer a Holden sphygmograph among its five models in 1893, long after Holden himself had abandoned the promotion of his sphygmograph.[52] The Holden model seems to have started and ended its career in the hands of its inventor.

Codman & Shurtleff, 1890), 92; Chas. Truax, Greene & Co., *Price List of Physicians' Supplies* (6th ed.) (Chicago: Chas. Truax, Greene & Co., 1892), 965.

[48] George Tiemann, *American Armamentarium Chirurgicum*, I:87 (illustration and description), 7 (price list); A. S. Aloe Co., *Aloe's Illustrated and Priced Catalogue of Superior Surgical Instruments, Physician's Supplies and Hospital Furnishings*, 6th ed. (St. Louis: A. S. Aloe Co., ca. 1893), 351. The date was in pencil on the catalogue in the collection of the New York Academy of Medicine.

[49] George Tiemann, *American Armamentarium*, I:82 (illustration), 7 (price list).

[50] Ibid., I:87.

[51] Shepard & Dudley, *Illustrated Catalogue of Surgical Instruments* (New York: Shepard & Dudley, 1878), 874, 877.

[52] A. S. Aloe, *Aloe's Illustrated and Priced Catalogue*, 351. It is possible that the St. Louis company was selling surplus instruments obtained from Tiemann or Shepard & Dudley in New York.

No instrument catalogues from Cincinnati—those most likely to offer the Keyt model—were located in the New York Academy of Medicine catalogue collection. Other Midwestern instrument companies—one from Chicago and another from St. Louis—did not offer a Keyt model. Because of his many articles in respected American medical magazines, the handful that he sold were likely made to order. One or more models reached the Marey group in France, possibly sent as a courtesy by Keyt.[53]

Dovetailing with the declining sphygmograph market was the exploding market in sphygmomanometers (blood pressure instruments). It took some time before blood pressure measurement was standardized and the modern "cuff" was universally accepted. Ten early models offered in 1917 by a Brooklyn supply company ranged from $13.50 to $27.50. The same catalogue offered only two sphygmograph models, both British (Dudgeon at $25.00 and Richardson at $27.50).[54] Unlike the sphygmograph, the sphygmomanometer, though it took several decades to mature and has been embellished by "upgrades" such as digital readout, remains a universal fixture in medical practice a century and more after its introduction. Its ubiquity is reflected in inexpensive self-monitoring models for home use. Even medically unsophisticated members of the general public, while they may have no undestanding of cardiovascular physiology (or familiarity with the word "sphygmomanometer"), easily converse about the numbers in the form of systolic pressure "over" diastoic pressure (e.g., 130 over 60)—whether ominous or reassuring—that comprise the "output" of the sphygmomanometer.

THE POLYGRAPH IN AMERICA

The polygraph, introduced by Mackenzie after the turn of the century, enjoyed a modest career in American; its high price and obvious research applications limited interest to cardiac physiologists and a few clinicians with specialized interests in cardiology. In 1912, T. Homer Coffen, an instructor at the New York Post-Graduate Medical School and College, reviewed the state of the art with respect to the polygraph. He concluded that the polygraph was "an indispensable aid in the accurate diagnosis of cardiac disease. It is now made in compact form and can be carried

---

[53] Asa B. Isham, "A Sketch of the Life and Work of Alonzo Thrasher Keyt," *Philadelphia Monthly Medical Journal*, 1 (1899): 729.

[54] Fred Haslam & Co., *Illustrated Catalogue of Surgical Instruments and Allied Lines* (Brooklyn NY: Fred Haslam & Co., 1917), 13, 16–19.

to the bedside. It gives information that can be obtained in no other way." It aided in diagnosis and prognosis of heart disease, but enhanced rather than replaced physical examination; the polygraph, wrote Coffen, can no more replace ordinary methods of diagnosis "any more than the stethoscope can be used to the exculsion of percussion [tapping with the finger] or inspection."[55] In 1915, a New York instrument supplier was offering Mackenzie's ink polygraph (introduced in 1908) for $84, probably prohibitively expensive for a general practitioner, but within reach of clinicians and researchers dedicated to the study and treatment of heart disease.[56]

THE RISE OF THE EKG AND THE ECLIPSE OF THE SPHYMOGRAPH AND POLYGRAPH

There is no doubt that instruments such as the laryngoscope and ophthalmoscope helped create medical specialties. As medicine moved from patients' homes to doctors' offices, clinics, and hospitals, interested physicians—"fortified with special tools"—began to focus their professional efforts on a single reasonably well-defined and manageable field of practice. The process was accompanied by tensions between specialists and generalists.[57]

In a 1920 discussion of modern cardiac methods, Harvey Ewing of Montclair, New Jersey, a clinician with an interest in cardiovascular diseases, acknowledged the invaluable advances made by Mackenzie through his polygraph studies, but devoted most of his discussion to electrocardiography, a new and exciting field. The polygraph did provide some slight advantage in rare cases. Otherwise, concluded Ewing, its portability—early EKG machines were massive—was its only advantage. In something of a requiem for the polygraph and a tribute to Mackenzie, Ewing remarked in 1920, "Historically, we owe much to it."[58]

---

[55] T. Homer Coffen, "The Clinical Value of the Polygraph," *Post-Graduate* 27 (1912): 173.
[56] Kny-Scheerer Co., *Illustrations of Surgical Instruments of Superior Quality*, 20th ed. (New York: Kny-Scheerer, 1915), 1085; James Mackenzie, "The Ink Polygraph," *British Medical Journal* 1 (1908): 1411.
[57] Audrey Davis, *Medicine and Its Technology: An Introduction to the History of Medical Instrumentation* (Westport CT: Greenwood, 1981), 240.
[58] Harvey M. Ewing, "Modern Cardiac Methods," *Journal of the Medical Society of New Jersey* 17 (1920): 256. The polygraph remained particularly useful in diagnosing *pulsus alterans*, a sign of heart failure. The term persists in modern cardiology.

As late as 1927, New York cardiologist Bishop, the early American adopter of the Mackenzie polygraph, observed, "While the polygraph is not used today as often as before the perfection of the electrocardiograph, it is nevertheless of value."[59] Mackenzie had some difficulty convincing American manufacturers to produce and sell his polygraph, but catalogues later offered an American model.[60] The Mackenzie polygraph lingered in American instrument catalogues well until the 1920s. A Rochester firm offered the "American Model" at $200 in 1925. Blood pressure cuffs in the same catalogue ranged from $15 to $30.[61]

TECHNOLOGY AND THE RISE OF SPECIALIZATION IN CARDIOLOGY

Cardiology was only gradually and unevenly defined as a specialty in America. The first generation of American cardiologists came of age in the second and third decades of the twentieth century, at a time when the sphygmograph was virtually forgotten, the polygraph waning, and the electrocardiogram in its robust youth. According to W. Bruce Fye, historian of the American College of Cardiology, the specialty was created by a small and diverse group of American doctors just prior to World War I. A number of these men were best described as physiological cardiologists, concerned with the transfer of medical instruments from the laboratory to the bedside. Equally important were overlapping categories of practitioner cardiologists, academic cardiologists, and public health cardiologists. The role of the practitioner cardiologists (often involved with general practice as well as clinical cardiology) vis-à-vis new technologies was one of diffusion into patient care.[62]

For the better prepared consultants such as Bishop, the early integration into practice of the electrocardiograph, the fluoroscope for evaluation of cardiac size and silhouette, the sphygmomanometer to record blood pressure, and the Mackenzie polygraph to evaluate pulse and cardiac pressure curves—in addtion to a term of study at a recognized European

---

[59] Louis Faugères Bishop and John Neilson Jr., *History of Cardiology* (New York: Medical Life Press, 1927), 70.
[60] Davis, *Medicine and Its Technology*, 130. The Mackenzie Ink Polygraph persisted in American catalogues well into the 1920s.
[61] R. J. Strasenburgh Co., *Catalogue of Surgical Instruments, Physician's and Hospital Supplies* (Rochester, NY: R. J. Strasenburgh Co., 1925), 7.
[62] Fye, *American Cardiology*, 13–14.

center of clinical or research cardiology—advanced the embryonic specialty of clinical cardiology in America.[63]

Joel Howell, a historian of medical technology, points out that the founders of the first cardiology societies did not consider technology to be the foundation of their expertise.[64] However, in Fye's analysis, the growing enthusiasm for technology not only distinguished them from general practitioners and general internists, but also helped such men be seen as specialists by generalists, colleagues, and patients.[65] To the extent that clinical cardiologists came together around technology, it was such early-twentieth-century instruments as the sphygmomanometer, electrocardiograph, and x-ray apparatus (including the fluoroscope) that dominated their practice.

Fye views the electrocardiograph (rather than the polygraph) as a "unique tool to differentiate" specialists in cardiology from the mass of general practitioners. Not only did the electrocardiograph contribute to the self-identification of aspiring cardiologists, but it also attracted patients to their practices and confirmed to their clientele (and referring general practitioners) their claims of expertise. In the decades before specialty regulation and board certification, the purchase of a pricey electrocardiograph machine and a short post-graduate course were sufficient to "transform [motivated general physicians] into cardiologists," at least in the eyes of some patients.[66]

The next chapter examines the successes and failures of the sphygmograph as a piece of technology that, in the course of a few decades, proved to be far more opaque and problematic than its initial enthusiastic reception seemed to promise.

---

[63] Ibid., 26–27.

[64] Joel D. Howell, "Introduction," in *Technology and American Medical Practice, 1880-1930; An Anthology of Sources* (New York: Garland, 1988), x.

[65] Fye, *American Cardiology*, 32.

[66] Ibid., 8.

Chapter 8

An Opaque and Slippery Technology: The Visions of the Sphygmograph Men

The limitations of the sphygmograph punctuate much of the narrative and commentary in this book. From the outset, doubts were raised by most of the early enthusiasts and persisted through the half-century trajectory of the sphygmograph. Judging by the number of entries in the *Index Catalogue of the Library of the Surgeon General*, interest in the sphygmograph in America peaked between 1875 and 1879.[1] Considering the difficulties in using the instrument and interpreting what Holden referred to as sphygmographic "hieroglyphics," many clinicians may have quickly relegated their hasty purchases of a convenient portable Dudgeon or Pond sphygmograph to a shelf.

Caveats, rationalizations, ambivalence, and a palpable sense of frustration seemed to be an intrinsic feature of the instrument itself,

---

[1] Robert G. Frank, "The Telltale Heart: Physiological Instruments, Graphic Methods, and Clinical Hopes," in *The Investigative Enterprise*, eds. William Coleman and Fredrick L. Holmes (Berkeley: University of California Press, 1988), 239. Using the *Index-Catalogue of the Library of the Surgeon-General's Office*, Frank found that there were over thirty articles on the subject of the sphygmograph between 1875 and 1879 and less than twenty between 1885 and 1889. However, many articles about sphygmography (or incorporating sphygmography) may have appeared under various other titles relating to cardiology or pulse study, thus calling into question the count used by Frank. For example, a good many articles by Keyt did not have "sphygmograph" in the title: for example, "The Influence of the Respiration on the Form, Rhythm, and Succession, of the Cardiac and Arterial Pulse Curves" (1879) and "Cardiography" (1885). However, the trend documented by Frank is unmistakable.

evident in much of the writing of the British and American sphygmograph men. This chapter examines the sphygmograph in light of the recent rich literature about medical technology.

Carl Ludwig's work with the kymograph and Étienne-Jules Marey's experiments with the prototypical sphygmographs created something of a technological imperative to move the graphic method out of the laboratory and into medical practice. All medical technologies have their growing pains, including many like the electrocardiograph and sphygmomanometer that would be considered resounding "successes" by physicians and medical historians alike. These two technologies evolved over a period of many decades; yet there was a sense of steady progress and increasing penetration into clinical practice. Complaints with respect to the sphygmograph were more persistent and insistent, and there did not seem to be a sense of progress.

The sphygmograph was the most important new cardiac diagnostic technology during much of the century following René T. H. Laennec's 1816 invention of the stethoscope in 1816, a profoundly simple technology. The stethoscope indeed *saw with a better eye*, a phrase introduced by Jean Nicholas Corvisart to characterize early advances in the diagnosis of diseases of the chest.[2] The sphygmograph was only marginally a "better eye," its trajectory much shorter than that of the stethoscope, a resounding and unqualified "success" for two centuries—uneclipsed by the sphygmograph, polygraph, sphygmomanometer, electrocardiograph, radiograph, echocardiograph, cardiac catheterization laboratory, and, very likely, other diagnostic technologies not yet imagined.

For three or four decades after its introduction in the 1860s, the sphygmograph and its various models and champions stood alone, sandwiched between the stethoscope (1820s) and the early blood pressure machines (1890s). Critics claimed that the sphygmograph added nothing to pulse palpation and they may have had a point. But they missed the magical, seductive vision of the future—the introduction of graphical representation of physiological events into clinical medicine. The sphygmograph men, for all their frustrations, saw the future and grabbed the only device yet invented that offered such a revolution. Those who championed the sphygmograph embraced the new graphic representation of the pulse—and in this they were visionary.

---

[2] Jacalyn Duffin, *To See with a Better Eye: A Life of R.T.H. Laennec* (Princeton, NJ: Princeton University Press, 1998), epigraph, 33.

THE FIRST DECADE: HOPEFUL PREDICTIONS AND GATHERING CAVEATS

In the 1860s, the application of the sphygmograph to clinical practice *seemed* self-evident to men who had little but their fingers and their stethoscopes to bring to the bedside. But the leap from laboratory to bedside would prove to be haphazard. British sphygmograph pioneer John Burdon-Sanderson anticipated that the sphygmograph "would create visible and permanent records of great precision, the factual contents of which, unlike the private knowledge of the pulse taker or the stethoscope user, would be so accessible to all that they would occasion no disagreement."[3] He predicted confidently in 1867 that the "use of the sphygmograph will tend to clear up all this uncertainty [in pulse palpation] . . . for, whatever else may be questioned, it cannot be denied that it is an impartial and consistent witness."[4] He admired the crisp objectivity that the sphygmograph brought to the murky subjectivity of traditional pulse study and proclaimed in 1866, "The utility of the sphygmograph as an instrument of physiological and clinical research is now so generally recognised that it is scarcely necessary to vindicate it."

But Burdon-Sanderson was a thoughtful physician who tempered his enthusiasm and urged caution, particularly with respect to the potential of the sphygmograph at the bedside. In an article in the *Lancet* in 1866, he warned that the sphygmograph was still a work in progress, writing in a "language which we are only beginning to understand." Even at this early date, it was clear that one must not expect the sphygmograph to give an exact diagnosis of a heart condition, but rather reveal information about the rather vaguely defined "state of the circulation." Cautious optimism was in order: "However imperfectly we may yet be able to interpret [the sphygmograph], we may confidently hope that it will some day help us to arrive at a more perfect knowledge of those individual peculiarities of healthy constitution which we now neglect for want of the means of appreciating them." Further, this was an instrument that could not be used by a mere mechanic: "Without a proper knowledge of the physiological facts, of which they are the transcript, the oscillations of the lever are quite as meaningless as the vibrations of the telegraphic needle to one who is not furnished with a proper alphabet."[5]

---

[3] Frank, "Telltale Heart," 212–13.

[4] John Burdon-Sanderson, "Lecture on the Characters of the Arterial Pulse, in Their Relation to the Mode and Duration of the Contraction of the Heart in Health and Diseases," *British Medical Journal* 2 (1867): 39.

[5] John Burdon-Sanderson, "On the Theory of the Pulse" (No. 1 in a series "On the

In an 1867 address to an audience of physicians at the Royal College of Physicians in London in 1867 and in his *Handbook of the Sphygmograph* published the same year, Burdon-Sanderson urged caution; the sphygmograph was no philosopher's stone.[6] On a positive note, He anticipated that the sphygmograph would contribute to a better understanding of cardiovascular physiology. The sphygmograph couldn't do *everything*—but perhaps it could do *something*: "Its value will, in my judgment, consist in the exactitude and precision which it will impart to the notions we at present possess as to the practical significance of the various forms of pulse."[7]

The laryngoscope (ca. 1855) and the ophthalmoscope (ca. 1851) fostered and revolutionized the specialties of otolaryngology and ophthalmology. Burdon-Sanderson specifically warned against putting the sphygmograph in the same revolutionary clinical category: "The sphygmograph is not to be regarded, like the laryngoscope or the ophthalmoscope, as an aid in the discovery and discrimination of organic diseases . . . Its use is to enable the physician to investigate the state of the circulation and circulatory organs in diseases of which the general nature is already recognized."[8]

CONFOUNDING THE CURVE: THE "DIARRHOEA PULSE"?

The pulse curve was a tricky business, dependent on the sphygmograph model, operator technique and experience, anatomy of the patient's wrist, pulse rate, and such picky factors as the time of day. Most distressing was the observation by Burdon-Sanderson and others that "very different tracings present themselves in morbid conditions which appear to be nearly the same, and similar tracings in states of the circulation which are entirely opposite." In today's terms, sphygmograms lacked both sensitivity and specificity.[9] The modern physician, with his multitude of tests, might

---

Application of Physical Methods to the Exploration of the Movement of the Heart and Pulse in Disease"), *Lancet* 2 (1866): 517–18.

[6] John Burdon-Sanderson, *Handbook of the Sphygmograph: Being a Guide to Its Use in Clinical Research, to Which is Appended A Lecture Delivered at the Royal College of Physicians on the 29th of March 1867 on the Mode and Duration of the Contraction of the Heart in Health and Disease* (London: Robert Hardwicke, 1867), 65.

[7] Burdon-Sanderson, *Handbook*, 65.

[8] Burdon-Sanderson. *Handbook* 27.

[9] Burdon-Sanderson, "On the Theory of the Pulse," 517–18. High sensitivity means few false negative results; high specificity means few false positive results. Ideal tests are

be more inclined to accept such disjunctions, using each test as but one more piece of evidence to be integrated with clinical findings. But Burdon-Sanderson had no other technologies beyond his stethoscope.

London medical writer and early sphygmograph adopter Francis E. Anstie found himself frustrated by variations in the pulse tracing caused by mundane confounding variables. As early as 1867 he complained that his own pulse tracing varied with the time of day. During a bout of diarrhea, Anstie found changes in his tracing, leading him to refer to the "diarrhoea pulse," while his state of fatigue resulted in a "fatigue pulse." The ingestion of a "hearty meal" was known to decrease the amplitude of the pulse wave, purportedly due to diversion of blood to the digestive organs. An article published in the *Lancet* and extracted for the *Medical Record of New York* listed Anstie's warnings: observations were "never to be taken" within two hours after dinner, one hour after breakfast, or fifteen minutes after an alcoholic drink; pressures taken too close to meals "are entirely worthless as a representation of the real conditions of the organs of circulation." Recordings, wrote Anstie, should never be taken during a state of "bodily fatigue from exertion," when the patient is "under cardiac excitement caused by muscular exercise," if the patient is "flushed with heat from external sources," or "under the influence of sudden emotional shock."[10] Anstie warned that a physician unwilling to invest "much training and practice," including repeated examinations of the pulses of particular persons," in learning to use the sphygmograph correctly would be rewarded with false readings and "disgust" with the instrument.[11] Such restrictions, if strictly applied, would certainly have tempered the enthusiasm of busy clinicians.

The pulse waves varied not only with the physiological status of the patient at the moment the tracing was made, but also with the construction of the individual machine, the perseverance and manual dexterity of the physician, and the soft-tissue anatomy of the subject's wrist. A clinician anxious to perfect his skills and extend his horizons might well be put off by such red flags from acknowledged, if self-appointed, authorities. In short, the sphygmograph was idiosyncratic—mastery tedious, interpretation tricky, and application to patient care uncertain.

---

both specific and sensitive.

[10] Francis E. Anstie, "Cautions in Regard to Use of Sphygmograph," *Medical Record New York* 2 (1867–68): 59; Francis E. Anstie, "On the Diurnal Fluctuations of the Pulse-Form, and on Certain Cautions Necessary to be Observed in Sphygmography," *Lancet* 1 (1867): 170–72.

[11] Francis E. Anstie, "Lectures on the Prognosis and Therapy of Certain Acute Diseases, with Specific Reference to the Indications Afforded by the Graphic Study of the Pulse," *Lancet* 2, 1867): 124.

In the early 1870s, research physiologist Alfred H. Garrod of Cambridge demonstrated that the shape of the pulse wave—the primary concern of the clinical sphymographer—was a function of the heart rate at the particular moment the tracing was made, although most sphygmographers ignored this point and the changes may have been subtle.[12]

Today, similar considerations (though easily resolvable with careful planning and technique) have a role in establishing a life-changing diagnosis of hypertension: arm position, emotional and activity states, dehydration, posture (recumbent vs. sitting), prescription or over-the-counter medication, and other factors can affect a baseline reading. So-called "white coat hypertension" (anxiety associated with a medical office visit) has become an important consideration. Of interest is Anstie's warning that palpable arterial rigidity "from atheromatous or calcareous change impairing the elasticity of the vessels" led to changes in the pulse tracing.[13] Today, physicians recognize that such a calcified artery may give a falsely high reading with the modern blood pressure cuff: so called "pseudohypertension."

"THE PERSONAL EQUATION"

In perhaps the strongest condemnation of the sphygmograph and particularly its less discriminating users, elite London hospital man and authority in the fields of cardiology and neurology William H. Broadbent, observed in 1890:

> It is not, therefore, from ignorance or want of familiarity with the sphygmograph that I have come to the conclusion that it is not especially useful in practice—that in any form known to me it is not a clinical instrument for everyday work. It is rarely necessary for diagnosis, and scarcely ever to be trusted in prognosis. The indications obtained from it are not like those of the thermometer, independent of the observer. Skill and practice are required in applying [the sphygmograph to the artery]; judgment is called for in determining the position

---

[12] Alfred H. Garrod, "On Sphygmography, Part II," *Journal of Anatomy and Physiology* 7 (1872): 104–5. Garrod derived an equation showing that sphygmosystole (the sphygmographic representation of physiologic cardiac systole) was proportional to the cube root of the pulse rate.

[13] Anstie, "Lectures on the Prognosis and Therapy," 124.

and pressure which give the best trace, and indeed in deciding which of the traces obtainable is the best representative of the particular pulse; the personal equation of the observer, therefore, comes in, and if any special result is expected or wished for, an enthusiastic investigator can obtain it, and may, without the least conscious intention, twist facts in the desired direction.[14]

Even Frederick Akbar Mahomed, the young British master of the sphygmograph and the man who, in the 1870s, brilliantly teased out the clinical entity of essential hypertension armed only with his modified Marey sphygmograph, was not above posthumous criticism. His memorialist in the *Lancet* (quite possibly his mentor Broadbent) hinted that his work and his enthusiasm were not transferable to his colleagues, many of whom must have been hospital men at Guy's in London:

> It must be twelve years ago that there appeared in the *Medical Times* that series of papers upon the sphygmograph which at once stamped him as an ardent and industrious student; indeed, he was characterised by an ardour and energy which often made him formulate propositions far in advance of the ideas of his more cautious comrades, and led him sometimes into mistaken inferences, but none the less honestly believed and advocated. It was a common saying that no one but Mahomed could interpret all the teachings of the sphygmograph, and it may be that this study of its records led him to place too strong a reliance upon the mechanical contrivance, without due allowance for its necessary imperfections. In spite of all that, it cannot be denied that his fervent advocacy did much to re-establish the sphygmograph in clinical estimation.[15]

PICTUREPHONE AND SPHYGMOGRAPH: FAILED TECHNOLOGIES?

Contested issues with respect to the sphygmograph included the undefined target audience for the technology, the overly-optimistic expectations of its champions, its place in the contemporary quest for

---

[14] William H. Broadbent, *The Pulse* (London: Cassell, 1890; Philadelphia: Lea Brothers, 1890), 32–33.

[15] "Frederick A. Mahomed" (obituary), *Lancet* 2 (1884): 973–74.

instruments of precision, the process of moving the technology from laboratory to clinic, the technological dialogue that shaped the use of the instrument, the critical problem of standardization, and the vexed issue of the role of the hallowed physician's art vis-à-vis technology. These are familiar themes in discussions of new medical technologies in our own times. While not simply a transitional technology, the sphygmograph filled a cardiovascular technology gap between the invention of the stethoscope (ca. 1820) and the introduction of the sphygmomanometer (blood pressure cuff) and the electrocardiograph (ca. 1895–1910). The apparent "failure" of the sphygmograph seems a stark contrast to the undeniable "success" of these two twentieth-century technologies.

The uneven fortunes of the sphygmograph can be examined in the context of a growing literature that investigates the problem of "failed technologies."[16] In 2003, historian Kenneth Lipartito revisited the notion of failed technology, using the unlamented Picturephone of the 1960s, a commercial disaster for Bell Laboratories, as a case study.[17] The Picturephone allowed users to transmit not only words, but real time images over telephone lines.

A key question about a new technology should be "Why was it invented?" rather than "Why did it fail?"[18] By the 1960s, the well-established telephone seemed to have created a "cultural imperative" that influenced imaginative inventors in the technology industry. In what proved to be a miscalculation, the addition of sight to sound promised by Picturephone seemed like an idea whose time had come.

Despite its commercial collapse (development expenses were astronomical, costs to the consumer at twenty dollars per minute were prohibitive, and sales quickly approached zero), Picturephone nevertheless "did not deflect technology from what [Bell laboratory engineers] confidently predicted was the road to the future."[19] Recent years have witnessed the (unacknowledged) reincarnation of the forgotten Picturephone in applications such as Skype and FaceTime. The personal computer created the cultural and social upheaval (as well as the free or low-cost access) that led to universal acceptance of—and increasing dependence

---

[16] Professor Richard Sher, Federated History Program, New Jersey Institute of Technology and Rutgers University, and Dr. Paul Israel, Edison Papers, Rutgers University provided helpful guidance to the recent literature of failed technologies.
[17] Kenneth Lipartito, "Picturephone and the Information Age: The Social Meaning of Failure," *Technology and Culture* 44 (2003): 50–81.
[18] Ibid., 63
[19] Ibid., 81.

on—face-to-face real-time long distance conversations, instruction, and interviews—just like Picturephone.

The practical life of the sphygmograph—some three or four decades—exceeded the brief trajectory of Picturephone. Like Picturephone, the sphygmograph added a "picture" (graphic representation over time) to a traditional "technology"—pulse palpation. Because technology is embedded in culture, apparent technology failures "are not inherent in hardware but constructed by contingent social conditions." In something of a feedback loop, the ways in which new technologies are used depends in part on expectations arising from previous experience.[20] The sphygmograph was used in ways that were intimately tied to traditional pulse lore as well as to evolving knowledge about cardiac physiology. The information the sphygmograph gave was marginal at best, in part because the pulse is more complicated than physicians of the day were able to appreciate; it did not prove to be the reliable window into the workings of the heart that early enthusiasts predicted.

But technology, as Lipartito reminds us, is not "a stable artifact but a system in evolution." Just as the Picturephone, which vanished quickly from the market and public memory, succeeded in "guid[ing] [future] innovators by helping to establish a basic paradigm for information services and technology," so the sphygmograph taught medical innovators to see the cardiovascular system in terms of graphical representations.[21] Dismissing a technology as a failure leads to historical lacunae, preventing historians from understanding the "ensembles, the systems, and the values embedded in machines."[22] The ambivalent experience with the sphygmograph did not discourage more successful efforts to create technology that could plumb the secrets of the cardiovascular system. Like Picturephone, the sphygmograph was—if not *the* road to the future—at least it was *a* road to the future.

Taking a nuanced view, historian David Pye suggests that no technology is failure-free. Every medical device produces its own learning curve, generates new questions, replaces something or someone else, finds new niches, and, in many cases, is superseded. Pye views at least partial failure as ubiquitous and "inherent in all useful design."[23] It would be a mistake, for example, to overemphasize the perfection of either the electrocardiograph or

---

[20] Ibid., 52, 54, 56.
[21] Ibid., 76–77.
[22] Ibid., 80.
[23] Commentary by David Pye, *The Nature and Aesthetics of Design* (London: Barrie & Jenkins, 1978) discussued in Graeme Gooday, "Re-writing the 'Book of Blots': Critical Reflections on Histories of Technological 'Failure,'" *History and Technology* 14 (1998): 277–78.

sphygmomanometer. Despite their relatively high sensitivity and specificity in many disease states, they each underperform in some circumstances and both have been superseded or complemented in special cases by newer more invasive or costly cardiac technologies. Intraarterial pressure monitoring is common in intensive care units, as it provides more exact and continuous blood pressure readings than the sphygmomanometer. Most people with abnormal electrocardiograms require further testing by invasive or non-invasive tests to define their cardiac pathology.

For any technology, there is a group of users who strive to "nourish a fledgling device." Such "initial adopters" are attracted to new technologies and are generally technologically savvy and capable of more complex operations than the potential end users. They serve as middlemen between inventors/manufacturers and the larger audience that will embrace future user-friendly models. Early users are attracted not only by the new technology, but also by the "the image of the future they represent." Lipartito uses the example of the early computer whizzes who helped take an exciting new technology from a complex device requiring multiple sophisticated inputs to the user-friendly omnipresent devices of today. [24] The initial adopters of the sphygmograph were only partially successful in making Marey's visionary invention convenient and practical for the general physician. The identity of the "end user" of the sphygmograph was never quite clear.

A dynamic that seems to have played a role in the trajectory of the sphymograph was "the ever more demanding expectations that human users impose upon their all-too-limited constructions."[25] Graeme Gooday, a historian and philosopher of science, believes that what fails is not technology, but rather human expectations.[26] Physicians expected that the sphygmograph would reveal much about the heart and circulation and in this they were disappointed.

CUI BONO? WHO BENEFITS

Audrey Davis, in *Medicine and Its Technology: An Introduction to the History of Medical Instrumentation*, explains the attraction of the sphygmograph and similar technologies. For the would-be specialist, instruments "offered those with manual dexterity a chance to excel as physicians in a profession that previously had favored individuals with good memories and a penchant

---

[24] Lipartito, "Picturephone," 74.
[25] Gooday, "Re-writing the 'Book of Blots,'" 278 (quoting Pye).
[26] Ibid., 286.

for theories."[27] In the hands of some physiologically oriented clinicians, both in Europe and America, the sphygmograph was a sign of expertise in diagnosis and a symbol of modernity. One thinks of elite physicians such as Burdon-Sanderson and Anstie who enjoyed an enhanced status among their peers as clinicians and sphygmographers; Burdon-Sanderson's early work with the sphygmograph may have been an important factor in his 1895 appointment to the post of Regius Professor of Medicine at Oxford, where he undertook basic research in physiology.

The sphygmograph could serve to refine the art of pulse study among clinicians. Broadbent, who harbored considerable doubts about the value of the sphygmograph in clinical practice, told colleagues at St. Mary's Hospital in 1875 that the sphygmograph was "a great means of educating us how to feel and properly appreciate the pulse [and] has, in fact . . . rediscovered for us the indications furnished by the pulse."[28] The sphygmograph could be a valuable learning tool for the student embarking upon the art of pulse palpation: "While, then, I think," Broadbent (who taught medical students at St. Mary's Hospital) told the Royal College of Physicians in 1887, "that every student ought to be familiar with the sphygmograph, and will gain from a study of its indications a comprehension of the pulse in its different forms obtainable in no other way, I am of [the] opinion that we learn by means of the educated finger all that the sphygmograph can teach, and more."[29]

Edgar Holden in Newark parlayed his sphygmographic studies, some quite sophisticated, into the prestigious Stevens Triennial Prize of the College of Physicians and Surgeons, and a published monograph that stands as the only American book-length work on the sphygmograph.[30] On the strength of his monograph, he was awarded an honorary doctorate from Princeton and was recognized as a consultant by his fellow Newark physicians. Some, like Robert Dudgeon in England and Erasmus Pond in the United States, enjoyed some financial gain from their popular portable sphygmographs. T. Lauder Brunton in Edinburgh established the value

---

[27] Audrey Davis, *Medicine and Its Technology: An Introduction to the History of Medical Instrumentation* (Westport CT: Greenwood, 1981), 233.

[28] William H. Broadbent, "The Pulse: Its Diagnostic, Prognostic, and Therapeutic Indications," *Lancet* 2 (1875): 549.

[29] William H. Broadbent, "The Pulse: The Croonian Lecture delivered to the Royal College of Physicians, 1887," *British Medical Journal* 1 (1887): 657; "Sir William Henry Broadbent" (obituary), *Lancet* 1 (1907): 126–29.

[30] Alonzo T. Keyt's book, *Sphygmography and Cardiography, Physiological and Clinical* was a compilation of his many articles about the sphygmograph, edited and published posthumously in 1887.

of amyl nitrate for angina pectoris with the aid of serial sphygmograms. Garrod in England and Keyt in Cincinnati advanced the study of time intervals between sequential events in the cardiovascular system. Keyt gained some recognition from Marey and his disciples in France. For Mahomed and James Mackenzie in England, the sphygmograph opened doors to hypertension and arrhythmias, respectively. For Marey, who started it all, the sphygmograph served as an intellectual and conceptual stepping-stone to later experiments in the space and time of human and animal locomotion through chronophotography. Mary Putnam Jacobi used the sphygmograph to make a powerful statement debunking the frailty of women.

For all these sphygmograph users, whether "initial adopters" and technical innovators or simply purchasers of standard machines, the sphygmograph was one of many exciting new "instruments of precision" that helped break the stranglehold of classical medicine on the imagination of clinicians and turn their gaze from the past to the future.

General practitioners—at least those who kept up with the medical literature—also benefited. As historian Robert G. Frank Jr. points out in "The Telltale Heart," the sphygmograph demonstrated to practicing physicians how *la méthode graphique* actually worked. Readers of medical journals and textbooks became accustomed to seeing sphygmographic tracings in print, even if they had never personally used a sphygmograph and could not interpret the relatively uninterpretable tracings. The jump from experiencing a patient's pulse as a palpable event to seeing the same pulse as a waveform on a piece of paper was easily made—the pulse moved up and down under the palpating finger and the wave tracing moved up and down on the recording surface. Physicians came to feel at ease with the notion of pulse tracings and were thus better prepared to accept later graphic representations such as that of the polygraph and the electrocardiograph. Today's physicians have "learned to write and read a Babel of new graphic languages, languages both created and taught by physiological instruments."[31]

LOSING THE BOOSTERS

A modern historian has suggested that the sphygmograph suffered partly because it lost its greatest champions.[32] By the late 1860s, Marey

---

[31] Frank, "Telltale Heart," 275.
[32] Ibid., 224.

was becoming interested in time and motion studies in animals.[33] In the 1870s, Burdon-Sanderson turned toward academic physiology, first in London and later at Oxford. Anstie died of sepsis in 1874 at age forty. Garrod died of tuberculosis in 1878 at age thirty-three. Mahomed in his last years turned to epidemiology, collective investigation, and studies of the "tuberculous diathesis" based on physiognomy before his death in 1884 at age thirty-five of typhoid fever.[34] Broadbent remained devoted to bedside pulse study. Thomas A. McBride of New York, who promoted the sphygmograph to general practitioners, died at age forty of kidney failure. Holden, who foresaw a "dictionary in which each individual tracing can be referred for interpretation," was disillusioned by the mid 1870s. Pond undertook little serious study of sphygmography, focusing his attention on designing, producing, and marketing his portable sphygmograph.[35]

Most of these men became disillusioned with the sphygmograph and did not die or abandon their investigations extolling its virtues. Alone of all the sphygmograph men discussed in this book, Keyt of Cincinnati maintained his faith in his careful metric sphygmographic studies until his death in 1885. But Keyt's elegant chrono-cardio-sphygmograph and his complicated analyses of tracings died with him. The reasons for the slow death of the sphygmgraph were complex and occupy much of the discussion in this chapter. Perhaps it might be more accurate to say that the sphygmograph drove away many of its early champions.

ELITE BRITISH MEDICINE AND THE CHALLENGE OF TECHNOLOGY

There were complex forces at work within elite British medicine at the turn of the twentieth century. Technology was a vexed question. Influential clinicians, while aware of the new laboratory medicine and often adopting such technology as might enhance their status, based their professional self esteem on the ingrained notion of a hallowed healing art, the gold standard

---

[33] Anson Rabinbach, *The Human Motor: Energy, Fatigue, and the Origins of Modernity* (Berkeley: University of California Press, 1990), 99–104.

[34] J. Stewart Cameron and Jackie Hicks, "Frederick Akbar Mahomed and His Role in the Description of Hypertension at Guy's Hospital," *Kidney International* 49 (1996): 1500–1.

[35] Edgar Holden, *The Sphygmograph: Its Physiological and Pathological Indications* (Philadelphia: Lindsay and Blakiston, 1874), 89.

of clinical experience, and, to some extent, the magisterial presence of the cultured physician.[36]

Medical gentlemen in Britain were skeptical of the role of diagnostic technologies in consultancy and hospital practices. The *art* of medicine—built on the hallowed sciences of anatomy and physiology and filtered through deeply ingrained social and bedside skills—as practiced by the classically educated and trained physician—remained a guiding principal and point of professional identification. Experience in practice fostered knowledge that defied simple transmission to younger physicians or less endowed practitioners; it was "incommunicable." The term is taken from pioneering British ophthalmologist William Bowman's address at King's College in 1851.[37]

Medical historian Christopher Lawrence, in "Incommunicable Knowledge: Science, Technology and the Clinical Art in Britain, 1850-1914," notes that the antipathy to technology went hand-in-hand with antipathy to specialization. The stethoscope, introduced into clinical practice by the 1820s, was not fully embraced by British practitioners until the 1880s. The ophthalmoscope, a German invention of the early 1850s, was somewhat neglected for two decades in Britain. The sphygmograph and later the sphygmomanometer

> ... had a very chequered career within English medicine until well into the twentieth century. Both of these instruments were essentially different from the foregoing [the stethoscope, ophthalmoscope, and clinical thermometer] in that they were tools developed within continental experimental physiology.... The [sphygmograph] was taken up in England by a small number of enthusiasts.... The [sphygmomanometer], too, found a few disciples in England.... The majority of the profession, however, were not impressed.[38]

The *British Medical Journal* had even more serious doubts about the value of the new instruments in measuring the blood pressure. In a 1905 editorial about the link between essential hypertension (high blood pressure

---

[36] Christopher Lawrence, "Incommunicable Knowledge: Science, Technology and the Clinical Art in Britain, 1850-1914," *Journal of Contemporary History* 20 (1985): 504–18.

[37] The quotation is from William Bowman, "An Introductory Address Delivered at King's College, London, October 1st, 1851," in *The Collected Papers of Sir W. Bowman, Bart., F.R.S.*, ed. J. Burdon-Sanderson and J. W. Hulke (London: Harrison and Sons, 1892), 2:61.

[38] Lawrence, "Incommunicable Knowledge," 514–16.

with normal kidneys) and cerebral apoplexy (stroke), the editorialist commented on Clifford Allbutt's elucidation of essential hypertension as revealed by newly introduced and still unstandardized sphygmomanometer models. Allbutt advised that the blood pressure should be "measured at regular intervals by means of the best instruments obtainable" in everyone over age forty; treatment would consist of what we could call today life style changes in the hopes of preventing apoplexy. On the future of technology, Allbutt got it right; the anonymous editorialist got it wrong:

> But it may reasonably be doubted whether instrumental research will ever be as useful in the investigation of blood-pressure in man as the fingers [to feel the pulse] and ears [to listen to the patient's recitation of symptoms] of a cultivated observer. There is a certain risk that the multiplication of instrument tends to pauperize the senses and to weaken their clinical acuity; even the sphygmograph is mainly used nowadays rather for the purpose of demonstration or of making a permanent record than for what it can tell us in diagnosis or prognosis.[39]

WHO WAS TO USE THE SPHYGMOGRAPH? THE BRITISH VIEW

The place of the sphygmograph in medical practice, whether with the urban elite or the provincial general practitioner, was never quite resolved. The problem was discussed in both America and Britain. When the sphygmograph was first introduced in Britain by Burdon-Sanderson and a handful of others, it seemed necessary to reassure even sophisticated clinicians that the instrument had a place outside the research laboratories on the Continent. To an audience of leading London physicians at the Royal College of Physicians in 1867, Burdon-Sanderson stressed that it should not be regarded as a mere dynamometer in the hands of the research physiologist. Stopping short of recommending the instrument to the general practitioner, he emphasized its value to the student of disease, the "pathologist," who was thereby "furnished with an instrument whereby he can investigate the mode, and measure the duration of the ventricular systole in disease."[40]

---

[39] "The Prevention of Apoplexy," *British Medical Journal* 1 (1905): 783.
[40] Burdon-Sanderson, *Handbook of the Sphygmograph*, 55.

In 1882, *Lancet* published an editorial plea for more general use of the sphygmograph under the title "The Sphygmograph in Private Practice." After observing rather tartly that "like everything else, sphygmography has been in turn recklessly extolled and unduly deprecated," the editorialist claimed for the sphygmograph "high practical value even to the busy practitioner." Further, "the discredit into which it has fallen has resulted from the not unnatural enthusiasm of its introducers, who made too much of it, and exaggerated the importance..." When "rightly" used, the instrument had much to offer. The *Lancet* editorialist saw the sphygmograph as an instrument that might potentially enhance the status of the profession: "[I]t is of interest to the progress of our art that it should be generally employed." The *Lancet* editorial was quoted in the *Medical and Surgical Reporter* (Philadelphia) and thus also reached an American audience.[41] General practitioners among the British and American readers probably paid little heed. Broadbent, who extolled the value of the sphygmograph in research, was convinced that it "will never come into use in general practice, for it demands not only time and care at each application, but also a careful preliminary training."[42]

THE AMERICAN RESPONSE A TOOL FOR THE GENERALIST?

Historian Joel Howell, in his introduction to *Technology and American Medical Practice: 1880–1930*, notes that, in general, American medical practice did not begin to take on modern trappings—and modern technology—until the end of the nineteenth century and the early years of the twentieth century. Notable exceptions were the adoptions of the ophthalmoscope and the laryngoscope, technologies of self-evident value to diagnosis and treatment; the specialties of ophthalmology and laryngology coalesced, in part, around these practical tools. Although some physicians in general practice embraced new devices, neither physicians nor their patients viewed technology as central to the practice of medicine or to the self-identity of practitioners.

A major impetus for the use of technology in clinical practice was the introduction, late in the nineteenth century, of laboratory work in the medical school curriculum. With work in the student laboratory came

---

[41] "The Sphygmograph in Private Practice," *Lancet* 1 (1882): 73; "The Sphygmograph" (editorial), *Medical and Surgical Reporter* 46 (1882), 378–79.

[42] Broadbent, "The Pulse: Its Diagnostic, Prognostic, and Therapeutic Indications," 549.

familiarity and some facility with physiological equipment. In a country eagerly embracing technology in all walks of daily life, students and general physicians saw value in developing practical skills ("craft knowledge") required to operate new devices that enhanced diagnosis and marked them as scientific physicians by colleagues and patients.[43]

There were isolated enthusiasts in America in the 1860s and 1870s who saw a place for the sphygmograph in general practice, though the more common view was that the sphygmograph was best left to the elite practitioner who alone could plumb its mysteries and cope with its idiosyncrasies. Austin Flint Sr., an American authority on cardiac diagnosis, concluded in 1873 that the "delicacy of the instrument, however, the nicety required for its employment, and the numerous incidental circumstances which are liable to affect its operation, must restrict very much its availability in the hands of the general practitioner."[44]

In contrast, French educated New York physician Édouard Séguin suggested somewhat counterintuitively in 1867 that far from being irrelevant to the ordinary practitioner, the very fussiness of the Marey sphygmograph presented an opportunity for general physicians to improve their skills in handling delicate instruments—the wave of the future—with ease and confidence.[45]

New York's McBride observed in 1879: "By most of the profession the instrument is looked upon as a toy, or as a piece of delicate and complicated machinery, which can only be operated by some specialist, whereas it is an instrument of very simple construction, which should be in every-day use, and which should be of the greatest value and assistance to the general practitioner." Its limited use, continued McBride, was due to "the great cost of the instrument," time expended in taking recordings, "apparently widely different traces obtained in the same pathological conditions by various observers," and the disparities in interpretation of the tracings. Once the novice came to appreciate the niceties of applied pressure on the artery, and the fact that "the pulse-trace is seldom pathognomonic or diagnostic of diseased conditions . . . the sphygmograph is proving to be of the greatest practical use in medicine.[46]

---

[43] Joel D. Howell, "Introduction," in *Technology and American Medical Practice, 1880–1930: An Anthology of Sources* (New York: Garland, 1988), ix–x.

[44] Austin Flint, Sr., *A Treatise on the Principles and Practice of Medicine; Designed for the Use of Practitioners and Students of Medicine*, 4th ed., (Philadelphia: Henry C. Lea, 1873), 117.

[45] É[douard] Séguin, "Sphygmometry," *Medical Record* (New York) 2 (1867/68): 244.

[46] Thomas A. McBride, "The Utility of the Sphygmograph in Medicine," *Archives of Medicine* 1 (1879): 184–85.

McBride's cheerful optimism aside, such a highly qualified encomium can hardly have been encouraging to busy general practitioners. For those general practitioners who kept up with the medical literature, sphygmographic tracings in medical articles might have appeared instructive and interesting, but hardly relevant to daily practice.

The voices of American boosters were little heard or heeded. In 1888, almost two decades after the United States first became (minimally) acquainted with the sphygmograph, Alfred Carroll, president of the Richmond County Medical Society (Staten Island) told an audience of medical men that care and discrimination were required: "We must guard against an over-estimate of its pretensions, bearing in mind that, like other instruments of medical inquiry, it is but an aid, not an all-sufficient means of diagnosis." He stressed the importance of weighing all findings in establishing a diagnosis. As an aid to diagnosis, sphygmographic tracings, "taken in conjunction with other sources of information, will often prove of the highest value, and sometimes afford the earliest indications of disease which we should otherwise have overlooked." Arterial tracings taken from subjects with diseased heart valves, for example, offered supportive rather than diagnostic information; in general, they were to be considered "only as indicating the extent to which the circulation is crippled."[47] The value of such supportive, but not diagnostic, tests should not be underestimated. Today, for example, echocardiography can be used to analyze reduced cardiac output, the common endpoint of *many* cardiac diseases. Such information carries diagnostic, prognostic, and therapeutic implications for modern cardiologists when used in the context of careful clinical evaluation and a selected suite of tests.

In the late nineteenth century, the quest for precision in diagnosis and treatment was accompanied by, and in part fueled by, a barrage of new "instruments of precision." This was one of the attractions of the sphygmograph to the self-selected men who embraced the new device. But some American physicians urged caution. In an 1884 challenge to the quest for new devices, Henry D. Didama from Onandaga County, the president of the New York State Medical Association, cautioned against what he saw as the dangers in "all the 'scopes,' all the 'graphs,' and all the 'meters'" that threatened "with unappeasable appetite [to] devour our substance." The ideal, in his view, was "conservative progress." Brandishing similes, he passionately declared:

---

[47] Alfred L. Carroll, "The Clinical Use of the Sphygmograph," *New York Medical Journal* 26 (1877): 255, 262.

> The innumerable instruments of precision, which promise to substitute mathematical accuracy for vague guesses and which are too often used, not to supplement but to supplant other and valuable methods of investigation, these, like the tribe of Abou Ben Adhem, will continue to increase till they become multitudinous, if not perplexing, like the grasshoppers of the West.[48]

S. Weir Mitchell, Philadelphia neurologist and physiologist, reflected more positively on the increasing role of instruments of precision in medicine. In his 1891 presidential address to the Congress of American Physicians and Surgeons, Mitchell advanced the counterintuitive notion that increased instrumentation might create, rather than save, labor:

> Thinking over the number of instruments of precision a single case may require you to use, it is clearly to be seen that no matter how expert we may be, the diagnostic study of an obscure case must to-day exact an amount of time far beyond that which Sydenham [seventeenth century physician known as the English Hippocrates] may have found need to employ.... These increasing demands upon us are due to the instruments of precision or to accurately precise methods.

This increased expenditure of time was, in Mitchell's view, worthwhile. Not only did medicine as a healing art and science advance, but the physician who took time to master the new technologies became a more acute observer. Whatever its failings—and the oft-mentioned time-consuming procedure needed to take a reliable tracing—the sphygmgraph brought new insights—a new mental image—to the time-honored ritual of simple pulse palpation:

> The use of instruments of precision . . . has tended to lift the general level of acuteness of observation. The instrument trains the man; it exacts accuracy and teaches care; it creates a wholesome appetite for precision which, at last, becomes habitual. The microscope, the balance, the thermometer, the chronograph [an instrument for recording time] have given birth to new standards in observation, by which we live, scarcely conscious of the change a generation has brought about.... If, indeed, you use

---

[48] Henry D. Didama, "The President's Annual Address: Conservative Progress," *Transactions of the New York State Medical Association* 1 (1884), 22.

the sphygmograph much, you get to making visual images of the pulse-curves whenever you very carefully feel a pulse.

Mitchell, however, stressed the risk posed by instruments such as the sphygmograph (and even the clinical thermometer) to the "lazy or unthoughtful" physician: "For unless men keep ahead of their instrumental aids, these, to coin a word, will merely dementalize them."[49]

STANDARDIZATION

The early sphygmograph men often found themselves dissatisfied with the sphygmographs and the sphygmograms of predecessors and colleagues. Even Marey was not above criticism. In 1867, Anstie found that "many of the tracings obtained by Marey, and recorded in his admirable work on the 'Medical Physiology of the Circulation' are inadequate, in consequence of neglect of these necessary measures [in positioning the instrument and recording the waves]."[50] Holden alluded to the "merits and defects of his [Marey's] invention," which he (i.e., Holden) ventured to correct.[51] The constant efforts by various inventors—Holden, Burdon-Sanderson, and Mahomed all introduced purported improvements—to redesign the Marey sphygmograph, while not in itself an unusual feature of medical technology, seemed to embody a sense of frustration rather than an air of progress. Pond and Keyt in the United States abandoned springs and looked to the sphygmoscope, a simple hydraulic design, as a model for their innovative sphygmographs.

Broadbent remarked of the sphygmograph in 1875, that the physician must not only know how to interpret the tracing, but he must also know "certain details respecting the sphygmograph producing it . . . and much experience is required to render the tracings by different instruments comparable."[52] Fifteen years later, he was more specific.

> It is necessary also before a trace can be interpreted with any degree of confidence to know what form of sphygmograph has been employed. Marey's is still, in my opinion, the best. . . .

---

[49] S. Weir Mitchell, *The Early History of Instrumental Precision in Medicine. An Address Before the Second Congress of American Physicians and Surgeons, September 23, 1891*, (New Haven: Tuttle, Morehouse, & Taylor, 1892): 8–9.

[50] Anstie, "On the Diurnal Fluctuations of the Pulse-Form, 172.

[51] Holden, *The Sphygmograph*, 18.

[52] Broadbent, "The Pulse: Its Diagnostic, Prognostic, and Therapeutic Indications," 549.

> English modifications of Marey's sphygmograph often magnify the pulsation too much, and in doing so introduce exaggerations due to the rapid movement of the writing lever. Pond's and Dudgeon's instruments are extremely handy and convenient, but a gratuitous provision for exaggerations and for extraneous vibrations exist in the loose and unmechanical way in which the motion of the intermediate lever is communicated to the writing lever, and in the weight which acts as counterpoise in this last-named lever.[53]

The desiderata of standardization and the related process of calibration of newly introduced medical instruments were critical to what was rapidly becoming a transatlantic pool of medical knowledge. For the clinical thermometer, the problem was rapidly solved. The inexpensive production of standardized thermometers was easily absorbed by a manufacturing sector that was accustomed to making thermometers for industry and other areas of science. A far simpler instrument than the sphygmograph, the medical thermometer played a key role in demonstrating to physicians that physiologic events in patients could be recorded and subjected to analysis that was applicable to therapeutic decision-making.[54] The stethoscope was improved over many decades, undergoing a fundamental transformation in the nineteenth from a monaural wooden tube to the binaural stethoscope with flexible tubing in use today. Although quality in the diaphragm, tubing, and earpieces was important, standardization and calibration were not necessary for an instrument that depended for its interpretation on what lay, so to speak, between the ears of the physician.

In contrast, there was never any move to standardize the sphygmograph. The multiplicity of "improved" instruments, each with unique idiosyncrasies, and the apparent opacity of the actual tracings contributed to problems with standardization. There was nothing to standardize the instrument *against*. For an instrument to be of practical value in medical practice, there must be some workable conventions that are based on sound premises and reproducible results. Without standardization, scientific dialogue was stymied.[55]

---

[53] Broadbent, *The Pulse*, 33. The mention of British modifications may have been a reference to the Burdon-Sanderson and Mahomed modifications of the Marey sphygmograph.

[54] Davis, *Medicine and Its Technology*, 85.

[55] Carita Constable Huang, "Instruments of Chaos: The Necessity and Impossibility of Standardizing the Sphygmograph in Late-nineteenth Century American Medicine" (abstract, Society for the History of Technology, ca. 2002). http://shot.press.jhu.edu/meeting/huang.htm. (no longer accessible in 2016).

"A VERY LITTLE PRACTICE"

When London homeopathic physician Robert Dudgeon introduced his portable sphygmograph in 1882, the accompanying pamphlet, *The Sphygmograph: Its History and Use as an Aid to Diagnosis in Ordinary Practice*, was addressed to practitioners intending to use the device in "ordinary practice," by which Dudgeon meant the well prepared and respected—but not necessarily elite—practitioner who might not be a "hospital man" or consultant. He advise those who were about to embark on sphygmography that "they should make themselves thoroughly acquainted with the pulse-tracings of healthy persons at all periods of life and under various conditions. . . . A considerable amount of practice is required in order to enable the operator to obtain the best tracing from every pulse." The last statement belies Dudgeon's earlier assurance that mastery comes with "a very little practice."[56]

Dudgeon reminded potential purchasers that the sphygmogram of a healthy person varies with rest and exercise, fasting and eating, stimulants, "mental emotions," fatigue, position, and changes in temperature—as well as variations in pressure upon the artery required to obtain the best tracing. In spite of these caveats, Dudgeon maintained, more optimistically than was warranted, that "the pulse of the same person in health under all circumstances will generally offer some more or less striking peculiarities that differentiate it from other pulses, so that we may almost recognise an acquaintance by his sphygmogram as surely as we can by the features of his face."[57] He observed, as had others, that the tracing could look perfectly normal even in the presence of significant organic heart disease. He did, however, reiterate the utility of the sphygmograph in determining the "soundness of the arteries" and "analy[sis] of the heart's actions in cases of tumultuous or excessively rapid action, which neither the finger [on the pulse] nor the ear [aided by the stethoscope] can properly judge."[58]

He assured his readers that the tedious process of correctly capturing a pulse reading was eased by the Dudgeon sphygmograph, for which he claimed "a decided superiority over all those hitherto in use." He was aware that the value of the Dudgeon sphygmograph in daily practice was as yet unproven, but was confident that with increased use, "its teachings will eventually be accurately appraised, and it will play as important a

---

[56] Robert E. Dudgeon, *The Sphygmograph: Its History and Use as an Aid to Diagnosis in Ordinary Practice* (London: Baillière, Tindall, & Cox, 1882), 64, 59.

[57] Ibid., 60–61.

[58] Ibid., 54–55.

part in clinical research as the stethoscope and the thermometer." But, he continued, "I must warn the practitioner against expecting too much from the revelations of the sphygmograph." Yet Dudgeon was guardedly hopeful that the sphygmograph, like the thermometer and the stethoscope, would become "pretty general" in daily practice. In particular, he hoped that *his* sphymograph, "hitherto mostly confined to hospital patients," would find a place in the "much more numerous patients of private practice."[59] The modern reader of Dudgeon's pamphlet might be left with the (unstated) impression that it would be more or less up to the purchasers of the Dudgeon sphygmograph to confirm its value.

Thus, the problems identified by the pioneers of the 1860s remained unsolved in the early 1880s. In retrospect, Dudgeon's intelligent and balanced monograph (written partly, to be sure, in pursuit of sales) might have dissuaded more potential buyers among private practitioners than it persuaded.

WILLIAM OSLER OF HOPKINS ON THE SPHYGMOGRAPH

One useful gauge of the importance of a medical trend to the turn-of-the-century American physician was the attention paid to it by William Osler of Johns Hopkins Hospital and the Johns Hopkins School of Medicine. Osler was the consummate bedside diagnostician, and the most influential American physician of his day. He was the sole author of several editions of his classic textbook, *The Principles and Practice of Medicine*. Although he relied a great deal upon his own vast experience, Osler collected and synthesized the work of the leading experts of Europe and America.

In the 1892 first edition of his textbook (a decade before the sphygmomanometer was introduced into clinical practice in America), Osler described palpation of the high tension pulse of arteriosclerosis, followed by a sentence on the sphygmographic pattern associated with the high tension pulse (sloping short upstroke, no percussion wave, and a gradual slow descent, with a "very slightly marked" dicrotic wave).[60] It seems likely, however, that Osler himself did not use the sphygmograph, nor did he expect his readers to use it in clinical diagnosis.

---

[59] Ibid., 65–66.

[60] William Osler, *The Principles and Practice of Medicine*, 1st ed. (New York: D. Appleton & Co., 1892) 668.

By the time the sixth edition of his textbook appeared in 1906, Osler had revised, though not rewritten, his paragraph on the symptoms of increased tension, replacing the reference to the sphygmograph with a reference to the sphygmomanometer: "The recent introduction of clinical instruments for measuring blood-pressure has been most useful. (Consult the work of T[heodore] Janeway on *Blood-Pressure*, 1904)."[61] In 1912, speaking to a medical audience in Glasgow, he gave the systolic pressure associated with various cases, noting "we have learnt to recognize an average pressure, as taken with ordinary instruments [i.e., the early sphygmomanometers], and the figures given are usually accepted."[62] There was no mention of the sphygmograph.

THE SPHYGMOMANOMETER AND THE SPHYGMOGRAPH

The sphygmograph was not conceived of as a blood pressure machine, but rather as a "pulse writer." The sphygmograph was already in decline when the earliest prototypes of blood pressure machines—sphygmomanometers—made their appearance in the 1880s. Practitioners and researchers were well aware by about 1870 that arterial tension was of critical prognostic and diagnostic importance. In the hands of a dogged researcher like Mahomed in London in the 1870s, the sphygmograph was literally forced to reveal insights into what would come to be known as essential hypertension. Both Mahomed, who died in 1884, and his sphygmographic studies of hypertension suffered almost instant obscurity. Mahomed's biographers suggest that the abandonment of the sphygmograph, "with its flawed technology in terms of diagnosing high arterial tension, perhaps also contributed to the abandonment of the revolutionary ideas Mahomed obtained by using it."[63] Twentieth-century men with sphygmomanometers would garner the credit for identifying and elucidating essential hypertension and its vascular and neurologic sequelae.

Scipione Riva-Rocci, the Italian professor whose revolutionary sphygmomanometer was introduced in 1896, reportedly dismissed previous

---

[61] William Osler, *The Principles and Practice of Medicine*, 6th ed. (New York: D. Appleton & Co., 1905), 851; for Janeway, see discussion later in this chapter.

[62] William Osler, "An Address on High Blood Pressure: Its Associations, Advantages, and Disadvantages: Delivered at the Glasgow Southern Medical Society," *British Medical Journal* 2 (1912): 1174. Osler was familiar with Allubtt's work using early sphygmomanometers to elucidate essential hypertension.

[63] Cameron and Hicks, "Frederick Akbar Mahomed," 1503.

sphygmomanometer designs as "no more than bad sphygmographs," hardly a tribute to that fading technology.[64] The key to accurate blood pressure measurement proved to be Riva-Rocci's concept of arterial compression by means of an inflatable cuff encircling the upper arm. The apparatus was connected to a calibrated mercury manometer. Air was pumped into the cuff by squeezing a rubber bulb, obliterating the pulse distal to the encircling. The cuff was gradually deflated until the pulse reappeared; the reading on the manometer at which the pulse reappeared was taken as the systolic blood pressure, read out in millimeters of mercury (mm Hg).[65]

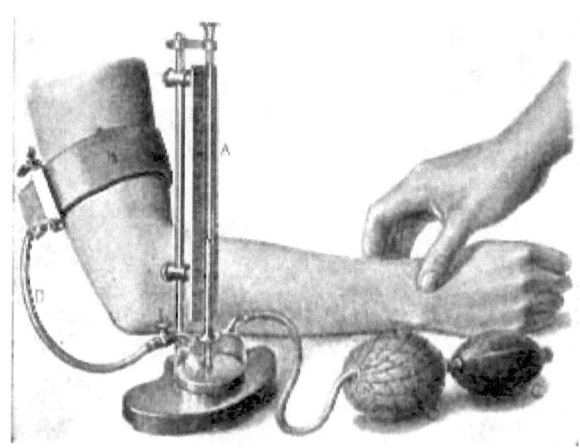

FIGURE 64: Riva Rocci sphygmomanometer. Note the thin inflatable cuff encircling the upper arm and the physician's fingers palpating the radial pulse as the cuff is deflated. Theodore Janeway, *The Clinical Study of Blood-Pressure* (D. Appleton and Company, 1904), figure 21, page 79.

The Riva-Rocci device, the prototype of all modern sphygmomanometers, was brought to the United States by Johns Hopkins neurosurgeon Harvey Cushing in 1901. Within months, Cushing demonstrated that the sphygmomanometer was easy to use, sufficiently quick to permit serial readings in the operating room, non-threatening to the awake patient, portable, and reasonably inexpensive. Although Cushing found that the Riva-Rocci sphygmomanometer was not always

---

[64] N. H. Naqvi and M. D. Blaufox, *Blood Pressure Measurement: An Illustrated History* (New York: Parthenon, 1998), 68.

[65] Ralph H. Major, "The History of Taking the Blood Pressure," *Annals of Medical History* 2 (1930): 54–55.

accurate or precise, its deficiencies were "more than compensated for by its ready applicability to most clinical demands."[66] Thus, from the outset, the reception of the sphygmomanometer stood in marked contrast to that afforded the sphygmograph. Compared to the subjective and vague information about high and low tension provided by the sphygmograph, the sphygmomanometer, with its numerical readout in millimeters of mercury, offered obvious advantages in precision, standardization, and practical utility.

A critical refinement in blood pressure determination appeared in 1905. As noted, the Riva-Rocci blood pressure cuff required only that the operator determine by digital pulse palpation the point on a mercury pressure gauge at which the pulse was obliterated—yielding a single number most closely corresponding to the systolic blood pressure (the upper number in the familiar "130 over 80" shorthand). This early technique resonated well with simple pulse palpation—the hallowed educated finger was still important. However, the introduction of auscultatory determination (the familiar application of the stethoscope over the brachial artery at the elbow fold as the pressure in the cuff encircling the upper arm is gradually lowered) by Russian surgeon Nikolai Korotkoff in 1905 added a new dimension to blood pressure determination in which the palpating finger was eliminated and both systolic and diastolic pressure readings determined. Historian of cardiology Louis C. Acierno considers Korotkoff's innovation as "one of the most outstanding events in the history of medicine," moving hypertension to a dominant place in the study, diagnosis, and treatment of human disease. The Korotkoff method, with minor modifications, remains the keystone of blood pressure measurement today.[67]

By the 1910s, using early modifications of the Riva-Rocci sphygmomanometer, Clifford Allbutt in Cambridge and Theodore Janeway in New York defined what we now call essential hypertension. Allbutt, writing in 1915, clearly carved out essential or primary hypertension—which he termed "hyperpiesia" (or "hyperpiesis"—*piesi* is Greek for pressure) distinguishing it from high blood pressure secondary to either kidney disease or arteriosclerosis.[68] Janeway, who had examined thousands of clinic and private patients with the sphygmomanometer

---

[66] Harvey Cushing, "On Routine Determinations of Arterial Tension in Operating Room and Clinic," *Boston Medical and Surgical Journal* (1903): 250–56.

[67] Louis J. Acierno, *History of Cardiology* (New York: Parthenon Publishing Group, 1994), 498–500.

[68] Frank S. Meara, "Hyperpiesia of Clifford Allbutt (Essential Hypertension)," *Medical Clinics of North America* 2 (1) (1918): 2–3.

over a period of years, concluded that the range of vascular lesions and clinical events found in such hypertensive patients (in the absence of primary kidney disease) was best unified under the term "hypertensive cardiovascular disease."[69]

Janeway, who appreciated the nuances and pitfalls of blood pressure determination with the sphygmomanometer, warned that technology could also be a trap. At a time in American history when technology carried enormous weight and promise, he took a page from the playbooks of the early British masters of the sphygmograph, warning physicians in 1906 against an uncritical and dangerous reliance on blood pressure readings without clinical acumen: "To those, however, who have not acquired the habits of painstaking observation and careful weighing of evidence, the little knowledge which the instrument can yield may, like other detached bits of information in these days of laboratory diagnosis, prove a really dangerous thing."[70]

The sphygmomanometer, despite the decade or so that it took to achieve at least partial standardization—in the device itself, in the technique of using the instrument, and in the interpretation of the somewhat complex Korotkoff sounds detected with the stethoscope over the artery—almost immediately produced valuable clinical information and avoided much of the fussiness and subjectivity that hampered the use of the sphygmograph and the interpretation of its graphic output.

Although the sphygmomanometer entered American medical practice relatively quickly, the decades between 1900 and 1920 were not free of controversy, confusion, and some resistance to the new technology. In a 1993 essay, "Losing Touch: The Controversy over the Introduction of Blood Pressure Instruments into Medicine," clinician and historian of science Hughes Evans found that "the introduction of blood pressure machines, and hence blood pressure measurements, caused an uproar in the American medical community." Physicians felt threatened by the apparatus and the implications of incorporating it into medical practice. As with the sphygmograph, the role of time-honored digital pulse palpation as it related to the determination of the blood pressure was a vexed issue in the years following its introduction into practice; some physicians viewed the sphygmomanometer as an "attack on one of the most basic and revered skills of the profession, that of palpating the pulse."[71]

---

[69] Acierno, *History of Cardiology*, 323–24.

[70] Theodore C. Janeway, "The Diagnostic Significance of Persistent Arterial Pressure," *American Journal of Medical Science* 131 (1906): 778.

[71] Hughes Evans, "Losing Touch: The Controversy over the Introduction of Blood

But in contrast to the trajectory of the sphygmograph, the technical problems and procedural details of the sphygmomanometer were largely solved over several decades. In 1921 and 1927, the Bureau of Standards in Washington issued detailed comparisons and recommended various standards for the sphygmomanometer.[72] The definition of what constitutes high blood pressure and how to use the information in various populations remains today, a century later, under periodic review by blue-ribbon multidisciplinary committees.[73]

The sphygmograph was not simply *replaced* by the sphygmomanometer. The sphygmograph and the sphygmomanometer asked different questions and gave different information about cardiovascular function. The sphygmograph literally "wrote" arterial or cardiac pressure waves, while the sphygmomanometer measured arterial pressure in numeric form. Although the sphygmograph proved inadequate as a practical blood pressure machine—a task for which it was not designed—it prepared the medical profession for the comparatively rapid adoption of the sphygmomanometer.

THE ELECTROCARDIOGRAPH AND THE SPHYGMOGRAPH

The sphygmograph recorded arterial or cardiac pressure waves, while the electrocardiograph read and recorded the electrical impulses of the conducting system of the heart. Both the sphymograph and the electrocardiograph transmitted their messages by *la méthode graphique*.

The electrocardiograph, first recorded in the frog and tortoise hearts in the 1870s by the omnipresent Marey and conceptually advanced by the capillary electrometer research of Burdon-Sanderson, was brought to practical clinical fruition by Augustus Waller in England in the 1880s,

---

Pressure Instruments into Medicine," *Technology and Culture* 34 (1993): 784, 801. The complexiry of the Korotkoff sounds led to confusion about whether to record the diastolic pressure as the point at which the audible sound is muffled or when it disappears entirely; Christopher W. Crenner, "Introduction of the Blood Pressure Cuff into U.S. Medical Practice: Technology and Skilled Practice," *Annals of Internal Medicine* 128 (1998): 492.

[72] J. L. Wilson, H. N. Eaton, and H. B. Henrickson, *Use and Testing of Sphygmomanometers* (Washington: United States Government Printing Office, 1927).

[73] For example, the Eighth Joint National Committee, with members selected from various professional organizations and institutes issues periodic guidelines, the latest in 2014 (http://sites.jamanetwork.com/jnc8/). The American Society of Hypertension also issues periodic guidelines (http://www.ash-us.org/Publications/ASH-Position-Papers.aspx).

Willem Einthoven in Holland in the 1890s, and Thomas Lewis in England after the turn of the twentieth century.[74] The electrocardiogram capitalized on newly discovered electrophysiological phenomena occurring within the conducting system of the heart, in essence a pacemaker and "wiring" system stimulating cardiac muscle contraction.

Frank contrasts the conceptual essences of the sphygmograph and electrocardiograph: "If the sphygmograph proved by the 1880s to be something less than the revolutionary device it had been touted to be, at least it operated on a set of physical principles that any clinician could understand." The electrocardiograph, in contrast, "recorded not something as obvious and palpable as the heart's beat, but a physiological signal imperceivable to human senses: the electrical wave that causes that heartbeat."[75] A leap of faith—another layer of imagination—was required to accept the physiological fact that muscle (myocardium) and collagenous tissue (valves) had an electrical conduction system invisible to the naked eye, and that the electrocardiograph could make an inscription of it. Three decades after the sphygmograph was introduced by Marey, curious physicians, already familiar with electricity in daily life and in medical applications such as neurophysiology, were prepared by their experience with sphygmographic tracings to accept the notion that squiggles and lines moving across a strip of paper truly recorded a physiologic event occurring within the human heart.

Paradoxically, the sphygmograph, built on simple mechanical principles (a "low" technology) produced complicated data that depended on both the heart and the arteries. In Frank's terms, there was "too loose and too adventitious a relation between picture and pathology." On the other hand, the electrocardiograph, a complicated construction not understandable to the average physician (a "high" technology) produced an essentially simple tracing of the electrical forces at work in the conduction system of the heart. The information was limited but precise; it told fundamental truths of great diagnostic and prognostic value.[76]

Graphic recorders like the sphygmograph and the electrocardiograph, if they are to make the move successfully from laboratory to clinic, must be affordable, usable by an intelligent though harried practitioner, practical to operate, "forgiving of mistakes," and acceptable to (human) patients.[77] The

---

[74] An excellent history of the development of the electrocardiograph is found in Frank, "Telltale Heart," 230–69.
[75] Ibid., 225–26.
[76] Ibid., 270-71.
[77] Ibid., 270.

electrocardiograph (once the ponderous six-hundred pound 1901 prototype was streamlined to a practical size), ultimately met all these criteria.

By the 1910s, and certainly the 1920s, interest in electrocardiography literally exploded. Lewis's primer of electrocardiography appeared in 1913. At that time, only three leads (I, II, and III) were recorded (today, the standard EKG has twelve leads beginning with the three Lewis leads). Lewis was able to identify characteristic patterns of a normal heart, ventricular hypertrophy, conduction disturbances and heart block, ventricular extrasystoles (premature beats), paroxysmal tachycardia and other atrial arrhythmias, and patterns reflecting valvular heart disease. Patterns consistent with coronary artery disease and myocardial infarction were not discussed in Lewis's book, *Clinical Electrocardiography*, although he did note that an inverted T wave (often seen with coronary artery disease in some leads) carried an ominous prognosis.[78]

As with the stethoscope and sphygmomanometer, all was not clear at first. However, there was a sense that knowledge grew with every passing year. The physiologic and pathologic correlations were worked out, and information was reproducible and easily communicated to other physicians. (Well into the twentieth century, the guidelines for interpretation of electrocardiograms required occasional tweaking.) A minimally trained technician could acquire (though not interpret) a reliable tracing, all properly built machines gave the same tracing, and cardiologists everywhere agreed on the principles of interpretation. The tracings had immediate clinical application to the study of cardiac arrhythmias; in time, anatomical disorders such as chamber enlargement and pathological events such as myocardial infarction were reliably diagnosed.

Progress with the sphygmograph was much more hesitant, even stagnant. Correlations between tracings and cardiovascular events were never satisfactorily worked out. A practiced and patient physician had to use a fussy, idiosyncratic instrument, often of his own design or tweaked to his satisfaction, to obtain a readable tracing. Tracings obtained by different machines were not interchangeable; and guides for interpretation were haphazard and incomplete. Knowledge and insight seemed to advance and retreat, with little reproducibility among operators. Clinical application was uncertain at best. And most of its early champions quickly grew discouraged. While there was some hesitancy about incorporating the electrocardiograph into practice, there was never a sense of discouragement;

---

[78] Thomas Lewis, *Clinical Electrocardiography* (London: Shaw and Sons, 1913); inverted T wave, 28.

once the electrocardiograph "took off," no physician could deny its power and utility.

It is instructive to look at the first published electrocardiograph tracing produced by Einthoven in 1902. A century later, any physician has but to glance at the tracing in order to make several valid diagnostic observations; except for some "static," the tracing might have been made yesterday. But few, if any, modern physicians could make much of the hundreds of "sphygmographic hieroglyphics" in Holden's monograph. Without helpful captions, the complex tracings and time intervals found in Keyt's articles seem dated and inaccessible to the modern physician. From the outset, the graphical representations of the electrocardiograph possessed a clarity and universality that was lacking in the sphygmograph. The output of the electrocardiograph, unlike that of the sphygmograph, entered the vocabulary of medicine clearly and indelibly.

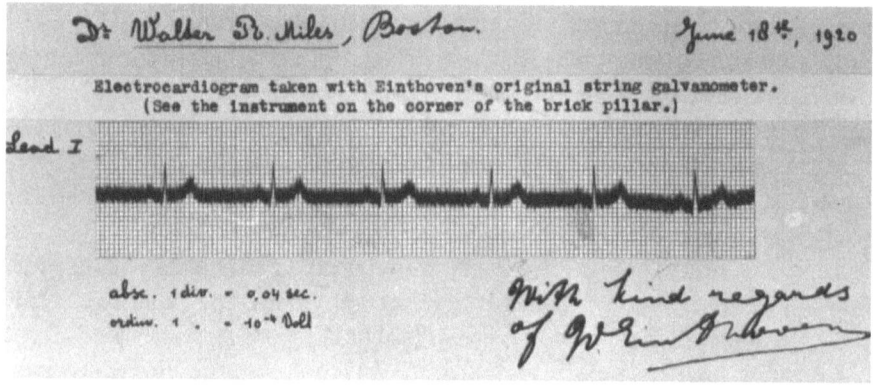

FIGURE 65: First published electrocardiogram with a single lead. The tracing from Einthoven, published in a Dutch journal in 1902, is online at the National Library of Medicine: Images in the History of Medicine, https://collections.nlm.nih.gov/catalog/nlm:nlmuid-101448113-img, accessed 8 September 2017. Probably from W. Einthoven "Galvanometrische registratie van het menschilijk electrocardiogram." In: *Herinneringsbundel Professor S. S. Rosenstein*. Leiden: Eduard Ijdo, 1902:101–7. The tracing appears to be a gift from Einthoven to a New York physician in 1920.

The functions—both realized and anticipated—of the sphygmograph were superceded rather than replaced by the agglomeration of the sphygmomanometer, electrocardiograph, fluoroscope, and forgotten devices such as the ballistocardiograph.[79] Today, ultrasound of the heart (echocardiography) and blood vessels (arterial ultrasound) answer many of the clinical questions that sphygmography asked but could not answer; perhaps ultrasound is the true heir of the sphygmograph.

MACKENZIE'S POLYGRAPH

What remained of the discrete identity of the sphygmograph was subsumed at the end of the nineteenth century into James Mackenzie's polygraph.[80] It was only after Mackenzie sharply narrowed the scope of arterial pulse study, while introducing the novel concept of simultaneous venous pulse study, that the sphygmograph (and then only as one component of the Mackenzie polygraph) yielded valuable information. Mackenzie transcended the hallowed expectations of pulse study that had gripped and ultimately hobbled the early sphygmographers.

But Mackenzie, like Broadbent a generation earlier, was loath to abandon clinical acumen. Mackenzie asserted in 1919 that his intense engagement with the polygraph "educated his senses" and particularly his finger upon the pulse—the hallowed *tactus eruditus* of the classical physician: "To one who takes a tracing of the pulse, the familiarity with the different kinds of artery and the different characters of the pulse, as perceived by the finger, yields a peculiar kind of knowledge . . . This familiarising of the doctor with the impressions given by the finger leads to the acquisition of a knowledge of real value."[81]

At the end of his brilliant career (1919), marked by application of his polygraph to elucidation of atrial fibrillation and right-sided cardiac pathophysiology and cardiodynamics, Mackenzie, like Janeway, warned against the seductive spell of medical technologies. For Mackenzie, the enduring tradition of British clinical medicine was too valuable to fall under the shadow of technology, particularly hastily adopted and unproven technologies. Technology, rather, should be seen as the servant of the

---

[79] The ballistocardiogram, conceived in the late 1870s and improved over the course of six decades, detected the vibrations of the body with each cardiac cycle, indicating, it was hoped, cardiac output. Louis J. Acierno, *History of Cardiology* (New York: Parthenon Publishing Group, 1994): 514–18.

[80] As discussed in Chapter 3, the Mackenzie polygraph combined a sphygmograph and a venous pulse wave recorder to investigate heart failure and the mechanism of cardiac arrhythmias.

[81] James Mackenzie, *The Future of Medicine* (London: Henry Frowde and Hodder and Stroughton, 1919), 185.

clinician, not his master. As with the stethoscope a century earlier and any number of promising laboratory tests and techniques since, the sphygmograph was, perhaps, too eagerly and quickly embraced. Mackenzie reflected: "Fifty years ago the sphygmograph came into use, and was hailed as another instrument for the better understanding of the heart's work. The character of the tracings of the radial pulse was found to vary, and speculation as to their cause became rife." Failure to fully understand the sphygmograph and other new devices led to mistaken diagnoses and false pathways in addition to distancing the physician from the patient he was attempting to diagnose and treat—or worse, leading to overreliance on specialists who provided a fragmented view of the whole patient.[82]

In a much-quoted remark, Mackenzie reflected that too much laboratory training "unfits a man for his work as a physician [i.e., clinician]." Not only does he fail to "educate his senses," but he comes to trust too much in "his mechanical methods" to the exclusion of intelligent clinical observation and judgment.[83] A century later, when clinical skills—time-consuming listening and examining and reflecting—have been overshadowed by technology in the eyes of many physicians, patients, and third-party payers, Mackenzie seems like less of a Luddite. Like the best of physicians today, the master sphygmographer never stopped being a clinician.

A SLIPPERY AND OPAQUE TECHNOLOGY

By 1900, it was clear that the sphygmograph "could make no claims to any exclusive spheres of knowledge."[84] It could not predict longevity, diagnose specific cardiac diseases, offer a prognosis, quantitate the blood pressure, or give much information about what nineteenth-century writers liked to call the "state of the circulation." The sphygmograph was, in the end, overshadowed by newer technologies. Certainly, its demise was hastened by its own insurmountable technical and interpretive difficulties.

Despite its almost complete disappearance from professional memory, the narrative of the sphygmograph lasted over forty years, and few historians of medical technology would deny that it was a lively narrative. The men who invented and perfected the polygraph, sphygmomanometer, and electrocardiograph had all grown up professionally in the sphygmograph era. To a greater or lesser degree, they benefited from some of the

---

[82] Mackenzie, *Future of Medicine*, 182–86; quotation 182.
[83] Ibid., 185–86.
[84] Frank, "Telltale Heart," 225.

information yielded by the sphygmograph. At the very least, the pitfalls and shortcomings of the sphygmograph contributed to a cautionary tale that helped shape new cardiovascular technologies. The sphygmograph was both a success and a failure, not simply because it was invented and then became outdated, but because it tapped into the medical and scientific temperament of its era.

Sphygmograms with their timed wavy lines introduced clinicians and engaged patients to the application of the graphic method to diagnosis and treatment. When the electrocardiograph, the fluoroscope, and the sphygmomanometer entered practice, not only the new specialists, but also generalists and their lay clientele, were prepared by this eclipsed technology for a new way of thinking about the heart and blood vessels. Despite the fears of some nineteenth and early twentieth century medical writers, the sphygmograph and other early "instruments of precision" did not "pauperize the senses." The art of physical diagnoses—feeling the pulse, applying the stethoscope to the chest wall—and the equally important art of listening to the patient's symptoms and impressions—were not entirely abandoned even as twentieth-century technologies such as echocardiography and cardiac catheterization opened new frontiers.

In the end, it was not the sphygmograph, but the essential power of the graphic method and the very notion and seductive allure of space and time machines that transformed physicians' experience of physical diagnosis, altered the ways in which they relied upon their own senses to know the workings of the body, redefined the nature of evidence in research and at the bedside, and recalibrated their mental images of disease.

The sphygmograph was a "time and space machine," the premier mid-nineteenth century medical instrument of precision. Marey used the expression in an 1876 talk to a medical congress in Brussels: "The graphic curve of a movement furnishes us with the double notion of time and space; it characterizes completely the act which it represents."[85] It drew much of its mystique from the *tactus eruditus* of the physician's ancient art. It taught a generation of physicians to "see with a better eye" the ancient "stirrings of the arteries."[86] The sphygmograph introduced *la méthode graphique*

---

[85] Étienne-Jules Marey, "Lectures on the Graphic Method in the Experimental Sciences, and on Its Special Application to Medicine," *British Medical Journal* 1 (1876): 1. The phrase "the time and space machines of medicine" comes from Stanley Joel Reiser, "The Technologies of Time Measurement: Implications at the Bedside and the Bench," *Annals of Internal Medicine* 132 (2000): 31–36.

[86] Jacalyn Duffin, *To See with a Better Eye: A Life of R.T.H. Laennec* (Princeton, NJ: Princeton University Press, 1998); Shigehisa Kuriyama, *The Expressiveness of the Body and the Divergence of Greek and Chinese Medicine* (New York: Zone Books, 1999), 18.

into medical practice and played a dominant role in the cardiovascular technology narrative of the last two centuries.

Interest in the sphygmograph tapered off in the United States in the 1880s, while, in Britain, it "remained the purview of a small group of urban consultant physicians" with an interest in physiology.[87] The occasional researcher continued to use the sphygmograph for quirky isolated studies. During World War I, for example, physiologist/psychologist Jean-Marie Lahy tested gunners for 'sang-froid,' by recording their response to the firing of a gun using a sphygmograph and a device for measuring respiratory rate.[88]

The sphygmograph of Marey and the British and American physicians who struggled to release its magic promised much but delivered less. Chronologically and intellectually, the sphygmograph bridged the long cardiovascular technology gap between the stethoscope and the sphygmomanometer/electrocardiograph. It was no mere transitional technology. If anything, it was quite unique, *sui generis*, an original technology that wrote its own epitaph.

---

[87] Frank, "Telltale Heart," 225.
[88] Rabinbach, *Human Motor*, 265.

BIBLIOGRAPHY

Acierno, Louis J. *History of Cardiology*. New York: Parthenon Publishing Group, 1994.

A. S. Aloe Co. *Aloe's Illustrated and Priced Catalogue of Superior Surgical Instruments, Physician's Supplies and Hospital Furnishings*, 6th ed. St. Louis: A. S. Aloe Co., 1893.

Allbutt, T. Clifford. *Diseases of the Arteries Including Angina Pectoris*. London: Macmillan and Co., 1915.

Allen, Timothy F., ed. *The Encyclopedia of Pure Materia Medica*. Vols 2 and 4. New York: Boericke and Tafel, 1875, 1876.

"Alonzo T. Keyt" (obituary). *Journal of the American Medical Association* 5 (1885): 615–16.

American Medical Association. *Code of Medical Ethics of the American Medical Association, Adopted May, 1847*. Philadelphia: P. K. and T. G. Collins, 1848. This booklet was printed privately for the Philadelphia Delegation to the National Convention in May, 1847. https://archive.org/stream/63310410R.nlm.nih.gov/63310410R#page/n7/mode/2up (accessed 9 September 2016).

Anderson, William Henry. "Report of the Committee on Education." *Transactions of the American Medical Association* 9 (1856): 552–62.

Anstie, Francis E. "Cautions in Regard to Use of Sphygmograph." *Medical Record* (New York) 2 (1867–68): 59.

⸺. "Lectures on the Prognosis and Therapy of Certain Acute Diseases, with Specific Reference to the Indications Afforded by the Graphic Study of the Pulse." *Lancet* 2 (1867): 35–36, 63–65, 123–24, 189–91, 385–87.

⸺. "On Certain Modifications of Marey's Sphygmograph." *Lancet* 1 (1868): 783–84.

———. "On the Diurnal Fluctuations of the Pulse-Form, and on Certain Cautions Necessary to be Observed in Sphygmography." *Lancet* 1 (1867): 170–72.

———. "The Sphygmograph in English Medical Practice." *Lancet* 1 (1866): 671.

Aronson, J. K. *An Account of the Foxglove and its Medical Uses, 1785–1985*. London: Oxford University Press, 1985.

Badham, David. "A Few Remarks on the Sphygmometer." *London Medical Gazette* 16 (1835–36): 265–68.

Bardeen, Charles R. "Oliver Wendell Holmes." In *A Cyclopedia of American Medical Biography*, edited by Howard Kelly, 419–24. Philadelphia: W. B. Saunders, 1912.

B[artlett], J. C. "The Profession in New York: Impressions of a Visitor." *Boston Medical and Surgical Journal* 58 (1858): 299–305.

Barton, W. H. H. "Sphygmophone, U.S. Patent No. 232,105, 14 September 1880." www.google.com/patents/US232105 (accessed 2 February 2017).

Beard, George M. *A Practical Treatise on Nervous Exhaustion (Neurasthenia): Its Symptoms, Nature, Sequences, Treatment*. New York, E. B. Treat, 1988.

Beasley, Henry, *The Book of Prescriptions*. Philadelphia: Lindsay & Blakiston, 1855.

Béhier, [Louis-Jules]. "A New Perfected Sphygmograph." *Bulletin de l'Académie Impériale de Médicine* 33 (1868): 962–64.

Benjamin, Dowling. "The Present Position of Antiseptic Practice." *Transactions of the Medical Society of New Jersey* (1887): 249–55.

Berg, Samuel, comp. *Medical Practice and Hospital Development in Newark, N.J., 1850–1887 as Reported in* Newark Daily Advertiser (ca. 1940). New Jersey Room, Newark Public Library.

Billings, John S. "An Address on Our Medical Literature." *British Medical Journal* 2 (1881): 262–68.

Bishop, Louis Faugères. *Heart Troubles: Their Prevention and Relief*. New York: Funk & Wagnalls, 1920.

Bishop, Louis Faugères and John Neilson Jr., *History of Cardiology*. New York: Medical Life Press, 1927.

Bittel, Carla. *Mary Putnam Jacobi and the Politics of Medicine in Nineteenth-Century America*. Chapel Hill: University of North Carolina Press, 2009.

Blundell, E. S. "Preface" and "Description of the Improvements of the Instrument." In Jules Hérisson. *Le Sphygmomètre: instrument qui traduit à l'oeil toute l'action des artères (The Sphgymometer, an Instrument Which Renders the Action of the Arteries Apparent to the Eye): Being a Memoir Presented to the Institute of France, by Dr. Jules Hérisson with an Improvement of the Instrument and Prefatory Remarks by the Translator, Dr. E. S. Blundell*, i–xvi; 42–45. London: Longman, Rees, Orme, Brown, Green, and Longman, 1835.

Blustein, Bonnie E. *Preserve Your Love for Science: Life of William A. Hammond, American Neurosurgeon*. Cambridge: Cambridge University Press, 1991.

Bonner, Thomas Neville. *American Doctors and German Universities: A Chapter in International Intellectual Relations, 1870-1914*. Lincoln, NE: University of Nebraska Press, 1953.

———. *Becoming a Physician: Medical Education in Britain, France, Germany, and the United States, 1750–1945*. Baltimore: Johns Hopkins University Press, 1995.

Borrell, Merriley. "Extending the Senses: The Graphic Method." *Medical Heritage* 2 (1985): 114–21.

———. "Marey and d'Arsonval: The Exact Science in Late Nineteenth-Century French Medicine." In *From Ancient Omens to Statistical Mechanics: Essays on the Exact Sciences Presented to Asger Aaboe*, edited by J. L. Berggren and B. R. Goldstein, 225–37. Copenhagen: University Library, 1987.

Bowditch, Henry P. (as H. P. B.). "Bibliographic Notice of *Handbook for the Physiological Laboratory*." *Boston Medical and Surgical Journal* 89 (1873): 360–61.

Bowman, William. "An Introductory Address Delivered at King's College, London, October 1st, 1851." In *The Collected Papers of Sir W. Bowman, Bart., F.R.S.*, edited by J. Burdon- Sanderson and J. W. Hulke, 2:51–67. London: Harrison and Sons, 1892.

Bramwell, Byrom. "Examination of the Pulse." *Edinburgh Medical Journal* 26 (1880): 520–32.

Braunwald, Eugene and Joseph K. Perloff. "Physical Examination of the Heart and Circulation." In *Heart Disease: A Textbook of Cardiovascular Medicine*, 6th ed. Edited by Eugene Braunwald. Philadelphia: W. B. Saunders, 2001.

Brieger, Gert. "*Annual Catalogue of the College of Physicians and Surgeons, in the City of New York, 1849-50.*" In *Medical America in the Nineteenth Century: Readings from the Literature*. Edited by Gert Brieger, 37–42. Baltimore: Johns Hopkins University Press, 1972.

Broadbent, William H. *The Pulse*. London: Cassell, 1890; Philadelphia: Lea Brothers, 1890.

———. "The Pulse: The Croonian Lecture Delivered to the Royal College of Physicians, 1887." *British Medical Journal* 1 (1887): 655–60.

———. "The Pulse: Its Diagnostic, Prognostic, and Therapeutic Indications." *Lancet* 2 (1875): 549–50.

Brodman, Estelle. "William Beaumont and the Transfer of Biomedical Information." *Federation Proceedings* (Federation of the American Societies of Experimental Biology) 44 (1985): 9–17.

Brunton, Thomas Lauder. "On the Use of Nitrite of Amyl in Angina Pectoris." *Lancet* 2 (1867): 97–98.

———. *Pharmacology and Therapeutics; or Medicine Past and Present*. London: Macmillan and Co., 1880.

Burdon-Sanderson, John. *Handbook of the Sphygmograph: Being a Guide to Its Use in Clinical Research, to Which is Appended A Lecture Delivered at the Royal College of Physicians on the 29th of March 1867 on the Mode and Duration of the Contraction of the Heart in Health and Disease*. London: Robert Hardwicke, 1867.

———. "Lecture on the Characters of the Arterial Pulse, in Relation to the Mode and Duration of the Contraction of the Heart in Health and Disease." *British Medical Journal* 2 (1867): 19–22, 39–40, 57–58.

———. "On the Theory of the Pulse" (No. 1 in a series "On the Application of Physical Methods to the Exploration of the Movement of the Heart and Pulse in Disease"). *Lancet* 2 (1866): 517–18.

———. "On the Varieties of Pulse in Disease" (No. 2 in a series "On the Application of Physical Methods to the Exploration of the Movement of the Heart and Pulse in Disease"). *Lancet* 2 (1866): 688–91.

Butler, Samuel W., comp. *Medical Register and Directory of the United States, 1878*. Philadelphia: Office of the *Medical and Surgical Reporter*, 1874, 1878.

Cameron, J. Stewart and Jackie Hicks. "Frederick Akbar Mahomed and His Role in the Description of Hypertension at Guy's Hospital." *Kidney International* 49 (1996): 1488–1506.

Carroll, Alfred L. "The Clinical Use of the Sphygmograph." *New York Medical Journal* 26 (1877): 254–65.

Caswell, Hazard. *Illustrated Catalogue of Surgical Instruments and Appliances*. New York: Caswell, Hazard & Co., 1874.

Chadwick, James R. "Proceedings of the Suffolk County District Medical Society: A New Sphygmoscope." *Boston Medical and Surgical Journal* 93 (1875): 740–42.

"Changing the Face of MedicineNational: Dr. Jacobi's Sphygmograph." National Library of Medicine, https://cfmedicine.nlm.nih.gov/artifact/jacobi.html (accessed 6 August 2017).

Chapman, Carleton B. *Order Out of Chaos: John Shaw Billings and America's Coming of Age*. Boston: Boston Medical Library, 1994.

Chas. Truax, Greene. *Price List of Physicians' Supplies*, 6th ed. Chicago: Chas. Truax, Greene & Co., 1892.

Clark, J. Henry. "The First Fifty Years of the District Medical Society of Essex County." *Transactions of the Medical Society of New Jersey* (1867): 77–181.

Clarke, Edward. *Sex in Education; or, A Fair Chance for the Girls*. Boston: James R. Osgood and Co., 1873.

Codman & Shurtleff. *Catalogue of Surgical Instruments*. Boston, Codman & Shurtleff, 1875.

_____. *Illustrated Catalogue: Surgical Instruments and Appliances*. Boston: Codman & Shurtleff, 1890.

Coffen, T. Homer. "The Clinical Value of the Polygraph." *Post-Graduate* 27 (1912): 168–73.

Coleman, J. P. "Reports of District Societies: Burlington County." *Transactions of the Medical Society of New Jersey* (1867): 223–27.

College of Physicians and Surgeons in the City of New York. *Catalogue of the Officers of the University and of the College and Annual Announcement of Lectures; Fifty-Third Session, 1859-60*. New York: Baker and Godwin, 1859.

Corvisart, J. N. *An Essay on the Organic Diseases and Lesions of the Heart and Great Vessels* (1806). Translated by Jacob Gates. Edited by C. E. Horeau. Philadelphia: Anthony Finlay; Boston: Bradford and Reed, 1812.

Council on Medical Education and Hospitals (American Medical Association), *Medical Colleges of the United States and of Foreign Countries*. American Medical Association, 1918, reprinted from *American Medical Directory*, 6th ed., 1918.

Cowen, David L. *Medicine and Health in New Jersey: A History*. Princeton: D.Van Nostrand, 1964.

Cranefield, Paul. "Foreword." In *Two Great Scientists of the Nineteenth Century: Correspondence of Emil Du Bois-Reymond and Carl Ludwig*, edited by Estelle Du Bois-Reymond and Paul Diepgen. Baltimore: Johns Hopkins University Press, ca. 1982.

Crenner. Christopher W. "Introduction of the Blood Pressure Cuff into U.S. Medical Practice: Technology and Skilled Practice." *Annals of Internal Medicine* 128 (1998): 488–93.

Cunningham, John T. *Clara Maass: A Nurse, A Hospital, A Spirit*. Cedar Grove, NJ: Rae Publishing, 1968.

Cushing, Harvey. "On Routine Determinations of Arterial Tension in Operating Room and Clinic." *Boston Medical and Surgical Journal* 148 (1903): 250–56.

DaCosta, Jacob M. "Clinical Notes on Chloral." *American Journal of the Medical Sciences* 59 (1870): 359–65.

———. "On Irritable Heart: A Clinical Study of a Form of Functional Cardiac Disorder and Its Consequences." *American Journal of the Medical Sciences* 61 (1871): 17–52.

Dalton, John Call. "How the Blood Circulates." *The Galaxy* 8 (1869): 667–77.

——— (as J. C. D.) *The Sphygmograph: Its Physiological and Pathological Indications* (review). *American Journal of the Medical Sciences* 67 (1874): 478–80.

———. *A Treatise on Human Physiology Designed for the Use of Students and Practitioners of Medicine*. 4th rev. ed. Philadelphia: Henry C. Lea, 1867.

Davis, Audrey B. "Life Insurance and the Physical Examination: A Chapter in the Rise of American Medical Technology." *Bulletin of the History of Medicine* 55 (1981): 392–406.

———. *Medicine and Its Technology: An Introduction to the History of Medical Instrumentation*. Westport CT: Greenwood, 1981.

[Davis, Nathan S.], "Original Investigations," *Journal of the American Medical Association* 1 (1883): 708–9.

"Death Comes to Dr. Holden." *Newark Evening News*, 19 July 1909 (annotated clipping).

Delp, Mahlon H. and Robert T. Manning, eds. *Major's Physical Diagnosis*. 7th ed. Philadelphia: W. B. Saunders, 1968.

Didama, Henry D. "The President's Annual Address: Conservative Progress." *Transactions of the New York State Medical Association* 1(1884): 18–32.

"Dr. E. A. Pond Dead." *Burlington Free Press*, 31 May 31 1889.

"Dr. Edgar Holden" (obituary). *New Jersey Historical Society Proceedings*, n.s. 1 (1916): 106–7.

"Dr. Edward J. Ill" (obituary). *Journal of the Medical Society of New Jersey* 39 (1942): 402.

"Dr. L. F. Bishop Dies; Heart Specialist" (obituary). *New York Times*, 7 October 1941.

"Dr. Thomas Alexander McBride" (obituary). *New York Times*, 7 September 1886.

Dougherty, Alexander M. "Observations on Glycosuria, Historical and Clinical." *Transactions of the Medical Society of New Jersey* (1878): 52–119.

Dubos, René and Jean Dubos. *The White Plague: Tuberculosis, Man and Society*. Boston, Little, Brown & Co., 1952. Reprint, New Brunswick, NJ: Rutgers University Press, 1987.

Dudgeon, Robert E. *The Sphygmograph: Its History and Use as an Aid to Diagnosis in Ordinary Practice*. London: Baillière, Tindall, & Cox, 1882.

Duffin, Jacalyn. *To See with a Better Eye: A Life of R.T. H. Laennec*. Princeton: Princeton University Press, 1998.

"Edgar Holden, M.D." (obituary). *Journal of the American Medical Association* 53 (1909): 474.

Edwards, A. Mead. "The Microscope in Gynecology." *Transactions of the Medical Society of New Jersey* (1875): 140–60.

"Erasmus A. Pond" (obituary). *Boston Medical and Surgical Journal* 120 (1889): 572.

Estes, J. Worth. *Hall Jackson and the Purple Foxglove: Medical Practice and Research in Revolutionary America, 1760–1820*. Hanover, NH: University Press of New England, 1979.

Evans, Hughes. "Losing Touch: The Controversy over the Introduction of Blood Pressure Instruments into Medicine." *Technology and Culture* 34 (1993): 784–807.

Ewing, Harvey M. "Modern Cardiac Methods." *Journal of the Medical Society of New Jersey* 17 (1920): 253–57.

Flint, Austin, Sr. *A Treatise on the Principles and Practice of Medicine; Designed for the Use of Practitioners and Students of Medicine*. 4th ed. Philadelphia: Henry C. Lea, 1873.

Floyer, John. *The Physician's Pulse-Watch*. London: S. Smith and B. Walford, 1707.

Forbes, W. A. "Biographical Notice." In *The Collected Scientific Papers of the Late Henry Garrod, M.A., F.R.S.*, ix–xxii. London: R. H. Porter, 1881.

Foster, Balthazar W. "Cases Illustrating the Use of the Sphygmograph and Cardiograph in the Study of Diseases of the Heart and Great Vessels." In *Clinical Medicine Lectures and Essays*, 267–330. London: J. & A. Churchill, 1874; Philadelphia: Lindsay and Blakiston, 1874.

———. "On the Use of the Sphygmograph in the Investigation of Disease." *British Medical Journal* 1 (1866): 275–78, 330–33.

———. *On the Use of the Sphygmograph in the Investigation of Disease*. London: John Churchill & Sons, 1866.

———. "The Sphygmograph in English Medical Practice" (letter). *Lancet* 1 (1866): 634.

"Francis Edmund Anstie" (obituary), *Lancet* 2 (1874): 433–34.

François-Franck, Charles. "Nerveux (Physiologie)." *Dictionnaire encyclopédique des idées médicales* (Paris: P. Asselin, G. Masson, 1878): 12:520–619.

Frank, Robert G. Jr. "American Physiologists in German Laboratories, 1865–1914." In *Physiology in the American Context, 1850–1940*, edited by Gerald L. Geison, 11–46. Bethesda: American Physiological Society, 1987.

———. "The Telltale Heart: Physiological Instruments, Graphic Methods, and Clinical Hopes." In *The Investigative Enterprise*, edited by William Coleman and Fredrick L. Holmes, 211–90. Berkeley: University of California Press, 1988.

Fred Haslam & Co. *Illustrated Catalogue of Surgical Instruments and Allied Lines*. Brooklyn NY: Fred Haslam & Co., 1917.

"Frederick A. Mahomed" (obituary). *Lancet* 2 (1884): 973–74.

Freeman, J. Addison. "Mercurial Disease among Hatters." *Transactions of the Medical Society of New Jersey* (1860), 61–64.

Fye, W. Bruce. *American Cardiology: The History of a Specialty and Its College*. Baltimore: Johns Hopkins University Press, 1996.

———. "Carl Ludwig and the Leipzig Physiological Institute: 'A Factory of New Knowledge.'" *Circulation* 74 (1986): 920–28.

———. *The Development of American Physiology: Scientific Medicine in the Nineteenth Century*. Baltimore: Johns Hopkins University Press, 1987.

———. "The Literature of American Internal Medicine: A Historical View." *Annals of Internal Medicine* 106 (1987), 451–60.

———. "T. Lauder Brunton and Amyl Nitrite: A Victorian Vasodilator." *Circulation* 74 (1986): 22–29.

Galishoff, Stuart. *Newark: The Nation's Unhealthiest City, 1832-1895*. New Brunswick, NJ: Rutgers University Press, 1988.

Garrison, Fielding H. *An Introduction to the History of Medicine*, 4th ed. Philadelphia: W. B. Saunders, 1929.

Garrod, Alfred H. "On the Mutual Relations of the Apex Cardiograph and the Radial Sphygmographic Trace." *Proceedings of the Royal Society of London* 19 (1870): 318–24.

──────. "On the Relative Duration of the Component Parts of the Radial Sphygmographic Trace in Health." *Proceedings of the Royal Society of London* 18 (1869): 351–54.

──────. "On Some Points Connected with the Circulation of the Blood, Arrived at from a Study of the Sphygmograph-Trace" (abstract). *Proceedings of the Royal Society of London* 22 (1873): 291–93. Full paper: "On Some Points Connected to the Circulation of the Blood, Arrived at from a Study of the Sphygmographic Trace." *Proceedings of the Royal Society of London* 23 (1874): 140–51.

──────. "On Sphygmography, Part I," *Journal of Anatomy and Physiology* 6 (1871–72): 399–404.

──────. "On Sphygmography, Part II," *Journal of Anatomy and Physiology* 7 (1872): 98–105.

Gazetteer and Business Directory of Rutland County, VT., for 1881–82. Syracuse NY: Journal Office, 1881.

Geddes, L. A. *Handbook of Blood Pressure Measurement.* New York: Springer Scientific, 1991.

Geison, Gerald L. "Divided We Stand: Physiologists and Clinicians in the American Context." In *The Therapeutic Revolution: Essays in the Social History of American Medicine*, edited by Morris J. Vogel and Charles E. Rosenberg, 67–90. Philadelphia: University of Pennsylvania Press, 1979.

George Tiemann & Co. *The American Armamentarium Chirurgicum.* New York: George Tiemann & Co., ca. 1879.

Gooday, Graeme. "Re-writing the 'Book of Blots': Critical Reflections on Histories of Technological 'Failure'" *History and Technology* 14 (1998): 265–91.

Grimes, David. "Technology Follies: The Uncritical Acceptance of Medical Innovation." *Journal of the American Medical Association* 269 (1993): 3030-33.

"The Haemodynamometer." *Lancet* 1 (1838–39): 278.

Hales, Stephen. *Statistical Essay Containing Haemastaticks: An Account of Some Hydraulic and Hydrostatic Experiments Made on the Blood and Blood-Vessels of Animals.* London: W. Innys and R. Manby, 1733.

Hammond, William A. "Cardine; The Extract of the Heart: Its Preparation and Physiological and Therapeutic Effects." *New York Medical Journal* 57 (1893): 429–31.

———. "A Further Contribution to the Subject of 'Animal Extracts.'" *New York Medical Journal* 58 (1893): 14–15.

———. "'The Sphygmograph as an Instrument of Precision' (With Apologies to Dr. Leonhardt)." *New York Medical Journal* 58 (1893): 588–89.

Hanna, Ibrahim R. and Mark E. Silverman. "A History of Cardiac Auscultation and Some of Its Contributors." *American Journal of Cardiology* 90 (2002): 259–67.

Hartshorne, Henry. "Memoir of Edward Hartshorne, A.M., M.D., (1818–1885), Read October 6, 1886." *Transactions of the College of Physicians of Philadelphia* (3rd ser.) 16 (1887): cdxxv-cdxxxiv (425–36).

Hérisson, Jules. *Le sphygmomètre: instrument qui traduit à l'oeil toute l'action des artères*. Paris : À la Librairie universelle de Bohaire : Chez Crochard, 1834. See bibliographic entries for Blundell, E. S. and Nancred, Joseph D. for English language translations and commentaries.

"History of the 'Ward' U.S.A. General Hospital." *Ward Hospital Bulletin*, 15 June 1865–10 August 1865.

"Holden" (obituary). *Journal of the Medical Society of New Jersey* 6 (1909): 137–38.

Holden, Edgar. "Anomalies in Cardiac Pathology." *American Journal of the Medical Sciences* 70 (1875): 92–99.

———. "The Availability of the Sphygmograph, with Description of a New Instrument." *Medical Record* (New York) 5 (1870–71): 9–10.

———. "Circulatory Physiology and the Sphygmograph." *Transactions of the Medical Society of New Jersey* (1871): 47–67; also published as a monograph: *The Sphygmograph and the Physiology of the Circulation: A Monograph Read Before the Medical Society of New Jersey, Upon Investigations Made Preparatory to a Larger Work on the Practical Value of the Sphygmograph*. New York: William Wood, 1871.

———. "Errors of the Sphygmograph." *New York Medical Journal* 26 (1877): 498–504.

———. "The Factors Which Govern the Acceptance of Risks after Middle Life." *Medical Examiner New York* 7 (1897): 143–45.

———. "The First Cruise of the 'Monitor' *Passaic*." *Harper's Monthly Magazine* 27 (October 1863), 577–95.

———. "Gelseminum for Hectic." *Medical Record* (New York) 15 (1879): 202–3.

———. "An Inquiry into the Causes of Certain Diseases on Ships of War." *American Journal of the Medical Sciences* 51 (1866): 75–84

———. *Mortality and Sanitary Record of Newark, New Jersey: A Report Presented to the President and Directors of the Mutual Benefit Life Insurance Company, January, 1880.* Newark: Mutual Benefit Life Insurance Company, 1880.

———. "On the Influence of Antecedent Disorders upon Organic Affections of the Heart and Brain." *American Journal of the Medical Sciences* 54 (1867): 54–67.

———. *The Sphygmograph: Its Physiological and Pathological Indications—The Essay to Which was Awarded the Stevens Triennial Prize, by the College of Physicians and Surgeons, New York, April, 1873.* Philadelphia: Lindsay & Blakiston, 1874.

———. "Successful (Internal) Use of Nitrite of Amyl in Dilated Heart with Aortic Regurgitation." *Medical Record* (New York) 13 (1878): 324–25.

———. "Tuberculosis—The Potential Factors in its Spread—Whether Hereditary Capacity, Inherited Bacilli or Transmission from the Lower Animals." *Transactions of the Medical Society of New Jersey* (1891): 83–107.

"Holden" (obituary), *Journal of the Medical Society of New Jersey* 6 (1909): 137–38.

"Holden, Edgar, M.D." In *Biographical Encyclopaedia of New Jersey of the Nineteenth Century*, 284. Philadelphia: Galaxy, 1877.

"Holden, Edgar, M.D." In *Cyclopedia of New Jersey Biography*. 330–31. New York: American Historical Society, 1923.

"Holden, Edgar." In *National Cyclopaedia of American Biography*. 15:91–92. New York: James T. White, 1916.

Horowitz, Helen Lefkowitz, "The Body in the Library." In *The "Woman Question" and Higher Education*, edited by Ann Mari May (Cheltenham, England: Edward Elgar Publishing, 2008): 11–31.

Howell, Joel D., ed. "Introduction." In *Technology and American Medical Practice, 1880-1930: An Anthology of Sources*, ix–xiii. New York: Garland, 1988.

Howell, Joel D. *Technology in the Hospital: Transforming Patient Care in the Early Twentieth Century.* Baltimore: Johns Hopkins University Press, 1995.

Huang, Carita Constable. "Instruments of Chaos: The Necessity and Impossibility of Standardizing the Sphygmograph in Late-nineteenth Century American Medicine." Abstract, Society for the History of Technology, ca. 2002. http://shot.press.jhu.edu/meeting/huang.htm (no longer accessible in 2016).

Hudson, Robert P. "Abraham Flexner in Perspective: American Medical Education, 1865-1910." *Bulletin of the History of Medicine* 46 (1972): 545–61.

Hunt, Ezra Mundy. "Origin of Disease and Micro-organisms as Related Thereto." *Transactions of the Medical Society of New Jersey* (1888): 95–111.

Hutchinson, John. "On the Capacity of the Lungs, and on the Respiratory Functions, with a View of Establishing a Precise and Easy Method of Detecting Disease by the Spirometer." *Medico-Chirurgical Transactions*, 2nd ser., 29 (1846): 137–252.

Hutchison, Joseph C. *A Treatise of Physiology and Hygiene for Educational Institutions and General Readers.* New York: Clark & Maynard, 1872.

"In Memoriam, Edgar Holden." *Circular No. 13, Military Order of the Loyal Legion of the United States.* New York: Military Order of the Loyal Legion of the United States, 1909.

[Isham, Asa B.]. "Alonzo Thrasher Keyt." In *Daniel Drake and His Followers—Historical and Biographical Sketches, 1785–1909,* edited by Otto Juettner, 463–65. Cincinnati: Harvey Publishing, 1909.

I[sham], A[sa] B. "Keyt, Alonzo Thrasher." In *A Cyclopedia of American Medical Biography,* edited by Howard A. Kelly, 2: 65–66. Philadelphia: W. B. Saunders, 1912.

Isham, Asa B. "A Sketch of the Life and Work of Alonzo Thrasher Keyt." *Philadelphia Monthly Medical Journal* 1 (1899): 726–29.

_____. "Value of Cardiosphygmography for the Determination of Cardiac Valvular Conditions and of Aneurism, particularly for Examiners of Life Insurance." *American Journal of the Medical Sciences* 84 (1882): 119–29.

Jacobi, Mary Putnam. *The Question of Rest for Women during Menstruation.* New York: G. P. Putnam, 1877.

_____. "Sphygmographic Experiments Upon a Human Brain, Exposed by an Opening in the Cranium." *American Journal of the Medical Sciences* 76 (1878): 103–12.

Janeway, Theodore C. "The Diagnostic Significance of Persistent Arterial Pressure." *American Journal of Medical Science* 131 (1906): 772–78.

J. E. N. "Dr. Edgar Holden" (obituary). *Transactions of the Thirty-First Annual Meeting of the American Laryngological Association* (1909): 393–95.

John Reynders. *Illustrated Catalogue and Price-List of Surgical Instruments.* New York: John Reynders & Co., 1884.

Johnson, W. O. "The Sphygmograph," *North American Review* 117 (1873): 1, 13–17.

Jordan, Furneaux. "On Shock after Surgical Operations and Injuries: The Sphygmograph in Shock." *British Medical Journal* 1 (1867): 192–93.

"Joseph William Stickler" (obituary). *Transactions of the Medical Society of New Jersey* (1899): 286–88.

Kelly, Howard A. and Walter L. Burrage. *American Medical Biographies.* Baltimore: Norman Remington Co., 1920.

Keyt, Alonzo T. "Cardiographic and Sphygmographic Studies." *New York Medical Journal* 26 (1877): 20–36.

———. "Cardiography." *Journal of the American Medical Association* 5 (1885): 141–45.

———. "Cardio-Sphygmographic History of Aortic Obstructive Lesion." *Medical Record* (New York) 19 (1881): 621–24.

———. "The Causes of the Variations of the Cardio-Aortic or 'Pre-Sphygmic' Interval (III)." *Journal of the American Medical Association* 1 (1883): 661–68.

———. "The Claims of the Graphic Method." *Cincinnati Lancet and Clinic* n.s. 8 (1882): 475–86.

———. "The Compound Sphygmograph." *Lancet* (London) 2 (1880): 50.

———. "The Compound Sphygmograph." *Boston Medical and Surgical Journal* 102 (1880): 484–85.

———. "Enormous Delay of the Pulse." *Medical Record* (New York) 17 (1880): 169–70.

———. "Experiments to Determine the Relative Merits of Water and Air as Media of Transmission for Sphygmographs." *Medical Record* (New York) 18 (1880): 479–82.

———. "An Experimental Inquiry into the Causes of the Variations of Pulse-Wave Velocity and Duration of the Cardio-Aortic or Presphygmic Interval Observed in Man (I)." *Journal of the American Medical Association* 1 (1883): 437–46.

———. "Facts and New Experiments in Illustration of the Variations of Pulse-Wave Velocity in Man, and Bearing Upon the Elucidation of the Causes Which Produce Them (II)." *Journal of the American Medical Association* 1 (1883): 605–12.

———. "The Influence of Aortic Aneurism and Aortic Insufficiency, Singly and Combined, on the Retardation of the Pulse." *Boston Medical and Surgical Journal* 103 (1880): 315–18.

———. "The Mechanism of the Cardiac and Arterial Traces, and Some of the Teachings of Cardio-Sphygmography." *Boston Medical and Surgical Journal* 105 (1881): 293–97.

———. "A New Interpretation of Flint's Mitral Direct or Presystolic Murmur without Mitral Lesions." *Boston Medical and Surgical Journal* 109 (1883): 30–31.

———. "A New Sphygmograph—Elastic Membrane and Liquids for Transmitting the Pulsations of the Artery" (Abstract of a paper read before the American Medical Association, May 1875). *Medical Record* (New York) 10 (1875): 365.

———. "The New Sphygmograph; Or, Instrument Adapted as a Sphygmograph, Sphygmometer, Cardiograph, Cardiometer, and to Other Uses." *New York Medical Journal* 23 (1876): 26–56.

———. "The New Sphygmograph" (Correspondence). *New York Medical Journal* 23 (1876): 506–7.

———. "Observations on Bertha Von Hillern's Pulse." *Cincinnati Clinic* (1878).

———. "O'Leary's Pulsations." [*Cincinnati*] *Lancet and Clinic* (1878).

———. "The Presphygmic Interval, or Time Required to Start the Arterial Pulse after the Beginning of the Systole of the Ventricle." *Boston Medical and Surgical Journal* 102 (1880): 409–13.

———. "The Sphygmographic Indications in Aneurism." *Medical Record* (New York) 16 (1879): 507–11.

———. *Sphygmography and Cardiography, Physiological and Clinical*, edited by Asa B. Isham and M. H. Keyt. New York: G. P. Putnam's Sons, 1887.

———. "Sphygmometer, U.S. Patent No. 203548, 14 May 1878," United States Patent and Trade Office, www.google.com/patents/US203548 (accessed 3 February 2017).

Klein, Edward, John Burdon-Sanderson, Michael Foster, and T. Lauder Brunton. *Handbook for the Physiology Laboratory*. Philadelphia: Lindsay & Blakiston, 1873.

Kny-Scheerer Co. *Illustrations of Surgical Instruments of Superior Quality* (Catalogue), 20th ed. New York, Kny-Scheerer Co., 1915.

Koschlakoff, D. K. "Untersuchungen über den Puls mit Hülfe des Marey'schen Sphygmographen." *Archiv für Pathologische Anatomie und Physiologie und für Klinische Medicin* 30 (1864): 149–76.

Kroker, Kenton. "From Reflex to Rhythm: Sleep, Dreaming, and the Discovery of Rapid Eye Movement, 1870–1960." PhD diss., Institute for the History & Philosophy of Science & Technology, University of Toronto, 2000. http://www.collectionscanada.gc.ca/obj/s4/f2/dsk2/ftp02/NQ53765.pdf (accessed 17 February 2017).

Kuriyama, Shigehisa. *The Expressiveness of the Body and the Divergence of Greek and Chinese Medicine*. New York: Zone Books, 1999.

Landois, Leonard. *A Text-book of Human Physiology; Translated from the Seventh German Edition*. Philadelphia: P. Blakiston, Son & Co., 1892.

Lawrence, Christopher. "Incommunicable Knowledge: Science, Technology and the Clinical Art in Britain, 1850–1914." *Journal of Contemporary History* 20 (1985): 503–20.

Lederer, Susan E. *Subjected to Science: Human Experimentation in America before the Second World War*. Baltimore: Johns Hopkins University Press, 1995.

Leonhardt, J. S. "Organic Juices in Therapeutics." *New York Medical Journal* 57 (1893): 641–43.

———. "The Sphygmograph as an Instrument of Precision." *New York Medical Journal* 58 (1893): 225–26.

Lewis, Thomas. *Clinical Electrocardiography*. London: Shaw and Sons, 1913.

Lipartito, Kenneth. "Picturephone and the Information Age: The Social Meaning of Failure." *Technology and Culture* 44 (2003): 50–81.

"Louis Faugeres Bishop Sr." (obituary). *Journal of the American Medical Association* 117 (1941): 1458.

Ludmerer, Kenneth M. *Learning to Heal: The Development of American Medical Education*. Baltimore: Johns Hopkins University Press, 1985.

Mackenzie, James. *The Study of the Pulse: Arterial Venous and Hepatic, and of the Movements of the Heart*. Edinburgh and London: Young J. Pentland, 1902.

———. *The Future of Medicine*. London: Oxford University Press, 1919.

———. "The Ink Polygraph." *British Medical Journal* 1 (1908): 1411.

Mahomed, Frederick Akbar. "On the Sphygmograph" (1871); unpublished essay presented to the Pupil's Physical Society, Guy's Hospital, London; first page reproduced in J. Stewart Cameron and Jackie Hicks. "Frederick Akbar Mahomed and His Role in the Description of Hypertension at Guy's Hospital." *Kidney International* 49 (1996): 1488–1506.

———. "Some of the Clinical Aspects of Chronic Bright's Disease." *Guy's Hospital Reports*, 24 (1879): 363–436.
Mair, Alex. *Sir James Mackenzie, M.D., 1853–1925: General Practitioner.* Edinburgh: Churchill Livingstone, 1973.
Major, Ralph H. *Classic Descriptions of Disease.* 3rd ed. Springfield, IL: Charles C. Thomas, 1945.
———. "The History of Taking the Blood Pressure." *Annals of Medical History* n.s. 2 (1930): 47–55.
Marey, Étienne-Jules. *La circulation du sang à l'état physiologique et dans les maladies.* Paris: G. Masson, 1881.
———. "Lectures on the Graphic Method in the Experimental Sciences, and on Its Special Application to Medicine," *British Medical Journal* 1 (1876): 1–3.
———. *Du mouvement dans les fonctions de la vie.* Paris: Germer Baillière, 1868.
———. *La méthode graphique dans les sciences expérimentales et principalement en physiologie et en médecine.* Paris: G. Masson, 1878.
———. *Physiologie expérimentale: Travaux du laboratoire de M. Marey.* Paris: G. Masson, 1876.
———. *Physiologie médicale de la circulation du sang.* Paris: Adrien Delahaye, 1863.
———. "Recherches sur le pouls au moyen d'un nouvel appareil enregistreur: le sphygmographe." *Comptes rendus des séances de la Société de biologie et de ses filiales*, 3rd ser., 1 (1859): 281–309.
———. "Recherches sur le pouls au moyen d'un nouvel appareil enregistreur (sphygmograph." *Gazette Médicale de Paris*, 3rd ser., 15 (1860): 225–26, 236–42, 298–301.
Marks, Harry M. *The Progress of Experiment: Science and Therapeutic Reform in the United States: 1900–1990.* Cambridge: Cambridge University Press, 1997.
McBride, Thomas A. "The Utility of the Sphygmograph in Medicine." *Archives of Medicine* 1 (1879): 184–98.
Meara, Frank S. "Hyperpiesia of Clifford Allbutt (Essential Hypertension)." *Medical Clinics of North America* 2 (1918): 2–3.
"Medical Patents" (editorial). *Medical Record* (New York) 11 (1876): 816.
Medical and Surgical Directory of the United States. Detroit: R. L. Polk, 1886.

Mitchell, S. Weir. *The Early History of Instrumental Precision in Medicine. An Address Before the Second Congress of American Physicians and Surgeons, September 23, 1891, by the President of the Congress.* New Haven: Tuttle, Morehouse, & Taylor, 1892; "The Early History of Instrumental Precision in Medicine. An Address Before the Second Congress of American Physicians and Surgeons, September 23, 1891, by the President of the Congress." *Transactions of the Congress of American Physicians and Surgeons* 2 (1892): 159–98.

———. "Memoir of John Call Dalton, 1825–1889: Read before the National Academy, April 16,1890." *Biographical Memoirs of the National Academy of Sciences* 3 (1890): 177–85.

Moss, Sandra W. *The Country Practitioner: Ellis P. Townsend's Brave Little Medical Journal.* Xlibris, 2011).

———. "The Doctor as Weatherman: Medical Topography in Nineteenth-Century New Jersey." *Journal of the Rutgers University Libraries* 62 (2006): 59–74.

———. *Edgar Holden, M.D., of Newark, New Jersey: Provincial Physician on a National Stage.* XLibris, 2014.

———. "Newark's Civil War Hospital." *New Jersey Heritage Magazine* 2 (2004): 18–28.

———. "Profiles in Cardiology: Alonzo Thrasher Keyt." *Clinical Cardiology* 29 (2006): 471–73.

———. "The Sphygmograph in America: Writing the Pulse." *American Journal of Cardiology* 97 (2006): 580–87.

Mumford, Lewis. *Technics and Civilization.* New York: Harcourt Brace, 1934; reprint New York: Harcourt Brace & Co., 1963.

Nancrede, Joseph G. "Preface," in Jules Hérisson. *The Sphygmometer. An Instrument which Exhibits to the Eye the Entire Action of the Arteries; The Usefulness of this Instrument in the Study of all Diseases; Researches on the Diseases of the Heart and on the Means of Discriminating Them: A Memoir Presented to the Institute of France by Dr. Julius [sic] Herisson, of Paris; Translated from the French by Joseph G. Nancrede, M.D.* Philadelphia: Grigg and Elliot, 1835.

Naqvi, N. H. and M. D. Blaufox. *Blood Pressure Measurement:An Illustrated History.* New York: Parthenon, 1998.

"Nécrologie—Marey." *Revue Scientifique* 1 (1904): 673–75.

"New Instruments: The Sphygmograph." *Medical Record* (New York) 1 (1866–1867): 580–81.

"The Newark City Almshouse—Description of the New Building," *Newark Daily Advertiser*, 15 July 1868.

Nuland, Sherwin B. "The New Medicine: Anatomical Concept of Giovanni Morgagni." In *Doctors: The Biography of Medicine*, 145–70. New York: Knopf, 1988; Vintage Books, 1989.

———. "Without Diagnosis There Is No Rational Treatment: René Laennec, Inventor of the Stethoscope." In *Doctors: The Biography of Medicine*, 200–37. New York: Knopf, 1988; Vintage Books, 1989.

O'Brien, Eion and Desmond Fitzgerald. "The History of Indirect Blood Pressure Measurement." In *Handbook of Hypertension*, edited by E. O'Brien and K. O'Malley, 14:1–54. Amsterdam: Elsevier Science Publishers, 1991.

"On the Use of the Sphygmograph in the Investigation of Disease, by B. W. Foster" (review). *Dublin Quarterly Journal of Medical Science* 42 (1866): 125–28.

"The Opening of the New City Hospital," *Newark Daily Advertiser*, 12 August 1882, 5 September 1882.

Osler, William. "An Address on High Blood Pressure: Its Associations, Advantages, and Disadvantages: Delivered at the Glasgow Southern Medical Society," *British Medical Journal* 2 (1912): 1173–77.

———. *The Principles and Practice of Medicine*, 2nd ed. New York: D. Appleton, 1892.

———. *The Principles and Practice of Medicine*, 6th ed. New York: D. Appleton, 1905.

Ozanam, Charles. *Le circulation et le pouls: histoire, physiologie, séméiotique, indications thérapeutic*. Paris: J. B. Baillière et Fils, 1886.

Pacey, Arnold. *Technology and World Civilization*. Cambridge, MA: Massachusetts Institute of Technology Press, 1990.

"Pancoast, Joseph." In *Appleton's Cyclopaedia of American Biography*, edited by James Grant Wilson and John Fiske, 4:641–42. New York: D. Appleton, 1888.

"Parisian Medical Intelligence." *Lancet* 2 (1860): 599.

Pennington, S. H., Newark, to Rev. Dr. McCosh, Princeton, 25 March 1874. Alumni Records, Class of 1859, Box 116. Seeley G. Mudd Manuscript Library, Princeton University, Princeton, NJ.

"Physicians and Physicists." *Lancet* 2 (1865): 599.

Pierson, William, Jr., "Case of Hydrophobia." *Transactions of the Medical Society of New Jersey* (1864): 100–1.

Poiseuille, J. L. M. "Researches on the Forces of the Aortal or Left Side of the Heart." *Edinburgh Medical and Surgical Journal* 32 (1829): 28–38.

Pond, Erasmus A. "Diphtheria." *Transactions of the Vermont Medical Society* (1864): 53–64.

———. "Pill Machine, U.S. Patent No. 9455, 7 December 1852," United States Patent and Trade Office, www.google.com/patents/US9455; "Pill Machine, U.S. Patent No. 12960, 29 May 1855," United States Patent and Trade Office, www.google.com/patents/US12960 (both accessed 2 February 2017).

———. *Pond's Improved Sphygmograph.* Pond Sphygmograph Company: Rutland: VT, 1877; Entry in *Index Catalog, Library of the Surgeon-General's Office*, Series 1, 11:493, 13:387.

———. *Pond's Perfected Sphygmograph.* Parke, Davis & Co. n.d.; Entry in *Index Catalog, Library of the Surgeon-General's Office*, Series 1, 11:493, 13:387.

———. "Sphygmoscopes, U.S. Patent No. 161821, 6 April 1875," United States Patent and Trade Office, www.google.com/patents/US161821 (accessed 2 February 2017).

———. "Sphygmographs, U.S. Patent No. 183205, 10 October 1876," United States Patent and Trade Office, www.google.com/patents/US183205; "Sphygmograph, U.S. Patent No. 205412, 25 June 1878," United States Patent and Trade Office, www.google.com/patents/US205412 (both accessed 1 February 2017).

Pond, Wallace R. "Correspondence." *New York Medical Journal* 23 (1876): 288–90.

———. "Sphygmoscope, U.S. Patent No. 167785, 14 September 1875," United States Patent and Trade Office, www.google.com/patents/US167785 (accessed 1 February 2017).

"Pond's Improved Sphygmograph" (advertisement), *The Country Practitioner* 3 (1881): np.

Porter, Roy. *The Greatest Benefit to Mankind: A Medical History of Humanity.* New York: W. W. Norton & Co., 1997.

"The Prevention of Apoplexy," *British Medical Journal 1* (1905): 782–83.

"Proceedings of the Sixty-fourth Annual Meeting [of the Vermont Medical Society] at Montpelier, October 11th and 12th, 1876." *Transactions of the Vermont Medical Society* (1864–1876): 421.

Proctor, L. B. "History of the Superintendents of the Poor for the County of Kings." In *The Civil, Political, Professional Record of the County of Kings and the City of Brooklyn N.Y. from 1683 to 1884*, edited by Henry R. Stiles 1:463–92. New York: W. W. Munsel and Co., 1884.

"The Pulse in Health and Disease." *Lancet* 2 (1866): 501.
Purdy, A. E. M., comp. *The Medical Register of New York and Vicinity for the Year Commencing June 1, 1871.* New York: William Wood, 1871.
_____. *The Medical Register of New York, New Jersey and Connecticut for the Year Commencing June 1, 1874.* New York: William Wood, 1874.
_____. *The Medical Register of New York, New Jersey, and Connecticut for the Year Commencing June 1, 1875.* New York: G. P. Putnam's Sons, 1875.
Pye, David. *The Nature and Aesthetics of Design* (London: Barrie & Jenkins, 1978). Cited in Graeme Gooday. "Re-writing the 'Book of Blots': Critical Reflections on Histories of Technological 'Failure.'" *History and Technology* 14 (1998): 277–78.
Rabinbach, Anson. *The Human Motor: Energy, Fatigue, and the Origins of Modernity.* Berkeley: University of California Press, 1990.
"Recent Deaths. (Erasmus Allington Pond)." *New York Medical Journal* 49 (1889): 635.
Reeds, Karen. *A State of Health: New Jersey's Medical Heritage.* New Brunswick, NJ: Rutgers University Press, 2001.
Register of the Commissioned, Warrant, and Volunteer Officers of the Navy of the United States to January 1, 1862 (1863, 1864, 1865). Washington: Government Printing Office, 1862–1865.
Registrar's Grade Books, AC #116, 1802-1906, Box 11 (1853 October–1863 June), Seeley G. Mudd Manuscript Library, Princeton University.
Reichert, Paul and Louis Faugères Bishop Jr., "Sir James Mackenzie and His Polygraph: The Contribution of Louis Faugères Bishop, Sr.," *American Journal of Cardiology* 24 (1969): 401–3.
Reiser, Stanley Joel. *Medicine and the Reign of Technology.* Cambridge: Cambridge University Press, 1978.
_____. "The Technologies of Time Measurement: Implications at the Bedside and the Bench." *Annals of Internal Medicine* 132 (2000): 31–36.
"Report from King's College Hospital: Large Aneurismal Tumour in the Posterior Triangle, Diagnosed by the Aid of the Sphygmograph; Haemorrhage from Rupture; Death; Autopsy." *Lancet* 1 (1866): 65–66.
Richardson, Benjamin Ward. "Note on the Invention of a Method for Making the Movements of the Pulse Audible by the Telephone. The Sphygmophone." *Proceedings of the Royal Society of London* 29 (1879): 70.
_____. "A Standard Sphygmograph." In *Aloe's Illustrated and Priced Catalogue of Superior Surgical Instruments, Physician's Supplies and Hospital Furnishings.* 6th ed., 351, 354–55. St. Louis: A. S. Aloe Co., ca. 1893.

Ringer, Sydney and William Murrell. "On Gelseminum Semipervirens." *Lancet* 2 (1875): 907–9.

R. J. Strasenburgh. *Catalogue of Surgical Instruments, Physicians' and Hospital Supplies 1925*. Rochester NY: R. J. Strasenburgh, 1925.

Rogers, Fred B. "Abraham Coles (1813-91): Poet Physician of New Jersey." In *Help Bringers: Versatile Physicians of New Jersey*, 72–80. New York: Vantage Press, 1960.

Rogers, Fred B. and A. Reasoner Sayre. *The Healing Art: A History of the Medical Society of New Jersey*. Trenton: Medical Society of New Jersey, 1966.

Romano, Terrie M. *Making Medicine Scientific: John Burdon Sanderson and the Culture of Victorian Science*. Baltimore: Johns Hopkins University Press, 2002.

Rosenberg, Charles E. "Social Class and Medical Care in Nineteenth-Century America: The Rise and Fall of the Dispensary." *Journal of the History of Medicine and Allied Sciences* 29 (1974): 32–54.

———. "The Therapeutic Revolution: Medicine, Meaning, and Social Change in Nineteenth-Century America." In *The Therapeutic Revolution: Essays in the Social History of Medicine*, edited by Morris J. Vogel and Charles E. Rosenberg, 3–25. Philadelphia: University of Pennsylvania Press, 1979.

Rosenbloom, Jacob. "The History of Pulse Timing with Some Remarks on Sir John Floyer and his Physician's Pulse Watch." *Annals of Medical History* 4 (1922): 97–99.

Rothstein, William G. *American Physicians in the 19th Century: From Sects to Science*. Baltimore: Johns Hopkins University Press, 1972.

"The Science Association." *Scientific American* n.s. 21 (1869): 162.

Scott Alison, Somerville (reported by G. O. Rees). "A Description of a New Sphygmoscope, an Instrument for Indicating the Movements of the Heart and Blood-Vessels; With an Account of Observations Obtained by the Aid of that Instrument." *Proceedings of the Royal Society of London* 8 (1856–57): 18–26.

———. *The Physical Examination of the Chest in Pulmonary Consumption*. London: John Churchill, 1861.

Seaverns, Joel. "Recent Advances in Medicine and Their Influence on Therapeutics." *Boston Medical and Surgical Journal* n.s. 8 (1871): 113–20.

Séguin, É[douard]. *Medical Thermometry and Human Temperature*. New York: William Wood & Co., 1876.

———. "Sphygmometry." *Medical Record* (New York) 2 (1867/68): 243–44.

"Self-adjusting Stethoscope of Dr. Cammann." *New York Medical Times* 4 (1855): 140–42.

Shaw, William H., comp. "The Medical Profession of Essex County." In *History of Essex and Hudson Counties, New Jersey*, 302–47. Philadelphia: Everts & Peck, 1884.

Sheehan, Helen and Richard Wedeen. "Hatters' Shakes." In *Toxic Circles: Environmental Hazards from the Workplace into the Community*, edited by Helen Sheehan and Richard Wedeen, 26–54. New Brunswick, NJ: Rutgers University Press, 1993.

Sheldon, Paul B. and Janet Doe. "The Development of the Stethoscope: An Exhibition Showing the Work of Laennec and His Successors." *Bulletin of the New York Academy of Medicine* 11 (1935): 608–28.

Shepard and Dudley. *Illustrated Catalogue of Surgical Instruments, Shepard and Dudley*. New York: Shepard and Dudley, 1878.

Shrady, John, comp. *Medical Register, New York and Vicinity, 1868*. New York: Baker and Godwin, 1868.

———. *Medical Register, New York and Vicinity, 1869–70*. New York: J. M. Bradstreet, 1869.

Singer, Charles. "To Vesalius on the Fourth Centenary of His *De Humani Corporis Fabrica*." *Journal of Anatomy* (London) 77 (1943): 261–65.

"Sir William Henry Broadbent" (obituary). *Lancet* 1 (1907): 126–29.

Smith, H. P. and W. S. Rann. *History of Rutland County, Vermont*. Syracuse NY: D. Mason, 1886.

Smith-Rosenberg, Caroll. *Disorderly Conduct: Visions of Gender in America*. New York: Oxford University Press, 1985.

Snellen, H. A. *E. J. Marey and Cardiology: Physiologist and Pioneer of Technology, 1830-1904: Selected Writings in Facsimile with Comments and Summaries, a Brief History of Life and Work, and a Bibliography*. Rotterdam: Kooyker Scientific, 1980.

Snowden, John. "The Advances Made in Medicine by Physical Diagnosis." *Transactions of the Medical Society of New Jersey* (1883): 56–78.

"Some Further Improvements in Medical Science: The Sphygmograph." *Boston Medical and Surgical Journal* 76 (1867): 359.

The Sphygmograph: Its Physiological and Pathological Indications, by Edgar Holden (review). *Canada Medical and Surgical Journal* 2 (1874): 492–95.

"The Sphygmograph, or Register of the Arterial Pulse." *Lancet* 1 (1860): 435.

Review of *The Sphygmometer: An Instrument Which Renders the Action of the Arteries Apparent to the Eye &c.* by Jules Hérisson. *Medico-Chirurgical Review and Journal of Practical Medicine* n.s. 27 (1835): 159–60.

Stevenson, Jonathan R. "Vital Statistics." *Transactions of the Medical Society of New Jersey* (1864): 145–53.
Stickler, Joseph W. "Foot and Mouth Disease as It Affects Man and Animals, and Its Relation to Human Scarlatina as a Prophylactic." *Boston Medical and Surgical Journal* 117 (1887): 607–9.
———. "Scarlet Fever Reproduced by Inoculation; Some Important Points Deducted Therefrom." *Transactions of the Medical Society of New Jersey* (1897): 201–12.
"The Sphygmograph" (editorial). *Medical and Surgical Reporter* 46 (1882): 378–79.
"The Sphygmograph in English Medical Practice" (editorial). *Lancet* 1 (1866): 579.
"The Sphygmograph in Private Practice." *Lancet* 1 (1882): 73.
"Sphygmography by Telegraph." *British Medical Journal* 2 (1869): 355–56.
St. Mary's Hospital: Aneurism of the Axillary Artery: Examination by the Sphygmograph." *Lancet* 1 (1866): 176.
Steell, Graham. *The Use of the Sphygmograph in Clinical Medicine*. Manchester: Sherratt & Hughes, 1899.
Stirling, William. *Some Apostles of Physiology: An Account of Their Lives and Labours*. London: Waterlow, 1902.
Stone, Mildred R. *Since 1845: A History of the Mutual Benefit Life Insurance Company*. New Brunswick, Rutgers University Press, 1957.
Taber, Sydney R. *Illustrations of Human Vivisection*. Chicago: Vivisetion Reform Society, 1906.
Tansey, E. M. "The Physiological Tradition." In *Companion Encyclopedia of the History of Medicine*, edited by W. F. Bynum and Roy Porter, 120–52. London: Routledge, 1993.
Townsend, Ellis P. "To Medical Practitioners." *The Country Practitioner* 1 (1879): 1–3.
Transactions of the Vermont State Medical Society (1864–1876): 421.
Transactions of the Vermont State Medical Society (1884): 4.
Turner, Thomas. "Annual Report of the Resident Physician of Kings County Hospital." In *Annual Report of the Superintendents of the Poor of Kings County, for the Year Ending July 31, 1861*, 49–64. Brooklyn, Daily Eagle Print, 1861.
Vanderbeck, C. C. "The Use of Ergot in Headaches." *Transactions of the Medical Society of New Jersey* (1873): 194–95.
Van Wagenen, George A. "Report of the Committee on the Blood Pressure Test," *Abstract of the Proceedings of the Annual Meeting of the Association of Life Insurance Medical Directors of America* (1912–1914): 239–46.

Vaughan, Charles E. "Middlesex South District Medical Society, October 14, 1868." *Boston Medical and Surgical Journal* 79 (1869): 232–33.
Vierordt, Karl. "Die bildliche Darstellung des menschlichen Arterienpulses." *Archiv für Physiologische Heilkunde* 13 (1854): 284–87.
_____. *Die Lehre vom Arterienpuls in Gesunden und Kranken Zuständen.* Braunschweig: Vieweg, 1855.
Vogel, Morris J. *The Invention of the Modern Hospital: Boston 1870-1930.* Chicago: University of Chicago Press, 1980.
Wailoo, Keith. "'Chlorosis' Remembered: Disease and the Moral Management of American Woman." In *Drawing Blood: Technology and Disease Identity in Twentieth-Century America*, 17–45. Baltimore: Johns Hopkins University Press, 1997.
Ward, Samuel B. "The Sphygmograph, and Some of Its Uses." *Medical Record* (New York) 3 (1868–69): 385–89.
Warner, John Harley. *Against the Spirit of System: The French Impulse in Nineteenth-Century American Medicine.* Princeton: Princeton University Press, 1998.
_____. *The Therapeutic Perspective: Medical Practice, Knowledge, and Identity in America, 1820–1885.* Princeton: Princeton University Press, 1997.
Watson, William P. "The Value of Creosote in Fifty Cases of Disease of the Air Passages." *Transactions of the Medical Society of New Jersey* (1889): 117–42.
Weatherall, Miles. "Drug Therapies." In *Companion Encyclopedia of the History of Medicine*, edited by W. F. Bynum and Roy Porter, 915–37. London: Routledge, 1993.
Weir, Robin A. P. and Henry J. Dargie. "Images in Clinical Medicine: Austin Flint Murmur." *New England Journal of Medicine* 359 (2008): e11; http://www.nejm.org/doi/full/10.1056/NEJMicm072437#t=article (accessed 27 January 2017).
Welch, William Henry. "Medical Education in the Unites States: The Harvey Lecture" (1916). In *Papers and Addresses by William Henry Welch*, 3:119–31. Baltimore: Johns Hopkins University Press, 1920.
_____. "Some of the Conditions Which Have Influenced the Development of American Medicine, Especially During the Past Century," *Bulletin of the Johns Hopkins Hospital* 19 (1908): 33–40.
White, Paul Dudley. *Heart Disease.* New York: Macmillin, 1931.
[Wickes, Stephen?]. "The Climatology and Diseases of Essex County." *Transactions of the Medical Society of New Jersey* (1887): 71–230.

Wickes, Stephen. *History of Medicine in New Jersey, and of Its Medical Men, From the Settlement of the Province to A.D. 1800.* Newark: Martin L. Dennis, 1879.

———. "Medical Topography of Orange, N.J." *Transactions of the Medical Society of New Jersey* (1859): 78–82.

Wickes, Stephen, Thos. Ryerson, and R. M. Cooper, "Report of the Standing Committee." *Transactions of the Medical Society of New Jersey* (1863): 20–37.

Wilmarth, Frank. "Reports of District Societies: Essex County." *Transactions of the Medical Society of New Jersey* (1874): 131–38.

Willms, Janice L., Henry Schneiderman, and Paula S. Altranati. *Physical Diagnosis: Bedside Evaluation of Diagnosis and Function.* Baltimore: Williams & Wilkins, 1994.

Wilson, J. L., H. N. Eaton, and H. B. Henrickson, *Use and Testing of Sphygmomanometers.* Washington: United States Government Printing Office, 1927.

Withering, William. *An Account of the Foxglove and Some of Its Medical Uses.* Birmingham: M. Swinney, 1785. Reprinted in facsimile with commentary in J. K. Aronson. *An Account of the Foxglove and its Medical Uses, 1785–1985.* London: Oxford University Press, 1985.

Woodbury, Frank. "Pond's American Sphygmograph." *Medical and Surgical Reporter* 38 (1878); 493–94.

Zumbruck, A. "The Sphygmograph or Pulse Writer." *Scientific American* 10, no. 28 (1855): 219.

INDEX

A

Aconite: Holden sphygmograph experiments with aconite, 156

Allbutt, T. Clifford: biography, 94; critique of sphygmograph, 94–95; eclipse of Mahomed as discover of essential hypertension, 95–96, 257–58; hyperpiesia, 94; use of sphygmograph, 95, 269

Allen, Timothy F.: homeopathic citation of Holden drug trials, 152–53

American sphygmograph men: comparison Holden, Keyt, Pond, 212–14; outside emerging American research establishment, 215; Yankee ingenuity, 213–15; see chapters 4 (Holden), 5 (Keyt), 6 (Pond)

Amyl nitrate: Brunton monitoring of amyl nitrate with sphygmograph, 78–79; in angina pectoris, 78–79

Anatomic pathology: see pathological anatomy

Aneurysm (aneurism, British spelling): use of sphygmograph to locate, 40, 70, 149, 181–82

Anstie, Frances: arterial rigidity alters pulse wave, 249; career and death, 69–70; confounding variables (fatigue, diarrhea, meals, time of day) 248; credit to Anstie, 79; demonstration of sphygmograph at medical meeting, 64; diarrhea pulse, 248; early use of sphygmograph, 62; "fever pulse," 72; hospital appointment, 62; *Lancet* article on technical expertise, 73; practice and training, 248; promotion of sphygmograph in *Lancet*, 63–64; sphygmograph as guide to therapy and prognosis, 71; sphygmograph in consultation, 69–70; studies on workhouse residents, 79

Antivivisectionists: Joseph Stickler's experiments criticized, 127; Mary Putman Jacobi's experiments criticized, 231–33

Arrhythmias: evaluation by sphygmograph, 96–97; Mackenzie polygraph and arrhythmias, 100–1; Steell identification of tachycardia,

bigeminy, trigeminy, atrial fibrillation (delirium cordis), alcoholic cardiomyopathy, 96–97
Art of the physician: contrast with technology technology, 6–7
Auenbrugger, Leopold: percussion of the chest, 7
Auscultation: mediate vs. immediate, 9; monaural vs. binaural, 9–10; see Stethoscope; see Laennec
Autopsy: confirm clinical examination, 5, 9; Hérisson confirmation of sphygmometer findings, 28; hypertensive changes at autopsy, 89; Laennec confirmation of auscultation, 9; "senile" vascular changes, 180; teaching exercise in New Jersey, 125–26

B

Badham, David: clinical application of sphygmometer, 30; critique of sphygmometer, 30–31
Beard, George Miller: mental fatigue and neurasthenia theories, 148
Beaumont, William: Alexis St. Martin research subject, 105; amateur medical science, 105–6; gastric acid studies, 104.
Béhier, Louis-Jules: modification of Marey sphygmograph, 57
Bernard, Claude: French physiologist, 14; leadership in physiology transferring to Germany, 106–7; vitalism, 41
Billings, John Shaw: diverse career, 118; *Index Catalogue*, 118; instruments of precision, 118
Bishop, Louis Faugeres: biography, 233–34; early adoption of Mackenzie polygraph for clinical cardiology practice, 234–35; early clinical cardiologist, 233–34; value to cardiac patients of sphygmographic examination, 222
Blood pressure: Allbutt hyperpiesia, 94; effect of arterial calcification, 249; Hales intraarterial cannulation, 19; Holden theories, 149–50; Marey early blood pressure device, 84; Riva-Rocci model, 93–94; Vierordt concept of blood pressure as pressure required to obliterate pulse, 84; von Basch and Potain models, 93–94; see sphygmomanometer; see hypertension
Blundell, E. S.: British translation of Hérisson's *Le sphygmomètre*, 28–29
Borrell, Merrilley: kymograph impact on physiology, 36; Marey sphygmograph as link between laboratory and clinical practice, 38; power of graphic method, 38; seeing the unobservable, 37
Boston Medical and Surgical Journal: report of early Boston demonstration of sphygmograph by Upham, 111; report of Pond sphygmoscope (sphygmometer) presentation, 194

Bowditch, Henry: French medical research eclipsed by German laboratories, 107; Harvard medical school, 108
Bramwell, Byron: warnings about misuse of sphygmograph, 77; patient discomfort and fear of Marey sphygmograph, 61
Bright's disease: chronic kidney disease, 86; study by Mahomed, 86; see hypertension
British Medical Journal: Balthazar publication on sphygmograph, 80; voice of provincial practitioner, 82
Broadbent, William: high tension pulse, 90; medical school lecturer, 77; persisting value of pulse palpation, 77–78; "personal equation" in sphygmograph technique and interpretation, 249–50; physician must know details of his own sphygmograph, 263–64; value of sphygmograph in teaching about the pulse, 77, 254; user must know details of sphygmograph model, 263–64
Brunton, Thomas Lauder: at Edinburgh Royal Infirmary, 78; bloodletting for angina pectoris, 78; introduction of amyl nitrate 78; monitoring drug effect with sphygmograph, 78–79
Burdon-Sanderson, John: advantages of sphymograph over pulse palpation, 65, 246; aneurysm location by sphygmography, 70; animal experiments, 68; author of *Handbook of the Sphygmograph*; capillary electrometer research leading to electrocardiograph, 272; carotid artery recording, 65; caveats and limitations of sphygmograph, 64–66; contribution to cardiac physiology knowledge, 247; disillusionment with sphygmograph, 68; doubts about classical pulse diagnosis, 14; early adoption of sphygmograph, 14, 62–63; experiments with model arteries using Marey sphygmograph, 62; later career and research, 68; London career, 61–62; modifications of Marey sphygmograph, 62–63; presentation to Royal College of Physicians, 67–68; redefinition of pulse palpation, 14–15; Regius Professor of Medicine at Oxford, 68, 254; sphygmograph useless in determining blood pressure, 85–86; student of Claude Bernard, 14
Burdon-Sanderson, wife (Gittel): comment on John Burdon-Sanderson experiments with the sphygmograph, 62

C

Camman, George: binaural stethoscope, 10
Cannabis: Holden sphygmograph experiments with cannabis, 154
Cardiac impulse: timing with arterial impulse by Scott Alison, 32; tracings with Marey sphygmograph, 54; use with Keyt sphygmograph/sphygmoscope, 172

Cardiac time intervals: Garrod cardiac contraction to radial pulse interval, 75; Garrod sphgmosystole and sphygmodiastole, 74–76; rate related changes in duration of sphygmosystole, 74–75
Cardiograph: apical pulsation recording, 172
Carroll, Alfred: caution in use of sphygmograph, 261; New York user of sphygmograph, 218; Pond best model, 218
La circulation du sang à l'état physiologique et dans les maladies: Marey monograph (1881), 49–50
Circulatory anatomy: early investigators Servetus, Cesalpino, d'Acquapendente, Malphigi, 5
Clock: reduction of human experience to numbers, 16; timekeeping in Western civilization, 16
Coles, Abraham: European training; 117; Newark practice, 117
College of Physicians and Surgeons, New York: attended by New Jersey students, 117; Dalton instruction in physiology, 129; Holden graduate, 129
College of Physicians of Philadelphia: collection of sphygmographs, 160
Congestive heart failure: Mackenzie polygraph and heart failure, 100
Consultation: role of sphygmograph, 70, 72
Corvisart, Jean Nicolas: Auenbrugger chest percussion popularizer, 7; French clinical school, 7; "see with a better eye," 43
Cowen, David: history of medicine in New Jersey, 116
Craft knowledge: learning to use new technologies, 165
Cullen, William: neurovascular tonicity theory, 5

D

DaCosta, Jacob Mendes: negative opinion of gelseminum, 155; use of sphygmograph at Philadelphia Hospital, 115, 210–11
Dalton, John Call: early use of sphygmograph, 113–4; European training, 108; Mitchell praise for Dalton's teaching, 108–9; physiologist at Columbia College of Physicians and Surgeons, 108; private research, 109; publication in popular press, 113–14, 220; review of Holden monograph, 159; vivisection demonstrations, 109
Davis, Nathan S.; praise for Keyt in *Journal of the American Medical Association*, 189
De humani corporis fabrica: Marey and the *"fabrica,"* 43; Vesalius and the workings of the body, 2–3; see Vesalius
Digitalis (foxglove): Mackenzie digitalis studies, 102; use in dropsy, 18; Withering application and trials, 18
Doyle, Arthur Conan: sphygmograph in fiction, xi

Dudgeon, Robert: British homeopath, 237; critique of Pond sphygmograph, 211; critique of Vierordt sphygmograph, 40; popularity of Dudgeon sphygmograph in U.S., 237; see sphygmograph (Dudgeon)

E

Einthoven, Willem: development of electrocardiograph, 272; first published tracing, 274

Electrocardiograph: compared to sphygmograph interpretation and clinical application, 273–74; development by Augustus Waller, Willem Einthoven, and Thomas Lewis, 272–73; early EKG machines, 241; Einthoven first published tracing, 274; graphic method instrument, 271; Marey and Burdon-Sanderson basic science of cardiac electrical impulses, 272; neuroelectrical infrastructure of heart, 47; overshadows polygraph, 241, 242; rapid advances in interpretation and clinical application, 273; rapid inclusion into practice, 273; role in development of cardiology specialization, 242–43

"Errors of the Sphgygmograph" (Holden): abandonment of and disillusionment with the sphygmograph, 163

Europe: destination for American medical students and physicians, 106

F

Fever: characteristic pulses (Latin), 13; "fever pulse," 72; redefinition as body temperature, 11–12

Flexner report: maturation of American medical education, 108

Flint, Austen Sr.; cardiopulmonary diagnosis and disease, 11; sphygmograph and general practitioner, 260; value of sphygmograph, 11

Floyer, John: pulse timing, 16–18; *Physician's Pulse-Watch*, 17; value of pulse rate in regulating the circulation, 18

Foster, Balthazar: controversy over right to publish, 81–82; *On the Use of the Sphygmograph in the Investigation of Disease*, 80, 82; "senile pulse," 79–80; sphygmograph in "the provinces" (Birmingham), 79–81; sphygmographic tracings during surgery, 81

François-Franck, Charles: cardiovascular and nervous system comparison, 47; praise of Keyt sphygmographic studies and instruments, 188; student of Marey, 47

Frank, Robert G.; sphygmograph demonstrated to clinicians how graphic method worked, 255; sphygmograph simple technology with complex output vs. electrocardiograph with complex technology and simple output, 272

French academic medicine: clinicopathological studies, 6–7; Corvisart and percussion 7; from clinical observation to laboratory, 41; vitalism of Bernard, 41

Fye, W. Bruce: cardiac specialization, 242; electrocardiograph adopted by early cardiologists, 243; Ludwig's kymograph, 37

G

Galen, Claudius: system of medicine, 2–3; pulse specific to disease, 15

Garrod, Alfred Henry; biography and career, 74, 77; cardiac to peripheral pulse intervals, 75; clinical value of sphygmograph is in measuring intervals, 76; dependence of pulse wave on heart rate, 248; inverse relationship of heart rate to sphysmosystole, 74–75; Keyt interest in Garrod study of cardiac-arterial intervals, 180; praise for Keyt's study of cardiac-arterial intervals, 189; time intervals of systole and diastole, 73

Gelseminum: Holden sphygmograph experiments with gelseminum, 154–56

General practitioner use of sphygmograph: Dudgeon sphygmograph in "ordinary practice," 237; Lancet editorial support for general use, 219; McBride support for general use, 218

Graphic method (*méthode graphique*): body as field of forces, 37; definition, 37; Ludwig kymograph as key invention, 35–37; role in physiology laboratory, 37; sphygmograph showed clinicians how graphic method worked, 255

H

"Haemastaticks": Hales' experiment, 19

Hales, Stephen: blood pressure measurement in horse, 19; "haemastaticks," 19

Hammond, William: career, 109–10, 222; disillusionment with sphygmograph, 224; early purchase of sphygmograph in Paris, 110; feud with Leonhardt over sphygmographic interpretation, 222–24; private physiologic research, 109–10

Handbook of the Sphygmograph: Burdon-Sanderson early British state-of-the-art text, 14, 66–67, 72–73

Hartshorne, Edward: Philadelphia physician purchaser of Holden book, 159–60

Harvey, William: circulation of the blood, *De motu cordis*, 2–3

Health and illness: natural vs. normal, 6

Helmholtz, Hermann von: body as a field of forces, 37

Hemocytometer: diagnosis of chlorosis (anemia) in women, 231

Hemodynamometer: application to Ludwig kymograph, 34; see Poiseuille
Hérisson, Jules: clinical application of sphygmometer, 28–30; sphygmometer invention, 26–31; *Le sphygmomètre*, 27; use in consultation, 29; see Blundell and Nancrede (translators)
Hippocrates: system of medicine, 2
Holden, Edgar: America's first sphygmograph man, 164; challenge to scientific elite, 106; childhood and Princeton, 129; Civil War naval service, 129–30; honorary doctorate, 161–62; house physician at King's County Hospital, 129; medical environment in Newark and New Jersey, 119–28; medical practice and specialization (insurance medicine, otolaryngology, cardiopulmonary medicine, tuberculosis), 131–32; medical publication, 133; modification of Marey sphygmograph, 58, 136–38; Mutual Benefit Life Insurance Company medical director, 141; physiology course with Dalton at Columbia College of Physicians and Surgeons, 129; use of sphygmograph in medical consultation, 160–61; Ward Army Hospital service in Newark, 130; see sphygmograph (Holden); see *The Sphygmograph: Its Physiological and Pathological Indications*; see *"Errors of the Sphygmograph"*
Holmes, Oliver Wendell: cautions about medical research, 123
Homeopathy: "provings" of drug effects, 152
Hospital use of sphygmgoraph: Massachusetts General Hospital, 219; Montreal General Hospital, 159; Philadelphia Hospital, 211–12
Hunt, Ezra Mundy: New Jersey not a "medical wilderness," 123
Hutchinson, John: spirometer invention and experiments, 20
Hyperpiesia (high blood pressure): use of term by Clifford Allbutt, 95
Hypertension: Allbutt rediscovery of essential hypertension, 93–95; Mahomed elucidation of essential hypertension, 86; system used to diagnose high arterial tension from sphygmograph tracing, 88–89; see Janeway

I

Ill, Edward: European training in medicine, 117; Newark practice, 117
Index-Catalogue of the Library of the Surgeon-General's Office: articles about sphygmograph, 244
Instrument catalogs offering sphygmographs: Brooklyn Fred Haslam & Co. 240; Keyt sphygmograph not found in U.S. catalogs, 240; New York George Tiemann Co. *American Armamentarium Chirurgicum*, 238–39; New York John Reynders, 238, New York Shepard and Dudley, 239; Pond sphygmographs), 238; St. Louis A. S. Aloe, 238–39

Instruments of precision: advances in diagnosis, 118–19; caution against overuse of all instruments of precision, 261–62; new technologies, 1–2; sphygmograph as instrument of precision, 74, 78

Insurance medicine: application of Keyt sphygmograph in life insurance, 190–91; Holden medical director at Mutual Benefit Life Insurance Company, 132; 141–42; use of insurance statistics, 132; see van Wagenen

Isham, Asa B.; application of Keyt cardiosphygmograph in life insurance risk assessment, 190–91; co-editor of collected works of Keyt, 189; commentary on Keyt's professional ethics, 209; family relation to Keyt, 166; Keyt biographer and posthumous champion, 188–89

J

Jackson, James: early adoption of stethoscope, 11

Jacobi, Mary Putnam: Boylston prize for study of menstruation effect on women's capacity for work, 226; conclusion that women do not require rest during menstruaiton, 230–31; experiments on brain blood flow, 232–33; fluid volume in menstruation, 230; Keyt comment on Jacobi experiments, 179; medical education, practice, professorship, 224–26; *The Question of Rest for Women*: dynamometer studies, 228; *The Question of Rest for Women*: laboratory studies, 227–28; *The Question of Rest for Women* sphygmographic studies, 228–29; *The Question of Rest for Women*: statistical evidence, 226–27; refutation of Edward Clarke's *Sex in Education*, 226; sphygmograph illustration, xiii; vivisection and antivivisectionists, 231–33; see sphygmograph (Jacobi); see Taber

Janeway, Theodore: sphygmomanometer to define essential hypertension, 269; "hypertensive cardiovascular disease" research, 270

Jordan, Furneaux: sphygmograph tracings during surgery, 81

K

Keyt, Alonzo Thrasher: biography and medical practice, 166, 191; *Boston Medical and Surgical Journal* publication, 184; criticism of Holden sphygmograph, 169–70; dedication to sphygmographic work, 191–92; deficiencies of Marey sphygmograph, 168–69; disinterest in financial gain, 209; Garrod notice of Keyt's work, 189; *Journal of the American Medical Association* publication, 189; Keyt–Pond priority controversy, 203–4; Marey group connections 187–88; modification of sphygmoscope, 167; numeric objectivity, 192; publications in medical journals, 185; sale of instruments, 189; sphygmoscope, 166–67; see sphygmograph (Keyt); see sphygmograph (Keyt chrono-cardio-sphygmograph); see Isham, Asa B.; see *Sphygmography and Cardiography, Physiological and Clinical*; see life insurance; see patents

King's County Hospital: Holden house physician, 129

Korotkoff, Nicolai: auscultatory method of blood pressure determination, 269

Koschlakoff, D. K.: early adoption of Marey sphygmograph in Russia, 60

Kuriyama, Shigahesa: pulse as sign of life, 12–13

Kymograph: application of graphic method to physiology, 35–36; application to study of nerve and muscle, 38; incorporation of Poiseuille hemodynamometer, 34; Ludwig kymograph design, 34; permanent record of physiologic events, 34–35; "wave writer," 33

L

Laennec, René T. H.: *De l'auscultation médiate*, 9; invention of stethoscope, 8–9, 43

Laboratory: source of pharmaceutical knowledge and authority, 153; transfer of knowledge from laboratory to bedside, 2

Lahey, Jean-Marie: application of sphygmograph to World War I military, 278

Lancet: Anstie on fever and technical expertise, 73; Anstie promotion of sphygmograph, 63; Brunton work on amyl nitrate; 78; Burdon-Sanderson review article, 64–65; challenge to provincial Balthazar Foster work with sphgymograph, 81; reviews of Marey sphygmograph and adaptations, 60, 63, 64; voice of London elite practitioner, 82

Landois, Leonard: haemautorgram, 25

Leonhardt, J. S.: dispute with Hammond over interpretation of sphygmograms, 222–24

Lewis, Thomas: electrocardiograph development, 272; manual of electrocardiography, 273

Lipartito, Kenneth: sphygmograph as failed technology, 1, 251–53

Ludmerer, Kenneth: European training and new view of medical science, 107–8

Ludwig, Carl: destination for American trainees in physiology, 107 groundwork for sphygmograph invention, 23; introduction of graphic method into physiology and medicine, 37; vivisection experiments, 36; see kymograph

M

Mackenzie, James: arrhythmia in pregnant women; 97; biography, 97–98; congestive heart failure, 100; development of clinical and ink polygraphs, 98–101; digitalis studies, 102; emphasis on clinical acumen, 275–76; failure to understand sphygmograph, 276; Knoll's polygraph, 99; polygraph and arrhythmias, 101–2; polygraph as aid to clinical bedside diagnosis, 100–1; polygraph in America, 240–41; venous pulse waves studied by polygraph, 98, 100; see polygraph

Mahomed, Frederick Akbar: abandonment of sphygmograph at Guy's Hospital, 86; American review by McBride, 87; biography, 86, 90; credit to Allbutt as discover of essential hypertension, 95–96; Broadbent comments on overinterpretation by Mahomed, 91, 250; eclipse of Mahomed's reputation, 90; eclipse of pulse study by stethoscope, 21–22; identification of essential hypertension using modified sphygmograph, 57–58, 86, 88–91; method of determination of high tension from pulse wave, 88–89; study of Bright's disease, 86; sphygmomanometer succeeded sphygmographic assessment of blood pressure, 267

Malphigi, Marcello: discovery of capillaries, 3

Marey, Étienne-Jules: application of physical science to physiology, 41–42; critique of constructivism, 45; early blood pressure device, 84; early life, 42–43; election to the Collège du France, 57; "engineer of life," 42; heart (pump) and arteries (tubes) as mechanical system, 45; graphic method and clarity, 45; graphic method deciphering "unknown language" of physiological time, 45–46; Helmholtzian identity, 38; model heart and blood vessels: 55–57; modernity, 24; movement as expression of life, 45; praise for Keyt's instruments and studies, 188; range of interests, 24; replacing vivisection, 44, 59; sphygmogram as graphic image of arteries, 43; time and motion studies of animals and humans, 58; vitalism, 41; see sphygmograph (Marey)

Massachusetts General Hospital: temperature charts, 12

McBride, Thomas A.; American champion of sphygmograph, 163–64; assessment of European and American sphygmographs, 217; comprehensive review of sphygmograph for American journal, 87; praise for Pond sphygmograph, 212; review of Mahomed's investigations into blood pressure, 87; value of sphymgograph for general practitioner, 164, 260

Medical education in New Jersey: fraudulent irregular schools in New Jersey, 121–22; lack of medical schools in New Jersey, 121; schools in New York and Philadelphia, 121

Medical journals in New Jersey; *The Country Practitioner*, 124; *New Jersey Medical Reporter*, 124; *Transactions of the Medical Society of New Jersey*, 124

Medical research (United States): "amateur" American nineteenth century research, 104–5; Beaumont gastric juice studies, 104–5; privately supported and conducted, 109; see Mitchell, Hammond, Dalton, Bowditch

Medical research (New Jersey): asymptomatic glycosuria, 126; autopsy, 124–25; chest expansion in glass blowers, 126; collective investigation, 125; creosote for tuberculosis, 125; electromagnetism for rabies, 125; ergot for headache, 125; Koch's tuberculin for tuberculosis, 127; mercurialism among hatters, 126; scarlet fever experiments, 127

méthode graphique: see graphic method.

Mitchell, Silas Weir: praise for instruments of precision, 262; private physiological research, 109

Montreal General Hospital: purchase of Holden sphygmograph, 159

Morgagni, Giovannia: *De sedibus et causus morborum* and pathological anatomy, 5; "suffering organs," 5

Mumford, Lewis: medieval timekeeping reduction to numbers, 16

N

Nancrede, Joseph: American translation of Hérisson's *Le sphygmomètre*, 29

Newark (Essex County): almshouse, 120–21; City Dispensary, 120; Civil War military hospital, 120; "golden age," 117–18; lag in building dispensaries and hospitals, 119–20; medical life mid-nineteenth century, 116–21; medical research, 122–23; municipal hospital, 121; Newark German Hospital, 121; New Jersey a medical backwater, 128; shadow of New York, 117; training of physicians, 117; St. Barnabas Hospital, 121; St. Michael's Hospital, 121

O

Osler, William: sphygmograph in Osler textbooks, 266–67; sphygmomanometer in textbooks, 267

P

Pacey, Arnold: timekeeping applied to pulse, 17

Paracelsus: challenge to classical medical systems, 2

Patent of sphygmoscopes and sphygmographs: American Medical Association proscription of patents, 204–7; Holden disinterest in financial gain from patent; 209; Holden rejection of patent, 161–62; Keyt defensive patent on chrono-cardio-sphygmograph, 207; Keyt ethical opposition to patents, 207; Pond patents, 195, 199, 204–6

Pathological anatomy: basis for proof of disease, 1, 2; Giovanni Morgagni and *De sedibus et causus morborum*, 56
Pathophysiology: disease in terms of physiological dysfunction, 5–6
Pennington, Samuel: recommendation of Holden for honorary Ph.D. from Princeton, 161
Percussion: Auenbrugger innovation, 7; Corvisart popularization, 7; Piorry immediate vs. intermediate, 7–8 ; pleximeter (plessimeter) for intermediate percussion, 8
Pharmacy and pharmaceuticals: Brunton sphygmograph and amyl nitrite, 78–79, 254–55; Holden sphygmograph and pharmaceutical trials, 151–57; state of the art in America, 151–54
The Physician's Pulse-Watch: see Floyer
Piorry, Pierre Adolphe: intermediate percussion, 7
Poiseuille, Jean: application of haemodynamometer to Ludwig kymograph, 3; invention of haemodynamometer, 34
Polygraph: aid to clinical diagnosis, 100–1, 103–4; arrhythmias studied by polygraph, 97, 101–2; Bishop and polygraph, 234–35; congestive heart failure and polygraph, 100; digitalis studies and polygraph, 102–3; "indispensible" at bedside, 240–41; Knoll's polygraph 99; Mackenzie studies with polygraph, 97–102, 275; offered in New York catalog, 241; overshadowed by electrocardiograph, 241; polygraph and neck veins, 98, 100
Pond, Erasmus Allington: commercial success of Pond sphygmograph, 209–10; diphtheria epidemic, 194; medical education and practice, 193, 210; patents, 195, 199, 204–6; praise for Pond sphygmograph, 210; presentation of sphygmoscope to Suffolk County Medical Society, 194; priority of Pond vs. Keyt sphygmoscopes and sphygmographs, 198–99; 203–4; publications: 216; see sphygmometer (sphygmoscope); see sphygmograph (Pond)
Pond Sphygmograph Company: establishment and marketing, 210
Pond, Wallace A.: sphygmoscope patent, 195
Potain, Pierre Carl Edouard: modification of von Basch blood pressure device, 93
Princeton University: Honorary doctorate to Holden for sphygmograph book: 161–62
Problems of the sphygmograph: see sphygmograph (assessments and problems)
Prognosis: sphygmograph as guide, 64, 65, 71–72, 240, 249, 276
Provincial British physicians: *British Medical Journal* as voice of provincial physician, 82; use of sphygmograph, 78–82

Public awareness of sphygmograph: Bishop supports public awareness of sphygmograph in cardiac consultation, 222; Dalton article in *Galaxy* magazine, 220; *North American Review* report of British lecture, 220; health book for schools and public use, 221; little general knowledge of sphygmograph, 220–21

Pulse palpation: advantages of sphygmographic tracings over pulse palpation, 65; "beacon of physicians," 13; Burdon-Sanderson pulse as guide to "condition of the circulation," 14–15; classical, 12; Corrigan's or "water-hammer" pulse, 22; "hard" and "soft" pulses, 83; modern eclipse of pulse study by stethoscope, 21–22; Latin names for pulse qualities, 13; modern clinical practice, 22; neglect of pulse study, 23; not displaced by sphygmograph, 77–78; "sign-bearer of disease," 13; sphygmograph educates the finger on the pulse, 92; sphygmology or pulse study by physician, 13; "stirrings of the arteries," 12; theory of pulse specific to disease, 15

Pulse rate: Floyer pulse watch, 16–18; pulsilogium of Sanctorius, 15

Pulse study (invasive): Hales intraarterial pulse of horse, 19; "haemautogram" of Landois, 25; intraarterial pulse during surgery, 25

Pulsilogium: see pulse rate.

Putnam Jacobi, Mary: see Jacobi, Mary Putnam

Q

Quinine: Holden sphygmograph experiments with quinine, 156–57

R

Rabinbach, Anson: "human motor," 23; *Kraft* (energy) linking social and scientific theories and practices, 37; Marey and modernity, 24; Marey as Helmholtzian, 38; Marey critique of constructivism, 45

Reiser, Stanley Joel: stethoscope and "translation," 9; temperature chart as technology, 12; time and space machines of medicine, 2

Richardson, Benjamin Ward: modified Dudgeon sphygmograph, 237–38; sphygmophone, 83

Riva-Rocci, Scipione: conceptual and technical development of modern sphygmomanometer, 267–69

Rosenberg, Charles: nineteenth-century understanding of drug therapeutics, 153

Rush, Benjamin: neurovascular tonicity theory, 5

S

Sanctorius of Padua (Santorio Santorio): pulsilogium, 15

Scientific American: erroneous claim for American invention of sphygmograph, 40–41

Scott Alison, Somerville: Pond priority controversy, 198; sphygmoscope, 31–33

Seaverns, Joel: scientific approach to pharmaceuticals, 153–54

Séguin, Édouard: pulse as "beacon of physicians," 13; reflections on the pulse, xi

"Senile pulse": Foster work with sphygmograph in Birmingham, 79–80; harbinger of progressive cardiovascular disease, 80

Singer, Charles: Vesalius' workings of the body, 3

Sinus arrhythmia (changes in pulse rate with respiration): detected by Marey, 53

Smith-Rosenberg, Carroll: theories of women's limitations, 226

Snellen, H. A.: Marey and neural influence on circulation, 47

Snowden, John: instruments of precision advancing medicine in New Jersey, 118–19; praise for Holden sphygmograph, 119

Sphygmograph (assessments and problems): American views of target users, 260–63; artifacts, 236; assessment of historical role in acceptance of graphic method, 277–78; assessment of historical role in cardiac instrumentation, 276–78; bridging technology gap between stethoscope and sphygmomanometer, 278; British views of target users, 258–59; Broadbent insists physician must know details of his own sphygmograph, 263–64; caution with overuse of "all scopes" and new technology, 261–62; complex timing of procedure, 248; confounding low sensitivity and specificity (different conditions produce similar tracings and same conditions produce different tracings), 247; contributions to development of cardiology and cardiological instrumentation, 274–75; deaths or abandonment of early sphygmographers, 256; deceptive simplicity of sphygmograph, 236; dependence of tracing on heart rate, 249; Dudgeon's cautions and preparation for using sphygmograph, 265–66; elucidates state of the circulation but does not identify diseases, 247; errors of comparison, observation, and of interpretation, 162; finicky and operator dependent, 247; frustration with technical details and "errors of the sphymograph," 162; hardening of arteries affecting pulse wave, 249; lack of standardization of sphygmograph models, 248; lack of supporting technologies, 248; Mitchell praise for sphygmograph and other instruments of precision, 262–63; need for clinical correlation and knowledge of physiology, 246; need for training and practice, 248;

peak and decline in, 244; persistent frustration, 244-45; positioned between stethoscope and sphygmomanometer, 245; technical problems with sphygmographs (Anstie observations in *Lancet*), 72; time and space machine, 277; too much expected of the sphygmograph, 162; unable to give exact diagnosis, 141, 246; value of graphic representation, 245; variables (fatigue, diarrhea, meals, time of day) 248

Sphygmograph (blood pressure): Broadbent and high tension pulse, 91; Burdon-Sanderson sphygmograph of no use in determining blood pressure, 85; caution with overuse of "all scopes" and new technology, 261–62; elucidating essential or primary hypertension using sphygmograph, 90; Mahomed methods of determining high tension pulse, 88–90; Mitchell praise for sphygmograph and other instruments of precision, 262–63; prepared physicians for sphygmomanometer, 271; pressure exerted on the artery to create a sphygmogram not the blood pressure, 84; Steele's features of high tension pulse, 92; Vierordt concept of pressure required to obliterate artery, 84

Sphygmograph (Dudgeon): application to "ordinary practice," 237; learning to use the Dudgeon sphygmograph, 265–66; popularity in US, 237; portable practical British model, 237; Richardson modification, 237–38; useful pamphlet, 237, 265

Sphygmograph (general): advantages over unaided observation of pulse and circulation, 46; arrhythmias, 96–97; Broadbent and problems of technique, 90; conceptual links to medical progress, 25; correlation with specific diseases, 64; Greek origin of word, 24; guide to prognosis, 72; guide to therapy, 71; Osler on sphygmograph, 266–67; patient discomfort, 61; portable and permanent written record of pulse, 46; smoked glass vs. ink and paper recording system, 72–73; specific to fevers, 72; technical expertise, 72; technological narrative, 24; technology of registration, 38; use in consultation, 69–70; use outside London, 78–82

Sphygmograph (Holden): artificial heart and arteries experiments, 139–40; atlas of sphygmographic tracings, 158; caveats about limitations of sphygmograph, 140–41; disillusionment with the sphygmograph, 163; early modification of Marey sphygmograph, 135; electrified sphygmograph, 136; familiarity with work of European and British sphygmographers, 135; guide to soundness, 141–42; large scale sphygmograph, 139–40; modification Marey instrument; 135–37, 138; motivation, 134; "sphygmographic hieroglyphics," 146–47; Stevens Triennial Prize monograph, 142–43; strapless model, 144, 146; see *The Sphygmograph: Its Physiological and Pathological Indications*; see "*Errors of the Sphygmograph*" *The Sphygmograph: Its Physiological and Pathological*

Indications; The Essay to Which Was Awarded the Stevens Triennial Prize, by the College of Physicians and Surgeons, New York, April, 1873 (Holden's book): aconite experiments, 156; arterial tension, 149–50; *Canadian Medical and Surgical Review* review, 159; cannabis experiments, 154; cardiac disorders, 148; components of pulse wave, 147; Dalton review, 159; details of publication, 144–45; diagnosis of mental fatigue, 148; ease of use, 146; gelseminum experiments, 154–56; homeopathic model of drug testing, 152–53; pharmaceutical self-experiments, 151–57; pulses in tuberculosis (phthisis),, 149; quinine experiments, 156–57; reservations and warnings about the sphygmograph, 157–59; sphygmographic hieroglyphics (confusing tracings), 146–47, 148; 149; value in prognosis and diagnosis, 148–49

Sphygmograph (Jacobi): antivivisectionist criticism of child drug studies, 231–33; characteristics of pulse waves in menstrual cycle, 229; detailed documentation and analysis of sphygmograms, 230; schematic operating sphygmograph, 50; sphygmographic studies of drug effects on cerebral pressure waves in child, 232–33; use of Mahomed modification of Marey sphygmograph, 228

Sphygmograph (Keyt): cardiograph application, 172; comparison of tracings with Keyt and Marey sphygmographs, 173; early model, 171; hydraulic system vs. air, 174; incorporation of sphgmoscope, 171–72; instrument used in Marey's laboratory in Paris, 240; paired arterial and cardiac recordings, 173; pneumograph application, 173; studies of athletic pulse in distance walkers, 179; vivisection experiments on turtle heart, 176; see also sphygmograph (Keyt chrono-cardio-sphygmograph)

Sphygmograph (Keyt chrono-cardio-sphygmograph); Austin Flint murmur, 184; cardiac impulse studies and apexcardiogrpahy, 185–86; clinical applications in cardiac patients 180–82; familiarity with work of Garrod, 180; fontanel studies, 178; never lost faith in sphygmograph, 256; *objet d'art*, 174; presphygmic interval, 180; role of mathematical/ numerical precision in medical diagnosis, 213; simultaneous cardiac and arterial tracings with time intervals, 174, 179–80; technique for cardio-arterial intervals, 176–77, 180; trials on normal child and adult, 177–78

Sphygmograph,(Marey): adoption of Marey sphygmograph in America and Britain, 57; advantages over Vierordt sphygmograph, 48; Burdon-Sanderson modifications, 72–73; comparison of tracings with Vierordt instrument, 51–52; demonstration for Napoleon III, 53; design and application of Marey's *sphygmograph élastique* in English translation, 48–51; early use in Russia, 60; graphic image of blood vessels, 43; Holden modification, 58; introduced 1859, 47; *Lancet* review, 60; limitations and caveats, 61, 64–65; Ludwig kymograph incorporated,

47; marketing Marey sphygmograph, 57; model heart and blood vessel design and experiments, 56–57; modifications, 57, 60; patient comfort, 61; replacing vivisection, 44; simultaneous pulse and cardiac impulse tracings, 54; sinus arrhythmia, 53; *sphygmograph à transmission* with longer tracings, 53; use by Mahomed to study blood pressure, 57–58; use in consultation, 58

Sphygmograph (Pond): Carroll claims Pond best available sphygmograph, 218; criticism of Pond sphygmograph, 211; design and development, 199, 202; Frank Woodbury trials of Pond sphygmograph, 211–12; hospital trials of Pond sphygmograph, 211–12; Keyt–Pond priority controversy, 203–4; Pond instrument in medical museums, 211; praise for Pond sphygmograph, 199200, 210, 211–12

Sphygmograph (standardization): Broadbent physician must know details of his own sphygmograph, 263–64; compare with thermometer and stethoscope, 264; Hammond-Leonhardt dispute over comparing output of different models, 223–24; lack of standardization, 219, 263–64

Sphygmograph (technology); British ambivalence about technology vs physicians' art, 256–58; elite physicians who benefit from early use of technology 253–55; European and American sphygmographers technology dialogue: 215–16; failure intrinsic in all technologies, 252–53; general physicians familiarized with instruments of precision and graphic method, 255; initial adopters of technology, 253; sphygmograph and Picturephone as "failed" technologies, 250–53; technological imperative, 245

Sphygmograph (Vierordt): comparison with Marey sphygmograms, 50–51; Dudgeon comment "meaningless tracing, 40first sphygmograph, 39–41; goal to measure blood pressure, 39; lack of detail in pulse waves, 40; overdamping of lever movement (isochronism), 40; *Scientific American* mistaken claim to priority, 40–41; tribute from Marey, 52

Sphygmographic hieroglyphics: Holden term for confusing tracings, 146–47

Sphygmography and Cardiography, Physiological and Clinical: collected works of Keyt, 189

Sphygmology: see pulse palpation

Sphygmometer (sphygmoscope): application to cardiac impulse, 31; clinical application and consultation, 29–30; criticism, 29–30; definition, 26; design and application, 31–33; evaluation of diseases heart valves, 92; Hérisson invention and application, 26–29; Keyt model, 166–67; limitation caused by lack of a permanent record, 33; Pond models application, 195–98; Pond models construction, 194; professional reception, 30; reinvention of Hérisson sphygmoscope, 167; Scott

Alison reinvention of Hérisson sphygmoscope, 31; timing of cardiac and arterial pulses, 32

Sphygmomanometer (blood pressure cuff): auscultatory method of Korotkoff, 269; Bureau of Standards report, 271; clinician anxiety and concern, 270–71; historical development, 267–71; Janeway hypertension studies, 269–70; Riva-Rocci cuff instrument, 267–69; standardization, 270–71; threat to traditional pulse study, 270–71

Sphygmophone: Richardson invention, 83; Barton American patent, 83

Sphygmoscope: see sphygmometer

Sphygmosystole and sphygmodiastole: see cardiac intervals; see Garrod.

Spirometer: Hutchinson's spirometer, 20; "time and space machine," 2

Steele, Graham: monograph on the sphygmograph, 91; sphygmograph as the "educator" of the examining finger on the pulse, 92

Stethoscope: Camman binaural stethoscope, 9; confirmation of clinical findings at autopsy, 9; Corvisart to "see with a better eye," 43, 245; early adopters, 11; Laennec invention, 8; monaural vs. binaural, 9

Stevens Triennial Prize (1873): essay topics, 142; Holden winner for sphygmograph essay, 141–42; role of Dalton in choosing sphygmograph as essay topic, 142

Stickler, Joseph: experiments with Koch's tuberculin, 127; experiments with streptococcus, 127

T

Taber, Sidney: criticism of Jacobi's studies of drug effects on cerebral pressure waves, 232

Tactus eruditus: see pulse palpation

Technology and the sphygmograph, see sphygmograph (technology)

Technology: conflict with physician's "art," 6–7

Temperature charts and graphs, 12

Therapy: Anstie guide to stimulant therapy, 71; sphygmgoraph as guide to therapy, 71

Thermometer: redefinition of "fever," 11–12

Timekeeping: applied to human health and disease, 17; see clock

Transmission of sphygmograms: Boston demonstration, 112–13, 199; erroneous claim for telegraph transmission, 40–41; Mahomed research misinterpreted re telegraphic transmission of sphygmograph, 220; see Upham

Tuberculosis: characteristic pulse, 13; Holden expertise, 133

U

Upham, J. B.: early demonstration of Marey sphygmograph in Boston, 111–13; priority controversy with Pond, 198–99; transmission by telegraph, 112–13

V

van Wagenen, George: early blood pressure cuffs (sphymomanometers) in insurance examination, 190–91; persisting "imperfections," 190l; successor to Holden at Mutual Benefit Life Insurance Co. in Newark, 190

Vesalius, Andreas: anatomic revolution, 2–3; *De humani corporis fabrica*, 2–3

Vierordt, Karl: concept of blood pressure as pressure required to obliterate pulse, 84; design faults in sphygmograph, overdamping, 39–40; erroneous American claim for priority, 40–41; invention of sphygmograph, 38–41

Vitalism: French academic medicine, 41–42

Vivisection: Jacobi and antivivisectionists, 231–33; Ludwig vivisection experiments, 36; Marey opposition to vivisection, 44, 59

W

Ward, Samuel: early demonstration of sphygmograph in New York, 113; possible influence on Holden, 134

Welch, William: European training, 107; future of American academic medicine, 107; physicians "better than the system", 133–34

White, Paul Dudley: deceptive simplicity of sphygmograph, 236; potential value of sphygmograph for cardiac arrhythmia diagnosis, 236; sphymgmographs and polygraph fallen into disuse, 236; use of Mackenzie polygraph, 236

Wickes, Stephen: climatology and medical topography, 122–23; history of medicine in Essex County, 116

Withering, William: foxglove (digitalis), 18; use of pulse watch, 18

Wunderlich, Carl: introduction of thermometer into clinical practice, 12

Wyman, Jeffries: early sphygmograph demonstration for Harvard medical students, 113

Z

Zumbruck, A.: *Scientific American* article claiming priority over Marey, 40

www.ingramcontent.com/pod-product-compliance
Lightning Source LLC
Chambersburg PA
CBHW020726180526
45163CB00001B/124